REPRODUCTION, GLOBALIZATION, AND THE STATE

/ CAROLE H. BROWNER AND CAROLYN F. SARGENT, EDITORS /

REPRODUCTION, GLOBALIZATION, AND THE STATE

New Theoretical and Ethnographic Perspectives

Duke University Press / Durham and London / 2011

© 2011 Duke University Press

All rights reserved

Printed in the United States of America on acid-free paper ∞

Designed by Heather Hensley

Typeset in Minion Pro by Keystone Typesetting, Inc.

Library of Congress Cataloging-in-Publication Data appear on
the last printed page of this book.

FOR RICHARD AND DAVID

Contents

RAYNA RAPP

Foreword

We anthropologists are astute observers of the local, trained to keep our ears to the ground. In countless villages, towns, and cities, we frequently report on the seismic jolts that globalizing projects necessarily entail for local social life. Processes like the uptake of pharmaceuticals, for example, play out with diverse consequences and appropriations in Delhi and Tokyo; Norplant and its iterations have been put to unanticipated ends in Brazil and Gambia; Thailand has become a hot destination for international medical tourism; and Ecuador funds its own in-vitro-fertilization industry in part through egg donations between women from the highlands who trust relatives more than anonymous producers, thus cheapening the cost of reproductive technologies. In cases like these, anthropologists have analyzed the constrained and exquisitely stratified agency that women and men exercise as their lives are shaped by international religious institutions, corporate markets, state policies, and multinational organizations.

There is, of course, more work to be done. We know, for example, very little about the reproductive aspirations and practices of men beyond *macho* stereotypes, as researchers now working in Mexico, the Caribbean, the Island Pacific, the Middle East, and elsewhere have recently shown us, even as masculinity is subject to globalizing forces with particularizing effects. And we are still caught in the conundrums of "letting the global in" to our understandings of the daily discourse and practice that our qualitative methods were initially designed to amplify and understand. What can our methods teach about the often invisibly present social relations of state, market, and activism woven into the concrete contexts in which our work is carried out?

The book you are about to read, *Reproduction, Globalization, and the*

State: New Theoretical and Ethnographic Perspectives, addresses these issues with intellectual and methodological creativity. It is especially welcome for its rich contributions to understanding the sexual and reproductive lives of women and men as they affect and are affected by gendered relations, legal frameworks, and health aspirations and dangers.

The authors whose work appears in this volume powerfully illustrate the globalizing forces that carve deep channels into daily practices in the realms of reproduction, reproductive politics, and reproductive health. Rapid socioeconomic change also involves the global circulation of reproductive technologies, the use of which may profoundly shape social relationships, as many of the chapters reveal. A pervasive question for many authors in this volume is how to conceptualize human agency—that of both women and men—in global anthropological studies of reproduction. Globalization may introduce heightened health perils for men as regional masculinities develop to their detriment, or render invisible the gendered violence to which women in highly compromised settings such as refugee camps or other forms of exile are deeply vulnerable. These incisive examinations of the unexpected consequences of globalizing forces in state, market, and international organizations on the sexual and reproductive lives of men and women constitute an excellent resource for thinking more thoroughly through the gendered dilemmas subjects often face.

This collection is also particularly strong in its contributions to methodological debates. Anthropologists have long taken up the call for multisited analysis, yet adapting our tools and techniques to this endeavor is often complicated by the very ethnographic skills that enable us to frame the local as if it were an antinomy of the global. The chapters of this book make a strong case for moving beyond the temptations of binary analysis, studying, for example, how questions of attachment between mother and child are measured by a double standard when applied to national citizens and to immigrants, reinforcing stereotypes of racial inferiority and superiority into a complex, contradictory, but unified system, or how men's behavioral repertoire may include performances of both public reputation and domestic respectability as they move through multiple economic and social contexts.

This collection is an important response to the call Faye Ginsburg and I issued to place reproduction at the center of social theory in 1995. In doing so, we surely intended anthropological research to use this sphere of quintessentially gendered social relations as an optic through which seemingly far-flung geopolitical structural forces would be made locally visible and their efficacy revealed. *Reproduction, Globalization, and the State* responds to that call by bringing the study of the globalizing forces and effects instantiated in the daily life of reproduction into the twenty-first century. The chapters that Carole Browner and Carolyn Sargent have assembled cover a broad range of timely topics, problems, and issues. Taken together, they help us to think through and scrutinize reproductive aspirations, ideologies, relationships, and oppressions with serious attention to their simultaneously transnational and specifically local realities.

Acknowledgments

This volume is, above all, a collective effort. We are deeply indebted to the Rockefeller Foundation, which funded a weeklong workshop in Bellagio, Italy, where the contributors presented early versions of their chapters. Invaluable additional funding was provided by the Wenner-Gren Foundation for Anthropological Research. The beauty of the Bellagio setting was surely reflected in the congeniality of our conference and the enduring bonds we established there. We thank the staff of the Rockefeller and Wenner-Gren foundations who facilitated the complex logistics, in particular Laurie Obbink of Wenner-Gren, and Rockefeller's on-site staff in Italy, who made our stay productive and memorable. We much regret that it was not possible to include contributions by our colleagues Azumi Tsuge and Oko Obono in this collection.

During the conference, the participants relied on support from doctoral students Lauren Gulbas and Stephanie Larchanche. In addition to taking exceptional notes on each day's discussions (which we were amazed to find in our in-boxes before breakfast), they produced a final wrap-up PowerPoint presentation and stupendous photographic slide show of our deliberations. We will always be grateful to Lauren and Stephanie for their grace, diligence, unflagging sense of humor, and extraordinary organizational abilities.

Marissa Strickland and Hanna Garth at UCLA made the process of preparing the manuscript for publication seem smooth and seamless. We appreciate their patient and meticulous attention to the details of copyediting, formatting, and tracking down, correcting and reconciling citations. We also thank Sondra Hale and Lynn Morgan for helping us get launched, the anonymous reviewers whose close readings of our manuscript led us to rethink the organization of the book and to strengthen our exposition of some of the volume's theoretical and ethnographic concerns, and Gail Kligman and Sherry Ortner for exemplary advice at critical points in writing the introduction. We are eternally grateful to Valerie Millholland, our editor at Duke University Press, for her enthusiastic support and encouragement throughout the long process of bringing this collection to fruition.

Toward Global Anthropological Studies of Reproduction

Concepts, Methods, Theoretical Approaches

Despite unprecedented levels of transnational migration and global flows of communication, commodities, and medical technologies, there remains a dearth of creative, new anthropological research investigating the impact of these processes on human reproductive activities (Barnard 2000; Ginsburg and Rapp 1995; Inda and Rosaldo 2002; Van Hollen 2003). To help ameliorate this situation, in June 2006 we convened a workshop with eighteen scholars from Asia, Africa, Western Europe, and the United States. Our objectives were to enhance understanding of the consequences for reproduction, reproductive health, and reproductive rights of escalating globalization processes as they intersect with state, regional, and local structures, policies, and practices, and to develop nuanced concepts and methodological approaches for investigating these interactions.

The chapters that follow show that the theories, concepts, and methods of global ethnography are particularly well suited for exploring these dialectical processes across a range of ethnographic contexts (Burawoy 2000b; Whiteford and Manderson 2000). Their aims are threefold: to better define and operationalize the concepts of global, state, local, and individual in relation to reproductive activities in the contemporary world; to achieve a more meaningful conceptualization of human agency through finely textured analyses of diverse facets of reproduction and reproductive health; and to move beyond the limitations of conventional methodology to develop better strategies for research in this domain.

Crosscutting the various chapters is a core question: to what extent might it be meaningful to conceptualize a global anthropology of reproduction and reproductive health? Over the past two decades, social scientists have convincingly shown that research on human reproduction, once disdained as marginal, is at the very core of social theory (Ginsburg and Rapp 1991; Browner 2000; Sargent 2005). This is because reproduction is inevitably shaped by and reflective of large-scale sociopolitical, economic, and ideological processes. Equally important, even in the face of efforts by the state and other institutions to intensify control over the bodies of women and men, individuals strategize through multiple forms of negotiation and resistance to circumvent these agendas. In this collection, we argue that by examining local, regional, state, and global structures as they shape and in turn are shaped by reproductive behavior, we gain new insight into the means through which women and men exercise initiative and intent. The following concepts provide the framework and orientation for the ethnographic chapters.

Why Reproduction?

Our aim is to understand the diverse consequences of interactions among global and state population politics and policies; public health, human rights, and feminist movements; religious doctrines and their manifestations; diverse medical systems and practices; and kinship relations, intimate personal relationships, and individual aspirations on the reproductive lives of women and men. In doing so, we build on thirty years of vital research (Franklin and McNeill 1988; Ginsburg and Rapp 1991, 1995; Pigg and Adams 2005; Sharp 2000; Browner and Sargent 1996, 2007).

Although anthropological interest in reproduction and childbirth dates from the earliest nineteenth- and twentieth-century ethnographies, it was not until the second wave of feminism began to transform academia in the 1970s that anthropological research on reproduction moved from descriptive to more analytical and began to focus on the multiple ways that broad structural factors in concert with different types of power dynamics shape reproductive experiences.

Ginsburg and Rapp's *Annual Reviews of Anthropology* article, "The Politics of Reproduction (1991), and the edited collection they published just a few years later (1995) were instrumental in this conceptual turn. Their objectives were to explicate the effects of global processes on women's reproductive experiences and, in so doing, argue for the necessity of placing reproduction at the center of social theory. Their brilliant, pathbreaking insight lay in unequivocally demonstrating that the social organization of reproduction was intrinsically linked to the production of culture, not a mere reflection of it (Ginsburg and Rapp 1995, 2). In addition they built upon and extended Shellee Colen's transformational concept of "stratified reproduction" to represent some of the diverse types of power relations brought to bear in certain reproductive sectors (Colen 1995). Ginsburg and Rapp were also among the first to explicate some of the kinds of social relationships created—or re-created—through reproductive technologies. Their book was broadly informed by an explicit political agenda: "Our interest in the agency of our subjects springs from our unapologetic concern with the political nature of both reproduction and research about it." Their express goal lay in the development of new theories and methods to enable researchers to discover unrecognized potential for innovation and activism (Ginsburg and Rapp 1995, 9, 12).

Conceiving the New World Order has remained a classic because of the high quality of its ethnographic chapters and its success at articulating how research and political agendas can be mutually informing and transformative. The collection also helped generate a spate of single-country monographs, including Kanaaneh's *Birthing the Nation* about Palestinians in Israel (2002), Kahn's *Reproducing Jews: A Cultural Account of Assisted Conception in Israel* (2000), Rivkin-Fish's *Women's Health in Post-Soviet Russia* (2005), Van Hollen's *Birth on the Threshold* (2003), Elizabeth Krause's *A Crisis of Births* (2004), Greenhalgh's account of science and reproductive policy in China (2008), Kligman's work on abortion policy in Ceauşescu's Romania (1998), Paxson's on family planning in urban Greece (2004), and Maternowska and Farmer's on poverty and population politics in Haiti (2006). These monographs are among the outstanding works that have added depth to our understanding of the ways in which reproductive processes are shaped through the confluence of historical, political economic, and social structural forces. Still, for the most part, they do not problematize globalization as a concept, explore methodological dilemmas associated with global ethnography, or examine the impact of global processes in concert with state policies for reproduction, as do the chapters in this book.

Since publication of Ginsburg and Rapp's collection, dazzling new developments have occurred in the field of reproduction, most notably a proliferation in technologies for assisted reproduction, far more sophisticated surrogacy practices, and a vast expansion of techniques to evaluate the health of a developing fetus and monitor childbirth. Growing movements promoting midwifery and more natural and lower-tech deliveries have arisen in counterreaction. Other important bodies of research on fetal subjectivity, DNA paternity testing, the consequences of the HIV/AIDS epidemic, and the dramatic growth of gay and lesbian families have also appeared (for a review see Sargent and Gulbas 2010).

At the heart of much of the earlier research was the insight that reproductive relations can generate conflict at every level of a society—from the cohabitating couple to contested efforts to enact state regulations and policies (Petchesky 1984; Browner 1986). As Kligman so eloquently writes:

> That reproduction has been politicized in all societies in one way or another is hardly surprising: reproduction provides the means by which individuals and collectivities ensure their continuity. . . . [Moreover] reproduction is fundamentally associated with identity: that of "the nation" as the "imagined community" that the state serves and protects, and over which it exercises authority; or that of the family and the lineage. . . . In view of the multiple interests and values attached to reproduction it is understandable that . . . individual, familial, and political interests in reproduction differ so dramatically. . . . [Reproductive] issues constitute a focus for contestation within societies as well as between them. (Kligman 1998, 5)

While a significant body of anthropological research on reproduction became increasingly more attentive to the political dynamics that inherently shape reproductive relations, relatively little anthropological attention has focused directly on the presence and role of the state (Greenhalgh 2003, 197). Instead research on this subject has generally been conducted by policy experts and demographers who tend toward top-down analyses of population as a vast field of power (for some exceptions, see Morsy 1995; Kligman 1998; Bledsoe 2002; Kanaaneh 2002; Greenhalgh and Winckler 2005). Furthermore, scholarly interest in the dramatic implications of globalization processes has marginalized research on the continued importance of the state in the management of reproduction. The authors in this collection seek to reinvigorate debates about the nature and consequences of these mutually reinforcing processes.

The chapters also build on earlier work to explicate how diverse political agendas may be served through reproduction. For instance, via negotiation or active protest, actors can establish new relationships between a state and its residents; they can redefine the categories by which inhabitants are classified or enumerated; reconstitute the political legitimacy of the state; redefine the category of nation with regard to which groups are included and excluded from it; and accept or deny women as particular types of political actors (Gal and Kligman 2000; see also Rivkin-Fish 2003).

Chapters by Carolyn Sargent and Carole Browner illustrate some of these dynamic issues. Sargent shows that reproduction among West African immigrants to France can produce multiple areas of conflict between spouses, among potentially rivalrous co-wives in polygamous marriages, between migrants in France and their families in West Africa, and between the migrant and biomedical communities. Browner analyzes the ambivalent reactions of pregnant recent immigrants from Mexico to California's state-mandated program of fetal diagnosis and reveals the immense "wild card" influence of untrained interpreters in these women's amniocentesis decisions. These two studies illuminate the range of broad structural factors and local, state, and global politics and policies that shape the everyday reproductive experiences of particular immigrant groups.

Similarly, Caroline Bledsoe and Papa Sow examine the impact of global humanitarian conventions, in this case, "family reunification" policies, on local reproductive life among African immigrants in Germany and Spain. They argue that in an age of transnationalism, attempts by immigrants to maintain family ties across national boundaries have drawn insufficient scholarly attention. Their chapter is a case study of how restrictive and contradictory family reunification requirements are increasingly shaping marital relations, reproductive decisions, and ultimately fertility patterns in some immigrant populations, as reproduction becomes one element in "immigration battlegrounds" that at once involve family, national, and global players.

Conceptualizing the Global, the State, and the Local

Intrinsic to global processes are reciprocal connections and consequent interactions across time and space. Accordingly, studying reproduction as a global process involves recognizing that the concepts of individual, local, state, and the global are mutually constituent forces that must be operationalized in relation to one another—and that these definitions are contingent on the specific topic, setting, and nature of the research in question.

To orient the reader and set the stage for our ethnographic chapters, we briefly define these concepts, as they will be used in this collection. We begin with globalization and its relevant constituent dimensions: global ethnography and the global assemblage. We then consider the concepts of the state, the local, and the individual, along with some productive intellectual frameworks for disarticulating their interrelationships, notably the concept of agency, practice theory, and co-production theory.

Globalization

Globalization is the term conventionally used to describe the movements—or flows—of information, products, commodities, capital, and people across national boundaries. Academics continue to debate the nature, origins, and consequences of these processes; whether on balance the outcomes are positive, negative, or both; and if it is even meaningful to ponder such questions. Anthropologists have been especially critical of the view that these movements are unitary processes with singular outcomes and the corollary that any global process will inevitably result in homogenization. Yet many consider the converse just as problematic: local formations are so unique, diverse, and particular that each can be understood only in its own terms. Stacy Pigg and Vincanne Adams offer a constructive exit from this conundrum: "It is necessary to replace vague, monolithic, and often hyperbolic references to the global with a more measured and empirical curiosity about myriad 'global projects' as specific, traceable networks of connection and exchange [which] would enable us to understand the effects of these networks on the people caught up in them (or bypassed by them)" (2005, 10).

Chapters in this collection adopt this more nuanced and situated perspective in their analyses of the making and remaking of individuals and social groups as they exercise diverse forms of agency in their everyday movements, relations, and shifting, competing agendas (Tsing 2000, 330). The specific issues that concern us are how global flows of people, technologies, and political agendas shape reproduction: for instance, how gender politics play out in reproductive arenas; how the reproductive behavior of immigrants comes to mirror that of women in a host society; and how state politics, policies, and institutions, which may at times be forged in the contexts of broader global political dynamics or processes, produce citizens who approximate certain ideal and idealized criteria (e.g., bearing children born without anomalies, pro- and antinatalist policies for different social groups, family "reunification" immigration policies, etc.). Chapters by Fonseca, Chen, and Gutmann, among others, address these issues.

Global Ethnography

Globalization studies are often criticized for being ethnographically thin, primarily because of the difficulties associated with conceptualizing and dealing with the intricate webs of articulations and disarticulations that exist between global, state, regional, and local levels (Gupta and Ferguson 1997; Burawoy 2000a, 2000b). The authors in this collection consider whether (and if so, how) standard ethnographic approaches (by which we mean the attempt to understand another lifeworld using the self as the main data-collecting instrument) can still be relevant in studying global processes of reproduction. Sherry Ortner has constructively argued that to the extent that the researcher maintains a commitment to producing understanding through richness, texture, and detail rather than parsimony, refinement, and mathematical elegance, "thickness" can remain at the heart of ethnographic research on global issues (1995, 173).

Still, researchers have been challenged to find ways to adapt standard ethnographic approaches developed to study territorially based social and political units (i.e., state, community, family) to contemporary globalized social life, where territorially based units are still meaningful but are not the only ones of consequence. Michael Burawoy offers the concept of *global ethnography* as a means toward advancing ethnographic studies beyond the boundaries of space and time. He urges ethnographers to investigate the constant movements of subjects, commodities, currencies, images, and technologies in relation to one another and to do so by incorporating perspectives "from singular but connected sites" (2000b, 4–5). Susan Erikson characterizes this type of ethnographic research as "iterative, involving a kind of snowball sampling of sites rather than of populations" (Erikson, this volume). Such a research strategy starts with human experiences, as defined in part by their spatial and temporal dimensions, such as regional migration patterns. These are then examined in the contexts of other levels of analysis (e.g., state, global) and particular domains—in our case, reproduction. Sites, then, take on relevance not necessarily in and of themselves but principally as manifestations of lived experience.

The promise of global ethnography is that it can provide a means to move beyond the static binaries of individual-social, local-global, structure-agency, structure-event, habitus-practice, subjectivity-objectivity, macro-micro, and so on, to a deeper and richer understanding. In addition, global ethnography offers a framework for examining tensions among state institutions and policies; individual, family, and community practices; and agency in the sense of initiatives, negotiation, complicity, and opposition. For the purposes of this collection, a global ethnographic approach offers insight into emergent social issues linked to macro-level demographic and other social policies and agendas, and reproduction, reproductive health, and reproductive rights initiatives.

Our broadest aims, then, are to articulate the connections among agency, structure, family, politics, and economy within the multiple dimensionalities of local, national, and global formations. Susan Erikson considers these linkages in her chapter on prenatal care and ultrasound imaging in Germany. She asks whether anthropologists can produce ethnographic narratives that are also global in scope and whether it is possible to transcend the conventional local-global binary. Her subtle analyses of women's lived experiences of pregnancy also suggest how anthropologists might reconceptualize ethnography to better capture the relationship between structure and agency. Linda Whiteford and Aimee Eden offer a rare and compelling analysis of the challenges faced by aid workers seeking to assist displaced women in need of humanitarian assistance. They illuminate the role of global forces in contexts where the authority of the state is nebulous at best, revealing the true magnitude of displaced women's reproductive health needs and how and why they might be either ignored or explicitly opposed in global humanitarian policies.

Ellen Gruenbaum draws on more than thirty years of research in the Sudan to examine the oftentimes paradoxical and contradictory interactions among global, state, and local discourses concerning female genital cutting (FGC) and the impact of these discourses on the forms and prevalence of such practices. She shows how the rhetoric of "eradication"—a term that robs social actors of their agency—reflects globalizing influences of Western feminism, public health, and human rights movements, all of which seek to free women and girls from harmful interventions. Yet global public health agendas also resonate with local struggles for change, thus refuting any notion of women's passivity with regard to the perpetuation of FGC. Gruenbaum's chapter reveals the multiplicity of ways that local orientations to FGC reflect these dynamics, even as they generate new perspectives and practices.

Global Assemblage

In employing global ethnographic techniques to investigate globalization processes, the concept of the *global assemblage* has been productive. A global assemblage is a collection of heterogeneous elements characterized by contingency, structure, organization, and change that reflect the manifestations, tensions, and contradictions intrinsic to global processes. Following Stephen Collier and Aihwa Ong, we define a global assemblage as "the convergence of scientific practices, material structures, administrative routines, value systems, legal regimes," and technologies of the self grouped together for purposes of inquiry (Collier and Ong 2003, 421). Examples of constituent elements include NGOs and multilateral donor agencies; treaties regulating population flows of refugees and migrants; and governance structures, global management practices, and transnational corporations, such as the biotechnology and pharmaceutical industries. Fluidity and open-endedness are essential features of the global assemblage, which references emergent forms rather than "a progression to some fixed state or new structural formation" (423; see also Fonseca, this book).

The concept of the global assemblage can be constructively employed in global ethnographic studies of reproduction because it can accommodate the partial, contingent, unstable, situated, and heterogeneous elements that constitute what Margaret Lock has termed "local biologies" (Lock 2001). Aditya Bharadwaj adds that it is in new, emerging, and dispersed biotechnological assemblages that "ethical ideologies, governance protocols, 'free' markets, venture capital, and geopolitical cultures of scientific research and application" intermingle (Bharadwaj, this book). Additional key features of global assemblages that serve to conceptualize links between reproduction and globalization processes include the commodification of the body and its parts, the manipulation of fertility, and transnational commerce in reproductive materials.

Marcia Inhorn's chapter, for example, examines the global movements of infertile women and men in pursuit of assisted reproductive technologies (ART). Based on ethnographic research in Egypt, Lebanon, and Arab America, she explores the political, social, and cultural factors that motivate this type of reproductive tourism. Chapters by Lisa Richey and Cecilia Van Hollen also examine global biotechnology flows and body commodification. Lisa Richey's study of antiretroviral treatment for HIV/AIDS in a township clinic in South Africa demonstrates the need for a genuinely integrated global concept of reproductive health that takes into account, among other things, the often contentious set of issues associated with efforts to integrate family planning technologies into HIV/AIDS treatment clinic protocols. Van Hollen, in also addressing the effects of HIV/AIDS on reproductive health, examines how globalizing policies and technologies intersect with local structures of kinship and marriage and with the organization of South Indian medical practices. The three case studies she offers of local programs designed to prevent mother-to-child HIV transmission vividly document the stigma and discrimination that seropositive women endure and the strategies they employ to pragmatically negotiate despite their stigmatized status.

The State

Anthropologists' efforts to formulate typologies of social organization have often yielded static and reified conceptualizations of *the state*. In reality, the term refers to a range of types of central governments whose scales, institutions, and forms of statecraft may differ vastly and may also vary in terms of their motivations for exercising power and integrating or excluding people (Covey 2007). Research on reproduction as a global process must therefore take into account the actual range of variation in state forms and processes (e.g., peripheral, central, weak, strong, absent, bounded, flexible), as well as the implications of this variation for lived experience. Chapters by Bledsoe and Sow, Chen, Sargent, and Van Hollen clearly illustrate this important point.

Claudia Fonseca further illustrates the diversity of ways that central state governments exercise power in the area of reproduction, and some of the factors that may limit their ability to do so. Fonseca presents the intriguing case of the astonishing popularity of DNA paternity testing in Brazil, offered by the government at no cost to a wide range of potential fathers. She traces the mix of gendered politics, national judicial policies, and transnational connections that are implicated in the routinization of DNA paternity tests in that nation-state.

Yet, despite significant variability in many particulars, states possess certain universal features. In addition to enumerating populations, one of the most significant functions of the modern state lies in its creation of cultural identities. James Scott refers to this as "the state's attempt to make a society legible," which he sees as taking varied forms, most associated with what he classifies under the category of high modernism: "The builders of the modern nation-state do not merely describe, observe, and map; they strive to shape a people and landscape that will fit these techniques of observation" (Scott 1998, 82; in this volume, see the chapters by Bledsoe and Sow, Browner, Chen, Erikson, Richey, and Sargent for illustrations). One principal means for achieving this is the census, whose purpose is not only to represent a state's aggregate populations but also to do so according to specific identity criteria (Kertzer and Arel 2002). Census practices enable states to aggregate information about social conditions while simultaneously developing empirically based plans for dealing with them. Michel Foucault regarded such practices as essential to the emergence of the modern state, in which populations are managed through increasingly sophisticated techniques of surveillance (Foucault 1977; 1978, 139–46).

A related core function of the modern state is protecting the health of its citizens. One of the ways this is accomplished is by establishing infrastructures and technologies for controlling the spread of disease and "producing sanitary citizens" (Briggs 2003, 288; see also Padilla, Sargent, Browner, this volume). Toward this end, state ideologies are deployed to encourage or impel immigrants and ethnic minority communities to adopt the lifestyles and values of the dominant society, at the same time as bodies and domestic spaces become identified as appropriate domains for such intervention. Efforts to control reproduction are an iconic example of these processes, as is illustrated in chapters by Chen, Gutmann, and Bledsoe and Sow, among others.

Whether the relationship between states and their citizens in contemporary society has assumed a different character than in the past has been of concern to social analysts like Nikolas Rose and Carlos Novas (Rose and Novas 2005; see also Petryna 2002). They suggest that advances in science, technology, and medicine, along with the complicated ethical dilemmas these advances can entail, require an educated and informed public of "biological citizens." In their view, biological citizens are characterized by particular types of subjectivities rooted in biological concepts and categories (e.g., regarding oneself as having a hereditary disposition for a particular disease or a certain specific kind of vulnerability to stress), and accordingly that the language with which individuals understand and represent themselves has become increasingly biological. According to Rose and Novas, these processes involve more than just changing subjectivities: they are also affecting how persons are understood by a wide range of authorities, including political, medical, and legal authorities, and even potential employers and insurance companies. Still, for now the relevance of the concept of biological citizen for different groups in any given society will necessarily vary, in that those most apt to perceive themselves in biological terms are generally educated, literate residents of industrialized nation-states. This, then, raises the intriguing question of how other groups (e.g., undocumented migrants relying on interpreters; or persons with little or no formal education) come to adopt and employ whole or partial representations of the biological subject based on popular discourse, interpretations of hearsay, and the like. Chapters by Richey, Fonseca, and Browner consider these dynamics in the global contexts of reproduction and reproductive health.

The Local

Just as the concepts of globalization and the state are often used in broad, imprecise ways, the same is true of *the local*—loosely deployed to encompass everything from conjugal intimacy to community politics (Pigg and Adams 2005). Authors in this collection argue that to better understand the local, the place to begin is with the lived experience of actual individuals—women and men—and from there to scale up to families, households, and domestic groups, and continue on to larger configurations including villages, neighborhoods, immigrant collectivities, refugee settlements, hospitals and clinics, and so on, and back again.

Mark Padilla's chapter is especially useful in this regard. He deconstructs some of the core processes through which social and contextual features of regions or spaces shape masculinity, and reveals ways that these "regional" masculinities may contribute to HIV/STI risks. In the course of ethnographic research among men who exchange sex for money in two cities in the Dominican Republic, Padilla discovered the limitations imposed by an overly bounded notion of the local in a context where a significant proportion of men migrate across Caribbean tourist sites in search of income. He develops a provocative model to move beyond population-based thinking in global reproductive health research that accommodates transnational migration, transformations in local economies, and shifting gender relations. Ethnographically, Padilla unpacks the set of specific meanings of the local as it is linked to regional variations that in turn produce reproductive and sexual health vulnerabilities among a group of men and their male and female sexual partners.

Agency and the Individual

Core problematics that concern us here are the nature of the individual in the context of globalization, the need for a theory of identity in this regard, and further how to conceptualize human agency in global anthropological studies of reproduction. Contemporary social theorists agree that agency is a fundamental human attribute (Sewell 1992). Without offering an exhaustive review of the many efforts to define the concept, for our current purposes, we define *agency* as the socioculturally mediated capacity to act. Broadly speaking, the term has been used to imply two different types of meanings: intentionality on the one hand and the exercise of power on the other. Interest in agency emerged largely in response to the limitations of a body of social theory that construed human behavior as shaped and defined by external constraint (Barnard 2000).

Most conceptualizations of agency assume an individual actor character-ized by self-reflection and the capacity to engage in the pursuit of goals (Ahearn 2001, but see Beldsoe's chapter for a discussion of social agency). Purnima Mankekar goes one step further to regard agency as "the ability to actively engage with, appropriate, challenge, or subvert" dominant dis-courses (Mankekar 1999). It is also the case that the constraints that bind people can become sources of creativity and transformation. Although many anthropologists have uncritically equated agency with empowerment, in reality exercising agency does not necessarily produce an unequivocally posi-tive outcome (Van Hollen 2007; Lock and Kaufert 1998). Strathern and Ong have each also added important complexity to the agency concept by offering instances in which individuals' actions may further the interests of a larger group while undermining their own (Strathern 1988; Ong 1990). Finally, in what sense is the term *agency* even meaningful when the very acts in ques-tion, although "agentive," may be destructive or rooted in the exigencies of survival (e.g., "survival sex," pressures to produce only sons, aborting female fetuses)? This last point has special relevance in research on women's lived experience including research on reproduction, in that their ability to act may be constrained by family obligations to a far greater extent than men's.

Despite its widespread use, the concept of agency has been critiqued for excessively reifying the individual (for a review, see Wardlow 2006, 6–8) and as being a product of Euro-American feminist preoccupations with agency as resistance. In addition, Mahmood, among others, reminds us that in addition to the more obvious and better-studied politically subversive forms that agency can take, we must not ignore its multiple other manifestations (2005, 153). We further take up this point later in the introduction. Moreover, integral for our purposes is to identify how the crosscutting dimensions of gender and reproduction complicate efforts to understand concepts of agency and to productively use them in global ethnographic analyses. Regardless of its definition, it is axiomatic that acts termed *agentive* are both culturally constituted and constrained and that in most societies those constraints take on different valences based on the individual's gender.

Sherry Ortner identified additional difficulties involved in conceptualizing the individual, the nature of identity, subjectivity, and agency within a global ethnographic framework. To her mind, the challenges are to find the means to "picture indissoluble formations of structurally embedded agency and intention-filled structures, to recognize the ways in which the subject is part of larger social and cultural webs, and in which social and cultural 'systems' are predicated upon human desires and projects" (Ortner 1996, 12). Following Anthony Giddens (1979), Marshall Sahlins (1978), and Ortner (2005), we regard humans as knowledgeable and intentional subjects with the capacity to reflect on their own actions, even as they perceive and experience larger forces impinging on them.

Pierre Bourdieu proposed a theory of identity and a framework for understanding individual subjectivity through his concept of habitus. Bourdieu, however, regarded individuals as principally the products of their class and collective history and not autonomous or self-generating to any meaningful extent. Moreover, Bourdieu's conceptualization cannot easily account for hybrid identities and shifting forms of subjectivity derived from experience (Reed-Dahanay 2005, 156).

Practice theory promises to move researchers beyond the arbitrary and sterile polarizations of structural determinists such as Karl Marx, Talcott Parsons, and Claude Lévi-Strauss, and pure constructivists like Louis Althusser, Jacques Derrida, and Michel Foucault. The pure constructivists regarded subjects as constructed by—and subjected to—historical, political, and other societal-level forces that provided the contexts for, and terms of, their survival. But neither the structural determinists nor the pure constructivists were especially interested in how actors enacted, resisted, or sought to negotiate change in their particular worlds. In contrast, a practice framework posits that although by their very nature sociocultural systems strive to constrain human action, that structure is itself the product of human action, which inevitably reproduces itself, transforms itself, or does both (Ortner 2006, chap. 6). Moreover, Jennifer Johnson-Hanks observes, "practice theory . . . proposes a constant interplay between structure and subjective disposition such that social structures are embodied by social actors as generative principles of action which guide actors' engagements with the world" (2006, 21). Practice theory, with its capacity to mediate rigid structuralist and extreme constructivist representations of social life, provides a useful theoretical framework for reading the chapters in this collection.

Deeper reflection on the concepts of agency, pragmatism, and resistance leads us to posit the human body as a uniquely rich domain for interrogating the dynamic interrelationships between individuals and larger structures (Browner, Ortiz de Montellano, and Rubel 1988). Yet as others have usefully observed, such a focus does not mean that we regard the body as "a privileged site . . . a supposedly evident and stable platform from which we can unproblematically speak" (Probyn 1991, 111, in Lester 1997, 483). Far from reifying the body as a source of absolute truth, the authors in this collection take it to be dynamically constructed by means of dominant discourses and societal constraints and structures. At the same time, we should not forget that the concept of the body does indeed reference actual physical bodies.

Several of our contributors further demonstrate the value of broadening the concept of site to refer not just to a geographic place but also to a subject (or body) where multiple social, cultural, political, and economic agendas converge. Matthew Gutmann's chapter is one of several to do so and also to consider reproduction and men (see also Browner, Padilla, Inhorn, Bledsoe and Sow, Fonseca). Using the example of Oaxaca, Mexico, Gutmann analyzes the global pharmaceutical industry, multilateral NGOs, national population control agencies, and the Catholic Church to reveal when, how, and why men became both excluded and absolved from responsibility for preventing pregnancy. His chapter is an exemplary case study of how interactions between state policies and institutions on the one hand and the global political economy on the other can play out in couples' intimate reproductive behaviors in a particular place and time.

Aditya Bharadwaj takes a different but related tack in his examination of

India's biocommerce in embryonic stem cells and his analysis of some of the consequences for women whose embryos are harvested and whose bodies can, in this way, be said to be serving the interests of the Indian state. His chapter illustrates the larger point that in today's world, body parts of poor people that would otherwise be considered expendable take on new meaning and value when profit can be derived from them. Although the Indian state has thus far avoided directly addressing the moral and public policy issues surrounding the commercialization of bioproducts like embryonic stem cells, Bharadwaj argues that the state cannot continue to do so indefinitely.

Co-production Theory

Several chapters also draw on *co-production theory* in developing their analytical frameworks (Jasanoff 2004; Thompson 2005). First developed by researchers in science and technology studies (Latour 1993; Lynch and Woolgar 1990; Latour and Woolgar 1979), co-production theory has been moving into other fields of inquiry, including medical anthropology, because co-production offers unique insights and tools for analyzing experience and the production of meaning across a broad range of contemporary global domains. Its main premise is to regard the natural and social orders as being produced together, in other words, as "co-produced."

Like practice theory, co-production theory is at its core deeply concerned with explicating links between culture, knowledge, and power. Through insights that derive from a rich synthesis of intellectual traditions, including history, politics, economics, philosophy, law, sociology, and anthropology, co-production theory offers a methodology for analyzing the nature and practice of science and technology at given historical, social, and cultural moments. As such it can offer tools for analyzing the nature of globalization processes in the modern historical period and, for our purposes, how the organization of reproductive practices takes a particular form (Cambrosio, Young, and Lock 2000).

Co-production theory assumes that any expert system of knowledge is in no way a detached, separate, or value-free reality but is fundamentally shaped by, and is itself capable of, shaping all that is cultural and social, including norms, conventions, identities, theories, and institutions (Hilgartner 1995; Rabinow 1999b). It follows, then, that the four main sites for co-production involve the creation of identities, institutions, discourses, and representations (Jasanoff 2004, 3, 7). It is important to remember, however, that co-production is not mainly about ideas, ideologies, and institutions but also about the creation and production of technologies and their associated practices. This is illustrated in Bharadwaj's chapter on India's embryonic stem cell industry, Fonseca's account of DNA paternity testing in Brazil, and Browner's contribution on the culture and politics of amniocentesis acceptance by a group of Mexican immigrant women in the United States.

Conclusion

The dialectical nature of the relationship between the individual and broader contexts and structures inevitably raises questions about subjectivity and intentionality. In acknowledging the fluidity of the processes associated with globalized forms of social life, we remain committed to the explanatory value of nuanced notions of structure(s) as they are transformed by human beings continually evaluating their circumstances, creating and pursuing strategies, and negotiating within and around larger constraints. It is by formulating and reenacting social projects that individuals sustain and transform themselves and their worlds. The challenge—and the reward—of global ethnographies of reproduction such as those in this collection, lie in their meticulous representation and analysis of these processes.

PART I

Global Technologies, States Policies, and Local Realities

Part I explores intersections of, and interactions among, local, national, and global influences on diverse reproductive practices. The chapters consider conceptual and methodological challenges anthropologists face when conducting global ethnography. In addition, they examine the impact of globalization processes on reproduction and the strategies that individuals and couples develop in response. Taken together, these chapters show that governmental policies and state power continue to have major impact on reproductive behavior in many parts of the world, even as global forces may to some extent eclipse them.

In "Global Ethnography: Problems of Theory and Method," Susan L. Erikson elucidates the complexities and principal dilemmas faced by anthropologists who seek to conduct global ethnography, and offers a model for conducting such research. Using the example of German prenatal care, Erikson identifies the complex network of actors (i.e., international corporations, private doctors' associations, insurance companies, medical practitioners, and pregnant women) who shape German practices associated with the use of fetal ultrasound technologies. Her chapter shows how an ethnographer can follow people, commodities, and concepts across the boundaries of nation-states, professions, and disciplines to apprehend the impact of the global flow of a medical technology as it is advanced by state and biomedical interests and the needs and desires of pregnant women.

Junjie Chen's "Globalizing, Reproducing, and Civilizing Rural Subjects:

Population Control Policy and Constructions of Rural Identity in China" shows that despite multiple changes in government policies and ideologies during the second half of the twentieth century, the Chinese state has consistently identified its peasant populations and their reproductive practices as directly opposed to the state's modernization agenda and therefore in need of "civilizing" state interventions. Rural women have been the main targets. After documenting the history of Chinese population policies and practices, including its highly criticized coercive aspects, Chen describes recent efforts to achieve a more internationally acceptable image by loosening some restrictions on individual reproductive choices. He argues, however, that these changes are largely cosmetic, aimed at the global community, and do not reflect any real change in policy.

Following Chen and paralleling some of his observations, in "Planning Men Out of Family Planning: A Case Study from Mexico," Matthew Gutmann documents the influences of global and national processes on the evolution of Mexico's population policy. He shows how men's reproduction and reproductive health needs have systematically been excluded from Mexican population policies over the past century, even as the government has shifted from a pronatalistic agenda to one of population control. Emergent from the similar themes evidenced in Chen's and Gutmann's chapters are the ideas that men, especially rural men, are barriers to responsible reproduction and therefore best excluded from state population policies, and that while international pressures may help shape state population policies, they do not entirely determine them.

Lisa Ann Richey's "Antiviral but Pronatal? ARVs and Reproductive Health: The View from a South African Township" explores the intersection of different histories and policies, at local, state, and global levels, on South African women being treated for HIV/AIDS. Richey uses the concept of the "therapeutic citizen" to discuss the transitive state that women occupy and enact while being treated with antiretroviral drugs (ARV). She argues that this concept needs to be reimagined and redefined in light of the seemingly contradictory stance of many women who are seropositive but want to become pregnant. ARV treatment is administered to these women, who, ironically, are encouraged to plan for future pregnancies—while also urged to have protected sex. Like both Chen and Gutmann, Richey describes the gendered nature of a medical intervention that once again systematically excludes men.

Whereas Richey's chapter reveals how many South African HIV/AIDS-positive women receiving ARV treatment hope to one day become pregnant, Cecilia Van Hollen's "Birth in the Age of AIDS: Local Responses to Global Policies and Technologies in South India" examines the social consequences for a group of Indian women who are already pregnant when they become aware of their HIV/AIDS-positive status. Van Hollen offers three case studies that illuminate how HIV/AIDS status is seen as a family—and hence a social—issue, as opposed to a private and personal one, as is generally the case in Western countries. The stigma attached to HIV/AIDS status in India and the related lack of enforced policies of informed consent create a milieu where doctors, patients, and family members engage in a web of duplicity, secrecy, and collusion. In the context of a weak regional state, Van Hollen describes the strategies that pregnant women have successfully used to navigate the Indian medical system, their individual kin, and larger social groups.

As with other chapters in part I, Ellen Gruenbaum's "Competing Globalizing Influences on Local Muslim Women's Reproductive Health and Human Rights in Sudan: Women's Rights, International Feminism, and Islamism" references a complex interplay of regional, national, international, ethnic, and religious policies and practices, in this instance to situate the contemporary history of female genital cutting (FGC) in Sudan. Recent debates about FGC have been shaped by globalizing influences in two seemingly opposite directions: on the one hand, Western feminism and human rights discourse, and on the other, that of various Islamist groups. Harking to themes introduced by both Chen and Gutmann, Gruenbaum shows how a state can interpret regional practices as appropriate or as backward at different points in its history, depending on multiple local and global dynamics.

The chapters that make up part I serve as a point of entry into the complex realities created by interactions among social, national, and global forces as they shape women's and men's reproductive experiences. In the context of these multiple, complex, and sometimes contradictory processes, these ethnographic accounts illustrate some of the creative means by which local actors navigate constraints and opportunities.

Global Ethnography

Problems of Theory and Method

Ingrid, a raven-haired twenty-nine-year-old medical student almost four months pregnant, strode gracefully into the ultrasound exam room, joining Dr. K and me.[1] Dr. K was the head obstetrician in the ultrasound department, and I had begun my fieldwork in an obstetric hospital in Germany only a few days earlier. Dr. K motioned for Ingrid to sit down in the empty chair on the other side of her desk for the pre-exam chat, and reached to take a blue, passport-sized booklet Ingrid was holding out to her. The booklet was the *Mutterpass* (literally, the "mother passport") that documented Ingrid's pregnancy and that all women in Germany are required to carry during their pregnancies.

Yes, it was true, Ingrid began slowly, answering Dr. K's question in a voice barely above a whisper. As her Mutterpass documented, she had spina bifida. Just a slight case, though, she added. She had been born with a small hole in the tissue at the base of her spine, and it had been surgically closed soon after her birth. But she was here now because she was concerned about her fetus. Her *Frauenarzt* (gynecologist or obstetrician in private practice) had recently given her the results from her amniocentesis, and the results for fetal spina bifida were inconclusive.[2] The Frauenarzt had recommended that Ingrid get an ultrasound in Dr. K's hospital department, where the machines produced better images and the doctors had special diagnostic training and experience. As Dr. K described how she would use ultrasound to look for an opening along the fetal spine, Ingrid closed her eyes and folded her tall, thin body forward in the chair, elbows resting on her knees, listening, but sitting very still. When Dr. K was done talking, Ingrid stood up and moved away from the desk like a sleepwalker. She climbed carefully onto the exam table and slowly lay down.

After almost thirty minutes of looking, first with transabdominal and then vaginal ultrasound, Dr. K abruptly gave up. She pulled the gel-covered condom off the vaginal transducer with a snap and told Ingrid she would have to walk around so that "das Kind"[3] would move into a better position for them to see. Ingrid dutifully consented.

Ingrid returned to the waiting room an hour later that morning and waited until after lunch for Dr. K to look again. After about fifteen minutes, Dr. K said it was still too hard to see with enough precision. She had been able to see more of the spine the second time, but the possibility for spina bifida still existed. Come back in a week, Dr. K told Ingrid, and we will look again to be sure. Later Dr. K told me that Ingrid, though she wasn't fat, "had the density of a fat woman." Some women's skin and tissues were just difficult to see through and that made looking for anomalies more difficult. Nothing to attribute the density to in this case; "Ingrid was just hard to see through."

I saw Ingrid three more times. Her boyfriend came with her for the next exam a week later. Sweet and gentle with Ingrid, he asked pointed questions of Dr. K and expressed exasperation at yet a third instance of "not being able to see 100 percent." The next time I saw Ingrid, she had received the same inconclusive news from Dr. K. She agreed to be interviewed that day, but the interview felt flat, and she wasn't particularly engaged or self-revealing.

My last meeting with Ingrid was by chance, and I wouldn't have recognized her if she hadn't greeted me first as I passed her in the hospital foyer. She looked different, transformed, downright bubbly, her dark eyes dancing. Ingrid was well into her fifth month, and her pregnancy was obvious now. She was just coming from an ultrasound exam with Dr. K, who had finally seen the entire spine clearly, top to bottom. It was completely intact. Ingrid's excitement, obvious in her face, was palpable. Then her face changed, becoming serious. Now, she said, she wanted to modify something that she had told me during her interview: when I had asked what she would do if the ultrasound detected a fetal anomaly, she had said something vague, on purpose, she added confessionally. But she wanted me to know that even then she had known: she and her boyfriend had already decided she would have had an abortion if Dr. K had found fetal spina bifida.

Going Global

Like much of the ethnography in this edited volume, Ingrid's experiences articulate interactions between agency, structure, state, market, biomedicine, disability, politics, and economy. In this chapter, I also situate her lived experience in relation to multiple local, national, and global dimensions. The aims of the chapter are ambitious, and I state them up front as a way to bring the problems of global ethnography into sharper focus: in global ethnography we try to do too much. The sheer number of dimensions we as anthropologists aim to negotiate is daunting. The theories we deploy as explanatory frames are multiple. The methodologies we must engage in to conduct research of both macro and micro forms are staggering in their breadth. How does a discipline embrace the global/macro and the local/micro theoretically and methodologically and make the results comprehensible in narrative form? How do anthropologists actually produce ethnographic narratives that are truly all-encompassing in the global sense? What is required of a social scientist collecting and analyzing data from so many different types of sources, from pregnant women like Ingrid to obstetricians like Dr. K, hospital directors, government bureaucrats, and vice presidents of multinational med-tech corporations? There are many answers to these questions in this book. In this chapter, I offer one way to try to get at the multiple ambitions of global ethnography, to transcend the micro-macro divide more inclusively and move more productively away from the local-global binary.

At first glance, Ingrid's personal narrative may not seem up to the task of global ethnography. Her narrative follows a fairly common trajectory: Ingrid gets pregnant, begins prenatal care, uses diagnostic technology, and (eventually) receives information about her future child. Compared with the other women I interviewed,[4] the specifics of Ingrid's case are compelling but not exceptional. (Many women reported receiving diagnoses during prenatal visits that made them extremely anxious, and which were not resolved as *unauffällig* [without pathology] until later exams.) More significantly for the purposes of global ethnography, though, even in this abridged version of Ingrid's story, the signs and symbols of much larger social, political, and economic influences weave throughout. Ingrid's use of ultrasound technology is shaped by her membership in various groups as well as by different types of governmentality. She is at once a pregnant female citizen of contemporary reunified Germany, a former West German, a woman labeled disabled by her society and thus automatically labeled a high-risk pregnant patient, and a smart and well-educated (soon-to-be) member of Germany's upper class. Additionally, Ingrid's use of prenatal diagnosis is shaped by several global or "universalizing" forces obscured at the narrative's surface. Government policies and corporate marketing strategies undergird Ingrid's prenatal care in ways that are invisible to most Germans. Many of the obstetricians I worked with did not seem to understand the full complement of government policies and corporate practices that shape Ingrid's prenatal care and their everyday praxis.

The theoretical and methodological tensions of global ethnography—agency-structure, micro-macro, local-global—are vexing, but they are also rich sources of ethnographic opportunity and complexity. Theoretical debates about how best to link individual experiences to large-scale structural factors have troubled anthropology for almost three decades now, dividing academic departments and the discipline itself. In studies of lived experience, what is the relationship between structure and agency? How do we describe universalizing effects of maternal-care policies at the same time that we embrace Ingrid's personal experiences of pregnancy as, for example, a first-time mother, a woman with spina bifida and labeled disabled, and a future doctor? My research points to the futility of claiming an overarching or irrefutable causality at one end of the structure or agency continuum. Further, it suggests that global ethnography needs to be reconceived in ways that simultaneously attempt to capture the more imposed (i.e., structured) aspects of people's lives while also capturing individual resistance, resiliencies, choices, and complicities.

If we use Ingrid's case as an opportunity to explore the tensions between agency and structure, we see the tension eases when we distinguish between Ingrid's *use* of prenatal diagnostic technologies and her *experience* of prenatal diagnostic technologies. Her use of prenatal diagnostic technologies was nested in large-scale infrastructures of medicine, technology, and knowledge practices, as well as the German government policies that guarantee her and every other pregnant woman living in Germany access to prenatal care. Her experience, though, was not *determined* by these infrastructures or by her membership in various social groups. Her decisiveness about having an abortion if prenatal scans revealed fetal spina bifida, for instance, was not consistent with what other former West German women said they would do with an anomalous diagnosis. Most women I interviewed in the former West Germany said they would not have an abortion.[5] Ingrid's decision was also contrary to the position some German disability rights advocates have taken about postdiagnostic abortion,[6] opposing such abortions on the grounds that they are an insult to individuals who live with disabilities. But while Ingrid's decision was contrary to the majority opinions of several of the groups to which she belonged, it was consistent with what most doctors think: anomalous results will be followed by an abortion. Capturing both Ingrid's individual experience of prenatal technologies as well as the policy structures, medical praxis, and social norms that make her use of technology highly likely in her pregnancy is one way of addressing issues of structure and agency. Aggregating multiple dimensionalities, with an emphasis on aggregating and collecting multiple and methodologically different types of research data, is one way to approach the challenges of global ethnography.

Starting with Ingrid

In my work, I have tried to move away from the binary of local and global that shaped globalization scholarship in anthropology in the 1990s. During the 1990s, when anthropologists contended with academics from other disciplines who insisted on the homogenizing effects of global forms, the local-global schema turned scholarly attention to more nuanced considerations of the heterodox ways in which global macro processes affected people's lived experiences at the local level. It was important to provide research that contested assumptions about globalization and homogenization. The downside of this, though, was that, in too many cases, this turn meant we gave short ethnographic shrift to the global in global ethnography, glad-handing the global in ways we would never tolerate at the local. We use words like *flows, circulation,* and *processes* to describe global phenomena but have been slow to design research projects that more fully contend ethnographically with macro forms of governance, institutions, and finance. What could a fuller complement of global ethnography look like?

My research suggests that we treat global ethnography constitutively as an aggregating process. Start with people like Ingrid and move through the various dimensionalities that *directly* affect their experiences. Move through the contexts of biomedicine, disability, politics, and the economy within which they live. Do research in those places. Follow the people, the thing, the conflict (Marcus 1998), and allow one site to lead to another. Pay attention to only those state and market sites that are actually relevant to lived experience. Using this approach, I met Ingrid and women like her in the hospitals, parents of children with disabilities, the German parliamentarians debating the ethics of prenatal diagnostic technologies in the Reichstag in Berlin, and vice presidents at Siemens Medical Solutions in California and Bavaria, interviewing almost three hundred people. I moved from village-scale (hospital) research sites to national-scale (government bureaucracies) and global-scale (multinational corporation) sites. This approach to ethnographic research is iterative, a kind of snowball sampling of sites rather than populations, rooted in the kind of commitments that brought Michael Burawoy and his students to operationalize "grounded globalizations" (2000a, 2000b).

Methodologically, such an approach has its challenges. It requires the relativity anthropologists have long employed in their research. Relativity is demonstrably more complicated for anthropologists, though, when the informants are bureaucrats, politicians, and corporate types. It also requires the flexibility to think about ethnography itself in more than one way, with multiple sets of design criteria. My research design included a large sample size at the lived-experience dimension (many women have ultrasound during pregnancy), but only a few people at the corporate level (there are only so many vice presidents). In the hospital stage of research, I could go and "take up residence" in conventional anthropological fashion (I lived in the hospital's fourth-floor doctors' quarters), but the governance and corporate stages of research required that I traipse all over the country. My mix-and-match methodological approach sometimes seemed suspect to those I consulted for advice, at some points too positivist, at others too poststructuralist, depending on the person's own orientation.

Theoretically there were challenges as well. Contemporary anthropology offers many theoretical tools to think with, but few are able to merge different types of data sets into one narrative stream. Quantitative results tend toward a particular narrative form; qualitative research toward several others. I found refuge in Collier and Ong's conceptualization of global assemblages—that is, the convergence of scientific practices, material structures, administrative routines, value systems, legal regimes, and more (Collier and Ong 2003, 3). Within this notion of assemblage there is room for the tensions and contradictions I found between the local, national, and global dimensionalities that shaped Ingrid's prenatal care, as well as the different types of data sets I had collected. Assemblage, as Ong and Collier (2005, 12) conceive it, accommodates the heterogeneous, contingent, unstable, partial, and situated elements that constitute prenatal diagnostic technology use in Germany. It makes room for critical perspectives of the state and market features that in conventional analyses tend to mask the interests and ambitions of administrations, corporations, institutions, and individuals. It provides a perspective on the "national and economic priorities, moral and civic values, and technoscientific institutional cultures" (Franklin 2005, 61) that constitute what Lock has called the "local biological" (Lock, in Franklin 2005). For this German case, a fuller complement of the global is not one true thing or one true group of people but rather a messy mix of rules and reactions, histories and habits, technologies and teleologies, that play out in the management of women's pregnancies.

Returning to Ingrid Again . . . and Again . . . and Again

When I asked Ingrid and other German women why they used ultrasound, most said they wanted to be safe and certain about the health of their fetus. They expected ultrasound to confirm that their child-to-be was healthy and developing normally. Getting a scan at every prenatal exam was just part of being pregnant in Germany, they said (few were aware that this is not the norm elsewhere). Individual experiences of ultrasound and other prenatal diagnostic technologies—like Ingrid's experiences during pregnancy of her own spina bifida as well as the possibility of finding the same condition in her fetus—are at the heart of this ethnographic project. But those narratives in and of themselves are not global ethnography, and they do not tell us much about the global circulation of prenatal diagnostic technologies. When I realized that Germany's high rates of ultrasound were a product of more than individual agency, patient demand, or obstetrician's self-interest, I faced a problem: if I were to turn my attention to the national and global phenomena that created a prenatal environment in Germany in which ultrasound "goes without saying," how would I keep Ingrid and other women from going missing in the ethnography? In a research endeavor that had decidedly federal and corporate components, how would I keep women center stage, as feminist anthropologists of reproduction have advocated (Ginsburg and Rapp 1991, 1995; Browner and Sargent 1996; Davis-Floyd and Sargent 1997; Browner 2000; Rapp 2001) and where my own commitments lie? How would I keep Ingrid central to more-encompassing ethnographic narratives of the social life of government policies and the state-and-market collusions that made Ingrid's use of prenatal ultrasound a taken-for-granted aspect of her prenatal care and create the context for this particular intersection of women and technology use?

The uneven distribution of ultrasound use in pregnancy throughout the world—in Germany a scan at every prenatal exam compared to no ultrasound use among uninsured women in the United States, for example—attests to ultrasound as a praxis requiring both societal cultivation and technological capacity. People are not born wanting ultrasound images of their future children, nor do all medical systems worldwide lie in wait ready to provide ultrasound scans. There is a social history to the ways technological, scientific, medical, and societal domains converged, in fits and starts, to support ultrasound's applications in prenatal care (see Erikson 2007).

In Germany, policy actually preceded patient demand for ultrasound when in 1979 two ultrasounds became a mandatory part of prenatal care in West Germany. The development of that policy, the first of its kind in the world, had a social life, one I elucidate later. The point is that the women whose lives I want to keep central to the ethnography were not aware of the federal policies and corporate strategies that shaped and in many instances endowed their prenatal-care regimes with ultrasound. The obstetricians could not fully articulate these, either. Conducting ethnographic research of policy and corporate interests meant that I had to leave the hospitals.

As I moved out of the hospitals and into government bureaucracies and corporations, I returned to Ingrid and her cohort again and again as a kind of homing activity. They were at the center of my research design and took on a mnemonic presence, continuing to bring my commitments as a feminist anthropologist to the forefront and keeping me focused on only those activities that affected them. As I began to move within the bureaucratic and corporate behemoths of German healthcare and Siemens Medical, respectively, I discovered that Ingrid's and other women's experiences were of some interest. Policymakers and salespeople did not actually know how their policies and machines affected women. Women like those I interviewed in the hospital were invisible to them. Many seemed shocked to learn that although women wanted ultrasound—they wanted to see and meet their babies, and getting the "first picture" was extremely important—women often also experienced increased anxiety from using ultrasound.

The Social Life of Policy

As convention has it, we anthropologists tend only to "name names" (albeit pseudonyms) and flesh people out at the local level. When our attentions turn macro, the people often go missing. But what if, in addition to designing research projects in which women are center stage, we applied the ethnographic conventions we use at the local level to bureaucracies and corporations?

In Germany there is an obstetrician, Dr. CC, who looms larger than life in the field of prenatal ultrasound. Women love him, midwives respect him, his fellows listen to him. He was a young research physician in the 1970s, specializing in the medical applications of ultrasound when the technology was first applied to pregnancy management. He is well known in both German and international prenatal ultrasound circles for his work to establish standards of care and doctor training for ultrasound diagnostics, and also for his personal bravado. When I met him for our first interview, he actually clicked his heels together, bowed deeply, and turned the hand I'd extended for a handshake over and kissed the air just above it. (This is an uncommon way to greet a stranger in Germany.) Without straightening and still holding my hand, he peeked at me over his très chic eyeglasses, said he had one more patient to see but would be with me in just one minute, and rushed off down the hall. One minute was fifteen, but when he finally entered the room where we did our interview, it was with a flourish. Our interview took an unexpected turn when I asked him about how ultrasound screening had become a mandatory protocol in Germany in 1979:

> I was called to Frankfurt in 1977 or 1978 and everyone else was in Japan at a conference, so I was asked to testify at the Motherhood Guidelines meeting. I gave a short introduction about using ultrasound in prenatal care, and, then, well, and then I made a lie. I said, "I am working now in Scotland—I said this even though I was not—and, I said, in Scotland they have introduced mandatory ultrasound screening." That was just a lie. Germans are very impressed if you come in and say, "In Scandinavia and in England and in Scotland, they do so and so. . . ." If you say, "In Germany . . . ," well, no, they don't care. But if someone else is doing something in medicine, then we have to do it as well. And I convinced them, and they made it the policy.

In 1979, West Germany was the first country in the world to make ultrasound a routine and mandatory part of maternal healthcare policy.

That policy—formalized in the *Mutterschaftsrichtlinien*, the "motherhood guidelines" that spell out not what mothers do during pregnancy but what obstetricians are obliged to do and how much they will be paid—was but an earlier version of the policy that ensured Ingrid would use ultrasound during her prenatal care. The policy keeps ultrasound in the hands of obstetricians rather than sonographers, as is the norm in the United States, and effectively ensures that all pregnant women in Germany experience ultrasound as part of their prenatal care or else their obstetrician will not be paid for any of the prenatal care they provide. At the policy's inception in the late 1970s, Dr. CC and only a few other obstetricians advised the Bundesausschuss, the quasi-government body tasked with making the official pregnancy care guidelines.[7] At that time, the power to influence policy lay in the hands of a small group of obstetricians whose specialization and research ambitions benefited from all German women having prenatal ultrasound paid for by the health insurance companies.

Fast-forward to 2000. When I asked German women who decided that they use ultrasound at every exam, about half the women said they really didn't know; about 32 percent said their insurance company decided, and about 20 percent said it was their doctor. "The *Krankenkassen* [health insurance companies] decide," many said.[8] But when I interviewed Krankenkassen administrators in Hamburg and Frankfurt, I was told that it is the Bundesausschuss in Cologne that determines which medical protocols are mandatory and reimbursed.

The Bundesausschuss is a small group of twenty-one people. Few Germans know it even exists. Even people who do know describe it as "a black box" or "a black hole," alluding to the mystery that they say shrouds its decision-making processes. In its official English-language brochure, it describes itself as the "little legislator," but there is nothing diminutive about the legally binding directives it produces, dictating pay and reimbursement for all healthcare provisions in Germany. The Bundesausschuss has a lot of power, and when I learned that its voting members are doctors and insurance company representatives, I wondered aloud to an older nurse at East Hospital about why Germany would allow two profit-seeking groups to set their own fees. "Well, my dear," she said slowly in simple German, as if she was talking to a child, "In Germany we had the good sense to make profit illegal for insurance companies." German health insurance companies merely manage the premium revenue; they are not profit making. But what about the doctors? Aren't they interested in guaranteeing a constant stream of patients who would use the technology of their specialty? The short answer is yes, and in Germany the doctors are the most powerful constituency in healthcare governance.

Most of the obstetricians in my study did not question the utility of ultrasound use in prenatal care. But for a minority, a tension resulted from the legally binding obligation to use ultrasound. I interviewed one well-known prenatal-care doctor in northern Germany who refused to provide routine prenatal ultrasound to his patients because he was unwilling to do the abortions that might result. He was unwilling to look for pathologies that he would not "take care of." Another obstetrician pointed out that ultrasound is "strange and special" because even though it is so widely accepted and such a normative part of prenatal care, she said ultrasound is the only diagnostic technology in all of medicine in which you search for something you cannot fix. "The normal 'cure' is death rather than life," she said. She regularly advised her patients "not to look too much."

What difference does it make when we identify the multiscalar, often manifold, and heterogeneous elements that create contexts of sociomedical likelihood? As we people the governmentality of prenatal care in Germany, we admittedly are moved by degrees away from women's direct experiences of ultrasound. But we stand to gain a broader understanding of how power, medicine, technology, and women's lives converge in reproductive praxis. Where is Ingrid in the governmentality of prenatal ultrasound? In relation to the organized practices and techniques governing women's care, the grim reality is that she is a mere abstraction, a recipient, the object body on which *Schwangerschaftskontrolle* (pregnancy surveillance), takes place. She is the ubiquitous German woman seen as having a health problem, pregnancy, to be managed. She is assumed to be ignorant about her body during pregnancy, even when she is a medical student. In the peopling of governmentality, Ingrid is a metaphor for political processes in which women are invisible. There is value in using the ethnographic method to produce narratives that documents this. For German reproductive health advocates there is value in research that finds that prenatal care protocols in Germany are decided by a small group of insurance company representatives and doctors, only one obstetrician among them.[9] Further, in the all-day Bundesausschuss meeting I attended, I counted three women among the twenty-one voting members. No woman spoke until well into the afternoon. The process that produces legally binding guidelines for German women using ultrasound in pregnancy is dominated by men and explicitly designed for the self-governing of doctors, not for the best antenatal experiences and outcomes.

Women Gone Global

A young woman lay on the exam table as the Siemens salesman scanned her pregnant belly with the ultrasound transducer again and again. Glancing infrequently at the screen, which pulsed with the beats of her baby's heart, she gazed off distractedly most of the time. Under the glare of the bright lights in the huge conference hall, she was playing the part of a patient in the staged marketing theater of the annual meeting of the German Society for Gynecology and Obstetrics (DGGG). It was the second day of the conference, markedly less busy than the first, and the salesman looked bored as he stood running the *Schallkopf* (ultrasound transducer or, literally, "sound head") back and forth while trying halfheartedly to catch the eye of a passing OB-GYN. After about an hour, the salesman stopped scanning and turned away without a word to his subject. She sat up on the patient table, wiped the transducer gel off her belly with paper towels, not seeming to care if she got all the sticky gel off. She edged off the table, stood up, and walked toward the back of the ministage. Through a half-closed curtain, I could see her sit down at a small table and begin to eat an apple.

In staged minitheaters throughout the cavernous convention center at this annual professional meeting in Berlin, Siemens and its major competitors— Phillips, GE, and Toshiba—were directing similar performance pieces with their salesmen's pregnant wives and girlfriends. Glossy floor-to-ceiling photos of beautiful couples gazing adoringly at ultrasound monitors provided backdrops to the live ultrasound demonstrations given by medical students-turned-salesmen. These ultrasound minisets were part of an opulent convention hall sales milieu in which medical devices and pharmaceuticals were plied in tandem with mimosas made with freshly squeezed orange juice and multisyllable coffee drinks from cafes. Gift bags were plentiful and overflowing. BMW had driven its latest model six-cylinder coupe into the convention hall, and a salesman encouraged passersby to sit down in its Italian leather seats. With a smirk, a midwife told me: BMW does not come to the midwifery conferences. Probably not, I thought. They are here to court the power and status of German OB-GYNS.

In the global circulations of ultrasound machines, pregnant women are props for sales pitches and not much more. Selling prenatal ultrasound in Germany casts pregnant women as no more than end users (obstetricians are the real consumers). A woman is the object body, necessary but taken for granted in the production of the fetal image. She and the machine are codependent, separately unable to deliver the image but together able to produce the image on which parental desires, obstetricians' responsibilities, and corporate profits are simultaneously projected. In this sphere of production, though, the textured personhood of a flesh-and-blood Ingrid is missing completely.

Moving from the intimacies of women's lives to the corporate milieu of companies like Siemens gave me pause as an ethnographer and forced me to think about how to expand methodological repertoires for keeping women center stage. Interviewing the pregnant women "performing ultrasound" in the Berlin convention center was one option. But as a result of my first visit to Siemens's global headquarters in California, I also became interested in understanding the culture at Siemens that *did not* put women at the center. How did they actually *not*? What was the culture of omission and erasure within transnational corporations like Siemens? I wanted to know what corporate insiders were doing *instead of* focusing on women.

In 2005 at Siemens's German headquarters in Erlangen, I met five senior marketing managers, all men, for a group interview. After the introductions, they asked me about my work, and I presented an overview of my research about women's experiences of ultrasound (using Siemens machines, in many instances). There was polite interest. During the interview, though, when my questions turned to policy, they became engaged and even animated. They understood German prenatal care policy intimately, better than most of the hospital doctors I worked with. They spoke expertly about German insurance payments and regulations and even waxed wistfully about a French insurance law that paid French doctors more for ultrasound images from newer machines, thus incentivizing the purchase of new machines. Central to these managers' concerns was selling as many machines as possible, and they knew sales were contingent on prenatal-care policy that favored high usage rates.

Collusion between state regulatory regimes and profit-making corporations is not new or unique to Germany, but the nature of these collusions differs around the world. In Germany, where lobbying negatively connotes secretive policy processes for attaining illegitimate influence (Ronit and Schneider 1998), Siemens does not directly lobby Parliament members for prenatal-care policy that mandates ultrasound use. Rather, they seek to influence doctors' associations, which are legally and socially sanctioned to make policy through the Bundesausschuss and other governance mechanisms. Siemens recognizes that governance structures place doctors (not women) at the center of prenatal-care policymaking, and the company makes the most of that fact.

Siemens's strategy for market dominion includes, in effect, "branding" doctors, and in this practice Siemens is not alone. Dr. CC, for example, was "a Phillips guy," one of Siemens's competitors. The approach is subtle. In a country where doctors do ultrasound (there are no sonographers), there is no residency component to doctors' training, and doctors can legally conduct ultrasound exams without a single day of ultrasound training (though few do). Siemens and its competitors influence obstetricians through continuing-education classes and special ultrasound training courses. In the all-day Siemens and Toshiba training sessions I attended, I learned that it was common for my fellow attendees, all doctors, to have taken all their ultrasound training from one corporate sponsor. These courses make it easy for doctors to develop brand loyalty; the courses familiarize them with keyboard and software features that they would have to learn anew if they switch to another brand. Senior obstetricians, the more famous of whom were being paid as much as €5,000 a day (about US$7,500) to teach junior obstetricians how to use Siemens's machines, usually had long-standing relationships with one company. The same obstetricians were also often heads of departments and thereby deciding which machines to buy for entire hospital departments. Instead of focusing on women, corporate insiders were pursuing and enhancing relationships with obstetricians, whom the companies viewed as the true consumers.

Women at the Center

Nesting the intimacies of women's lives within rich political, economic, and social contexts deepens our understandings of the multiple and scalar contexts shaping reproductive experiences. It gives us something else as well:

maps with which we can strategize how to undo socially constituted arrangements that hurt people or impinge on people's reproductive choices. Germany's high rate of prenatal ultrasound use in and of itself is mostly innocuous, compared with other reproductive health challenges facing women and men around the world. But cultivating a global ethnography flexible enough to bring anthropological theory and method to government agencies and corporate boardrooms in tandem with what we already do so well could help us think further about the relations between global assemblages and the disenfranchisement of reproductive agency.

Notes

1. All names are pseudonyms.
2. No conclusive test for fetal spina bifida (FSB) exists, but probability testing for FSB is based on elevated levels of alpha-fetoprotein (AFP) in amniotic fluid. If there is reason to suspect FSB, ultrasound is often used to check for visual confirmation or refutation of a FSB diagnosis.
3. English translation: "The child." I am aware of the reproductive politics that inform abortion rights critiques of this usage, but I default to its actual usage in the situation I describe.
4. This chapter is based on an ethnographic research project conducted from 1998 to 2008. In 1999–2000, during the first stage of this research, I observed 449 ultrasound exams in two obstetrical hospitals in Germany and interviewed 111 women. Latter research stages were focused on the politics and economics of ultrasound use.
5. What women said as well as what they did when actually faced with having to make postdiagnostic decisions about continuing or terminating their pregnancies is explored more fully in Erikson 2003.
6. Defined as abortions that take place after results of a prenatal diagnostic test has been returned to the parents.
7. I describe here the history and process in West Germany. East Germany had a different process, though many of the prenatal-care protocols were similar in intent, if not practice.
8. As a point of clarification, *Krankenkassen* literally translates to "sickness funds." In brief, they are nonprofit entities that manage healthcare spending rather than maximize profit.
9. Feminist reproductive health advocates have expressed this position. Many German researchers have been denied access to Bundesausschuss meetings.

Globalizing, Reproducing, and Civilizing Rural Subjects

Population Control Policy and Constructions of Rural Identity in China

In 2002, I conducted fieldwork on population control in the village of River Crossing in Liaoning, China.[1] During an informal conversation, a county official told me that nowadays, local population control policy was increasingly centered on providing high-quality services (*fuwu*) for rural citizens to cover a variety of issues such as childbearing and child rearing and informed options about contraception, abortion, and women's reproductive health. Since the nation has entered the age of the market economy, the state's local agent explained, peasants were coming to expect more caring services from the government. This, the official further added, is an "inevitable" historical process that has already been accomplished in Western societies, and China is now speeding up steps to get closer to this goal.

Now widely recognized, population control efforts in rural China have been an integral part of the state's modernization project since in the early 1970s, and they have equally widely been criticized as notoriously draconian (Anagnost 1997). Yet my opening narrative suggests a rather different scene, at least as claimed by the Chinese government: that around the turn of the new millennium, the postsocialist state's imagery of modernity undergirding its population policy in rural areas has experienced a discursive transformation—from its previous harsh appearance, which is now implicitly acknowledged as coercive, toward constructing an internationally acceptable image through the recent promise to offer various services that are now officially advertised as more "humane and caring" (Gu 2002).

Based on twenty-three months of ethnographic research in the village of River Crossing in Liaoning (in northeast China) in 2002 and 2004–5 and in the village of Yue in Zhejiang (on the nation's southeast coast) from 1992 to 1994 and in 1995, I examine major shifts in China's population policy in rural areas over the past three decades. During my fieldwork, I also collected data on population statistics, policy documents, and governmental publications on fertility and reproductive issues in both Beijing and local government offices in Liaoning and Zhejiang. My objective was to explore the changing terrain of state-local entanglements and fraught state-villager dynamics over the three-decade history of population control in rural China.

In the pages that follow, I argue that population control in rural China has been integral to the state's shifting images of modernity since the 1970s. To facilitate its population control efforts across the vast expanse of rural areas, the Chinese state has constructed a malleable rural identity, an image of the Other that, while somewhat variable, is nevertheless always seen as lacking something "good" and hence needing the state's incessant guidance, discipline, and efforts at "civilization" (Said 1978). Positioning rural subjects as deficient vis-à-vis the state's discourses of modernity, the Chinese state positions itself as invariably progressive, responsible, and promising in its quest to legitimize its hegemonic population policy and thereby discursively transform peasants—especially women—into docile instruments of its modernity project (Ferguson 1990; Horn 1994). By interrogating the three-decade trajectory of population control in rural China, I further suggest that the Chinese state's creation of the notorious one-child policy in the late 1970s, as well as its subsequent shifts, speaks actively to China's remarkable socioeconomic transformation from Maoist socialism to globalizing postsocialism (Gal and Kligman 2000; Hann 2002; Rofel 1999; Verdery 1996; Yan 2003).

As a theoretical strategy, I also aim to intentionally reify the state insofar as I emphasize ideological discourses that have shaped the Chinese state's population control policy in rural areas. Yet I simultaneously undercut this seeming reification by historicizing these discourses, documenting dramatic changes over the past three decades with the nation's remarkable transformations from Maoist socialism to postsocialism.

Maoist Modernity and the Formulation of China's
Population Control Policy in the 1970s

Reproduction is always entangled in complicated ways with various forms of politics (Ginsburg and Rapp 1991). Over the past three decades, China's population control policy has engaged in a dialogue with a set of shifting images of modernity fashioned by the state (Greenhalgh 2008). During the early and mid-1950s, shortly after the establishment of the People's Republic, some liberal activists tried to promote a birth control policy that would give women access to contraceptive methods and loosen official restrictions on abortion and sterilization (Shao 1954). Yet for a variety of reasons, these population control initiatives did not become widespread during the 1950s and 1960s.[2] As a result, China's population grew quickly. From 1962 to 1970, for example, China saw a net increase of 170 million people, with an average total fertility rate of 5.91 children per woman (Chu 1995, 75). By the 1970s, however, after the initial nationwide turmoil brought about by the Cultural Revolution had to some extent subsided, state leaders, including Mao, began to recognize that such rapid population growth was incompatible with the nation's planned economy (Yang, Liang, and Zhang 2001, 41–42). Grave socioeconomic realities further propelled state leaders to code their concern with population issues as a *problem* (Anagnost 1995). By the early 1970s, for example, the living standard for most Chinese was no better than in the 1950s.

On July 8, 1971, the State Council (China's central government) released Decree 51 (Peng et al. 1996, 64–65), stating that henceforth "mankind should not let anarchism dominate human reproduction; they also need birth planning." It proclaimed that by 1975, the nation's annual population growth rate would be reduced to around 10 per-thousand in cities and no more than 15 per-thousand in rural areas.[3] Subsequent birth policies increased the legal age for marriage, specified minimum birth intervals, and required couples to bear no more than two children (called *wan, xi, shao*—"later" [marriage], "sparser" [longer spacing between births], and "fewer" [births]—respectively) (Yang, Liang, and Zhang 2001, 51).

As a result of the state's population control policy, in the township containing the village of Yue in southeastern China where I conducted fieldwork in the 1990s, the annual crude birth rate plummeted from 35.9 per-thousand in 1971 to 13.7 per-thousand in 1979. Characteristic of the late Maoist era, the state claimed the slowdown of the local population growth rate as a "great success" of the Maoist ideology of "class struggle movement."[4] Aiming to repudiate "dregs of feudalism" that had been deemed influential in shaping peasants' reproductive practices, the birth control campaign was said to "demolish old ideas and foster new, prevailing [socialist] customs (*pochu jiu guannian, shuli xin fengshang*)."

Four Modernizations, the One-Child Policy, and the
Discursive Construction of a Backward Rural Identity

In the late 1970s, especially after Deng Xiaoping returned to power as China's de facto supreme leader in 1978, a burgeoning population was further diagnosed by the post-Mao state as a national "chronic illness" impeding the realization of "Four Modernizations"—a modernity now reenvisaged as "industry, agriculture, national defense, and science and technology" (Greenhalgh and Winckler 2005; White 1990). To rapidly achieve these sought-after modernizations, the post-Mao state became increasingly obsessed with controlling its population growth rate, and a more rigorous birth control program became a "fundamental national policy" (*jiben guoce*) (Greenhalgh 2008; Peng et al. 1996, 272–73). As Raymond Williams has argued in *The Country and the City* (1973), a "statistical mode" was invoked by the Chinese state to create an illusion of control in response to the extreme complexity the nation had to face in pursuit of its reconfigured post-Mao modernity blueprint. Indeed, following Williams, one might argue that the lower the targeted population growth rate, the more it was fetishized.

In 1979 "Cutting the [Annual] Population Growth Rate Down to Below 1%" became a nationwide propaganda slogan (Peng et al. 1996, 14) as the state set specific goals for annual population growth rates (Yang, Liang, and Zhang 2001, 73). The state's ultimate objective was to achieve zero population growth by 2000. Considering that the actual population growth rate was 12 per-thousand in 1978 and 11.61 per-thousand in 1979 (Yao and Yin 1994, 9), one can perceive how radical the population plan of 1979 was.[5] To achieve such ambitious goals, in 1979 the Chinese state began to promote a one-child policy. In 1980 this policy became mandatory in both urban and rural areas. On December 4, 1982, the one-child-oriented family-planning program was further written into the constitution (Peng et al. 1996, 16–17, 19, 43).

To achieve the radical goal of the one-child policy, the post-Mao state had once again to invoke a familiar political process from the Maoist period: mobilizing both the Party and its rank-and-file members to eschew old routines and adopt new ones (White 1990, 74). Accordingly, rural people's intimate reproductive practices came to further intersect discursively with valences of state notions of "backwardness" (*luohou*) that—ironically—were reminiscent of earlier Maoist language. In both campaigns, villagers were depicted as suffused by backward ideas embodied in their childbearing practices. In 1983 the state asserted:

> The old ideas left over from the feudalist past, such as "the more the sons, the higher the happiness" and "boys are superior to girls," are still dominating to varying degrees [and causing] a number of people to have "blind" (i.e., unchecked) childbirth. (Peng et al. 1996, 403–4)

From the official state perspective, such backwardness was most fully embodied by rural women. Thus in the same government file just cited, rural women were implicitly denounced as barbarous because of their continual potential for fertility:

> A woman will generally have about thirty years of fertility—from getting married, and starting to have babies, to menopause. [Meanwhile] human fertility is not affected by season and weather—it [conception] is always possible at any time of the year. (Peng et al. 1996, 403–4)

To the state, the potentially year-round nature of rural women's fertility defined them as having an even lower level of *animalness* than other mammals, whose fertility is largely governed by being in season only once or twice a year. During my fieldwork in Yue and River Crossing, I found this attitude still widely shared by the state's local agents. For example, Huang, the female director of the Family Planning Office of the township containing Yue, remarked in 1995:

> Peasants usually have a low level of understanding [of the population control policy]. [Village] women are especially short-sighted—they only care about their immediate desires and interests. If you do not exert direct control [over their fertility], they would keep on producing babies like hens lay eggs.

Huang's statement is reminiscent of how Edward Said has discussed the production of the Other. As Said has argued, the making of the Other is productive, and what are produced are ideas and statements that constitute a hegemonic description of the object—in this case, the "backward" Chinese peasants, especially women (Said 1978, 3).

Said further suggested that the production of an Other always implies a simultaneous creation of Self. By fashioning and mobilizing discourses of modernity and projecting a series of "despicable" backward models to rural subjects, the Chinese state constructed a progressive, responsible, and promising image of itself. In so doing, the state not only justified its modernity-promoting project but also effectively legitimized its sustained intrusion into rural citizens' private sphere of reproduction. In this regard, the Chinese state's discursive constructions of backward rural (female) identity became mutually constructive of its images of modernity (Barlow 1991; Gilmartin et al. 1994; Rofel 1999).

In the northeastern village of River Crossing, since implementing the one-child policy in 1980, local (female) officials regularly inquired about married women's monthly periods, even going so far as to verify the women's claims by inspecting their used menstrual pads (usually folded toilet paper strips attached to a handmade cloth sanitary belt). Usually women threw these pads in the outdoor toilet at the corner of a family's courtyard, and officials inspected them to make sure that women were not pregnant at a time that was deemed "outside" the population plan formulated for the village. Such surveillance was also common in the southeastern village of Yue. By exerting a veritable disciplinary panopticon surrounding rural women's bodies (cf. Foucault 1977, 206–7), the one-child policy, as the idealized embodiment of modernity, was entrusted with a mission of changing peasants' so-called backward reproductive ideas and practices.

During the implementation of the one-child policy, however, the state encountered varying degrees of resistance from rural citizens—including the majority Han as well as large ethnic minorities such as the Manchu—owing to the continuing cultural significance of these groups' long-standing patrilineal ideology and its attendant patrilineally oriented system of ancestor worship (Anagnost 1988; Chen 1995). To cite just one case: In 1979, a woman in the village of Yue was found to have violated the one-child policy shortly after it was announced, having become pregnant just two years after she gave birth to a girl. Local officials had hoped that, by persuading the woman to terminate her second pregnancy, they could not only accomplish the yearly population plan but also establish a behavioral model for local women to follow. However, believing her mother's prediction that the fetus she was carrying would be a boy, the woman refused to have an abortion. With her husband's assistance, she hid herself in a relative's house in another township area until her second baby—a *son* indeed—was born. Returning to Yue with a newborn son, the woman and her family were fined 200 yuan (about US$140 in 1979)—about one-third of an ordinary village family's annual income. Then the woman was forced to undergo tubal ligation to further pacify local authorities.

Compared with other rural women and their family members' reproductive experiences in the following years, this woman was fortunate in the sense that local officials did not exert direct physical violence to force her to terminate her second pregnancy. In 1979 the one-child policy was just advocated—not required—by the state. After 1980, however, when the one-child policy came to be mandatory nationwide, more draconian measures of enforcement, including various acts of violence against rural citizens, became more and more common.

Beginning in the late 1970s in the township containing Yue, all married women under forty-five who had not been granted permission to have a child (by being assigned an official birth quota by the local authority) were required to use contraception, generally an IUD. For twelve consecutive years, from 1980 to 1991, the township was categorized as an "advanced area for population control." During my fieldwork in the 1990s, township officials told me repeatedly and proudly that the population control effort was so successful during those twelve years that there had been not a single "out-of-plan" birth for a total of five years. Yet such an impressive record was primarily achieved through physically and emotionally harsh measures: induced abortions of all out-of-plan pregnancies. According to the statistics of the township government, from 1987 to 1991, the annual ratios of births to abortions were 1:0.22, 1:1.65, 1:0.73, 1:0.58, and 1:0.56, respectively. In explaining the statistics, a female township official told me that sometimes an out-of-plan pregnancy occurred because of contraception failures such as "IUDs falling out." Yet, as the official discovered, other unplanned pregnancies were largely intentional. For example, the official added, a village woman might stop taking pills or might try to remove an implanted IUD without official permission, leading to a pregnancy outside the local authority's annual birth plan. Considering that contraception has been virtually mandatory for every village woman, from the birth-abortion ratios just cited, one can perceive how the one-child policy has been fiercely contested between the state and its rural citizens.

In the township containing River Crossing, the local administration sought to rigorously implement the one-child policy by establishing the "Small Shock Brigades of the Family Planning Program" (*jihua shengyu xiao fengdui*) to "catch big wombs." The job of these officials was to detect "unexpected" pregnancies that occurred outside the commune government's annual population plan in village after village—largely through unannounced examinations—and then to require illegally pregnant women to have abortions. As a local female township official recalled in summer 2002, during the early 1980s, on average every brigade—an administrative unit immediately below the commune (renamed as a "township" in 1984)—had about eight to ten out-of-plan pregnancies a year. Sometimes women with "big wombs" (*da duzi*) escaped to the house of relatives or friends. In such cases, like Holmesian detectives, members of the Small Shock Brigade would "spread dragnets" (*sa wang*) for days and nights until the "big wombs" were caught. In a few cases, if a woman managed to have a baby out of plan, her family had to pay a fine—about 100–500 yuan—to the commune government, an enormous sum given that the annual income per capita at the time there was only about 120–150 yuan.

In River Crossing, to force pregnant women who violated the one-child policy to undergo an abortion, it was not uncommon for local officials to ask male militia and male government staff members to use their physical strength in subduing resistant women and their family members. To punish some unyielding villagers, local officials and militia even went so far as to remove tiles from the roofs of recalcitrant villagers—an action locally considered a severe symbolic humiliation to a family. In the local context, pulling down an old house usually begins with tearing tiles off the roof. Consequently, the act of removing tiles from the roof of one's house and smashing them on the ground signifies destroying the entire house as well as the family's symbolic integrity and fortune. Moreover, from the perspective of the state's local agents, it also symbolizes the state's continued assessment of rural subjects as backward people who follow old, unenlightened ways in an outdated house. Stripping the tiles from the roof of a disobedient villager's house was thus a further assertion of the state's modernity and rural subjects' *lack* of modernity.

Yet even with such draconian measures, in reality the one-child policy could still not be achieved in most areas because many villagers persisted in trying to bear a son if their first pregnancies had produced girls. Consequently, "more and more local officials had to make false reports to the state" if they themselves wished to evade criticism from the higher authorities (Liang, Tan, and Jing 1999, 33).

The Market Economy and Deficient Rural Subjects

To make its population policy acceptable to peasants, the post-Mao state of the mid-1980s started to soften its stringent policy. By 1984, the state accorded a larger birth quota to some rural women: about 10 percent of women whose first child was female were allowed a second birth, and second births were also granted to accommodate various special cases (e.g., if the first child died or was disabled after an accident) (Peng et al. 1996, 24–27). Since 1987, the state further softened its birth policy, according a second chance to bear a son to all rural women whose first births had produced girls. The local government generally granted this official approval only after a four- to six-year birth interval in most rural areas (including River Crossing and Yue) (Peng et al. 1996, 344–46).

Concurrent with villagers' fierce resistance, the changing post-Mao political economy in rural China also facilitated the gradual loosening of the state's one-child rule. Shortly after the implementation of the one-child policy, China launched a rural reform that tectonically transformed the contours of rural society by redistributing collective farmlands to individual households. As a result, by the mid-1980s, the Maoist commune system had effectively been dissolved. To many local governments, the dissolution of the commune system vitiated to varying degrees the state's ability to exert effective control over rural subjects' behavior, including reproduction (Chen and Mu 1996; Liu 2000). One recent ramification of this reorganization was apparent in the quality of the 2000 census, where the accuracy of numbers in many rural areas was seen as problematic because quite a few rural governments were to some extent paralyzed or otherwise rendered dysfunctional after the post-Mao reform. Consequently they were unable to register the exact number of family members, especially when a family had out-of-plan birth(s) and tried to hide them (Yu 2002).

Along with post-Mao reform, the Chinese state was pushing the entire nation toward a capitalist market economy and in doing so became increasingly postsocialist (Nee 1989). As the softened birth policy came to accommodate patrilineal gender stereotypes, the state virtually abandoned its mission of remolding peasants' backward patrilineal ideology. With this shift during the early 1990s, the discourse of modernity undergirding the state's population policy became largely material, centering on economic development.

In a 1996 report, the State Commission of Family Planning acknowledged that "peasants have some practical difficulties" in complying with the population control policy, and "many are worried that they could not become economically well-off quickly after having fewer children" (EDCPP 2000, 89–93). Nevertheless the state alleged that peasants' problems were mainly due to their poor accommodation to the growing market economy. To this end, the state promised its rural citizens a utopian scenario epitomized by the motto "Have less children, prosper quickly" (*shaosheng kuaifu*). That is, as a constituent part of its reconfigured image of modernity, the state now claimed that its population control policy entailed a mission of helping peasants develop their currently deficient understanding of economic rationality. As peasants saw their material conditions improve, the state alleged, they would become convinced that controlling population was not only essential for the nation's modernization but also beneficial to individual families (EDCPP 2000, 90). In so doing, the postsocialist Chinese state has redefined the ideal model of rural identity as epitomized by an *economic* desire for material prosperity—a desire that most peasants are now said insufficiently to possess. The current birth policy therefore embodied government efforts to prompt rural residents to adapt to market reforms by linking prospects for economic prosperity to birth regulation.

During my research in River Crossing, a female official told me that since the mid-1990s, through the coordination of the township government, hundreds of local women have been subcontracted to manually assemble cheap handicrafts such as silk or colored paper flowers for outside entrepreneurs.[6] This, the governmental agent alleged, was an exemplary form of how to connect the family planning program with the goal of fostering women's economic rationality by "enabling women to make a fortune." Yet after having interviewed eleven village women involved in the new project, I found that none of them linked the economic benefits of their manual labor with state family planning goals. Indeed, the reality was rather gloomy: local officials were taking advantage of these women and profiting through coordinating the subcontract; by contrast, a typical hardworking woman could hardly make a fortune from her meager earnings of about $1.50 per day for ten to twelve hours' labor. And because working conditions were harsh, stress injuries were common. Hu Lili, for example, was an outstanding worker in the new silk flower assembly plant in 2004. She earned about $400 for her first six months of work. In her neighborhood, no young woman could match her record. Unfortunately, after six months, the repetitive stress of flower assembly resulted in swelling and bruising of her wrists and finger joints—a common complaint among women assemblers. Even after a lengthy break, she could no longer be as productive as before because, in her words, "My hand is no longer skillful." Stories like Hu Lili's have led to a further irony: these women's difficulties in achieving "a relatively comfortable life" (*xiaokang shenghuo*) in turn contribute to reinforcing the state's teleological claim of women's deficiency in possessing market shrewdness.

The implication of this circular reinforcement is grim: rural women themselves should be blamed for their failure in the present era of a market economy because of their lack of economic rationality. Accordingly, rural citizens need the state's sustained guidance and discipline—via its population control efforts—to gradually reduce their various "lacks." These lacks include feudalist ideas embodied in their childbearing practices (especially during the 1970s and 1980s), their "low level of understanding" (Huang 1995) of the state's modernizing population policy, and their insufficient accommodation of the state's newly fashioned ideal model of rural identity as epitomized by an economic desire for material prosperity.

Producing Globalized Rural Subjects

Concomitant with this critique of rural identity as defined by a series of presumed deficiencies, the postsocialist Chinese state became preoccupied with constructing an internationally acceptable image of modernity at the turn of the new millennium. After the 1994 UN Cairo Population Conference and the subsequent Fourth World Conference on Women in Beijing (1995), the Chinese state began to transform its population policy from the virtually coercive "administrative measures" to more "humanistic services" (Peng et al. 1996, 252–54). In 1998 the local authority in both Yue and River Crossing, like many other local governments across China, banned violence and the confiscation of property in implementing population policy. In Deqing, a showcase county on the nation's southeastern coast, where the service for family planning has been well developed, the state even invited foreign scholars to conduct joint research (Gu 2002). By late 1999, over six hundred county-level units across the nation claimed to have joined the "high-quality service" (*youzhi fuwu*) project (Yang, Liang, and Zhang 2001, 465). As governmental officials have stated, the service would help to establish an amiable and acceptable image of the postsocialist Chinese state to international audiences (Zhong, Lai, and Shi 1998).

As an integral part of this globalized reform, the postsocialist Chinese state has also tried to disseminate new and "civilized" notions of family and childbearing practices among its rural subjects. On March 2, 2000, a "Resolution of the Central Committee of the Communist Party of China and the State Council on Reinforcing the Work of Population and Family Planning and Stabilizing the Low Level of Fertility" was released (EDCPP 2000, 43–52). It declared that one of the major goals in the first decade of the new millennium was to "form a preliminary new notion of marriage and childbearing as well as a new fertility culture" (45).

Following this lead, the state-run China Population Press soon published the two-volume, 977-page *Introduction to China's Fertility Culture* (Pan et al. 2001). These two edited volumes—written mostly by university professors, edited by high-ranking officials, and bearing a foreword by the minister of the State Commission of Family Planning—focused on advocating how to "build a new fertility culture" in the new millennium. In December 2001, the government legislated a national law on state planning of population and birth,[7] intended to further stabilize its population control efforts and provide rural people, especially women, with more "high-quality [reproductive health] services" (Gu 2002). To the postsocialist Chinese state, the goal of population control in rural China has become

> [to] promote well-coordinated development and sustainable development among population, economy, society, resources, and environment, and to create a favorable population environment for the [cause of] "Reform and Open" as well as the development of modernization. (EDCPP 2000, 99)

In these few lines, one can discern the major themes that are now being widely circulated globally: market economy, sustainable development, environmentalism, et cetera. In addition to its sustained obsession with economic growth, the postsocialist Chinese state has also constructed a highly globalized image of modernity to transform its population policy into a "civilized service." In this respect, the state's modernity project undergirding its population policy has now been speaking actively with and dialogically shaped by global society.

Along with this series of seemingly liberal reforms, the state endeavored to produce civilized rural subjects who were once again diagnosed as deficient. This time, the lack has been discursively located in the need for a more "scientific, civilized, and progressive notion of marriage and childbearing" (Yang et al. 2000, 164–65). Predictably, perhaps, the cure for this freshly identified deficiency is to transform the old "fertility culture" into a new, "civilized" one. In March 1999, the State Commission of Family Planning and the Propaganda Department of the Communist Party's Central Committee jointly launched another three-year-long campaign: "Letting the New Customs of Marriage and Childbearing Flow into Myriads of Families" (Yang, Liang, and Zhang 2001, 438). Designed to popularize "scientific, civilized, and progressive notions of marriage and childbearing," the campaign's goal was to raise public consciousness in such a way that peasants would feel motivated to voluntarily conform to the state's population policy (Shi 2001). In July 1999, the state further promoted the campaign nationwide at the rural grassroots level (Yang, Liang, and Zhang 2001, 446).

Yet my ethnographic observations belied the state's progressive claims. During my fieldwork in River Crossing, I witnessed several local events revealing how these so-called high-quality services have been administered. One Saturday morning, for example, a township official told me that a medical team from the county seat would be coming to offer free diagnoses, mainly for women, and would bring free medicines to the morning farmer's market. But it was near noon by the time a van carrying the medical team finally arrived; the morning market had been closed for over an hour, and everyone on the medical team was hungry. After a banquet provided by the township government, the team members got back in the van to return to the county seat without having diagnosed a single patient. The caring commitment that the local authority had claimed to demonstrate toward its village subjects eventuated in a hollow promise.

As for the new plan called "Letting the New Customs of Marriage and Childbearing Flow into Myriads of Families," local officials told me that they had promoted the policy for several years. Yet like the services I witnessed in River Crossing, this was largely performative. When I asked the daughter of my host family, the mother of a seven-year-old boy, if she knew about the plan, the daughter replied dismissively: "Why do you bother asking this?" As far as she knew, "activities" such as those existed in "newspapers and the mouths of the local officials."

Contrasting the state's progressive claims with my fieldwork experience, I conclude that an irony has persisted in the postsocialist Chinese state's pursuit of a globally acceptable model of modernity around the new millennium. According to the classic economic doctrine, the essence of an ideal market economy is to give individuals free choices to swim in the ocean of the market (Becker 1976)—although such an ideal or utopian situation has not yet been produced across the span of capitalist history (Lemke 2001). In any case, even with its seemingly liberal undertaking, China's population policy has left little space to allow rural people to have truly free choices in childbearing. After redefining rural subjects once again as deficient Others, the seemingly liberal, caring gestures that are discursively apparent in the state's recent population policy have also remained largely performative.

Conclusion

In rural China over the past three decades, population control has been dialogically premised on the state's discursive constructions of rural identity—constructions that have shifted significantly since the 1970s, along with metamorphoses in state images of modernity. Yet I have suggested that remarkable continuity lies behind these shifts in population policy. I maintain that the pursuit of modernity by the Chinese state entails a sequential, somewhat paradoxical, dual process: objectifying rural subjects as backward Others and locating these subjects as targets of a state-sponsored civilizing process—both of these eventuating in the state's regulation of reproduction (Horn 1994). As such, controlling the rural population arguably lies at the very core of the Chinese state's pursuit of modernity.

Indeed, I would situate China's recent shifts in population policy as integral to its yearning to join the capitalist world economy. I would further suggest that China's postsocialist transformation—especially since the early 1990s—has intersected with broader processes of globalization and transnationalism as China has endeavored to tailor its state discourses of reproduction to the global discursive marketplace.

Notes

I am deeply thankful for insightful comments from participants of the Bellagio workshop where this paper was presented, and especially from Carole Browner and Carolyn Sargent, organizers of the workshop. In preparing this paper, I benefited enormously from comments by Alma Gottlieb, Matti Bunzl, Andrew Orta, Janet Keller, Paula

Treichler, Gale Summerfield, Ann Anagnost, Gerald Creed, and the late Daphne Berdahl. The research and writing have been generously supported by the Chinese National Foundation for Social Sciences Research Grant (1992–94), a Predissertation Travel Grant from the Graduate College of the University of Illinois, Urbana-Champaign (2002), two Rita and Arnold Goodman Fellowships from the Women and Gender in Global Perspectives Program at UIUC (2002–3, 2004–5), a Doctoral Dissertation Fieldwork Grant from the Wenner-Gren Foundation for Anthropological Research (2004–5), and a Charlotte W. Newcombe Doctoral Dissertation Fellowship from the Woodrow Wilson National Fellowship Foundation (2006–7). I am deeply grateful to all these individuals and institutions for their support.

1. Pseudonyms are used to protect all informants and places.

2. Due to space limits here, I cannot offer a comprehensive investigation of the Chinese state's shifting, sometimes contradictory, attitudes toward birth control in the 1950s and 1960s.

3. The state did not achieve the goal of 1971. In 1975, China had an overall population growth rate of 15.69 per-thousand (Yao and Yin 1994, 9).

4. Although Mao died in 1976, Maoist policy and ideology continued to influence the government to a large extent until Deng Xiaoping returned to power in late 1978 (MacFarquhar 1997; White 1990).

5. In fact, the state never achieved its ambition of 1979—even with the ensuing stringent one-child policy in the early 1980s. From 1980 to 1985, the annual population growth rates were, respectively, 11.87 per-thousand, 14.55 per-thousand, 15.58 per-thousand, 13.29 per-thousand, 13.08 per-thousand, and 14.26 per-thousand (Yao and Yin 1994, 9). Instead of becoming zero growth in the new millennium, the annual growth rate was 7.58 per-thousand in 2000 (SCPFP and CPDRC 2005, 94).

6. The development of the silk and paper flower assembly industry in River Crossing, however, was much more complicated than the local official had presented. Because of space limits, I am not able to offer an in-depth examination here; for details see Junjie Chen, "While the State Claims the Intimate: Population Control Policy and the Makings of Chinese Modernity" (Ph.D. diss., Department of Anthropology, University of Illinois, Urbana-Champaign, n.d.).

7. After the 2001 National Population and Family Planning Law, in both Yue and River Crossing, provincial governments updated their regulation on population control in early 2003. Villagers were still strongly discouraged from having unapproved pregnancies; if they insisted on such pregnancies, they were required to pay the standardized Social Nurturance Fee (*shehui fuyang fei*) to the county government instead of being compelled to pay arbitrary fines or having family property confiscated.

Planning Men Out of Family Planning

A Case Study from Mexico

Family planning in Mexico has always been driven by public-sector institutions, meaning federal and state governments and health centers. Nongovernmental organizations, the pharmaceutical industry, and the church have played a role in promoting or opposing governmental policies, but at no time have their efforts been comparable in scope or impact. In the first decade of the twenty-first century, medical personnel in government institutions provided most contraceptive devices in Mexico, with private pharmacists acting as the second most significant group of providers, and the number-one group for first-time users. And in line with a local application of the female contraceptive culture (Viveros 2002), women were the main targets of all public efforts from the outset of Mexican government family planning programs in 1973. Although men were formally mentioned in certain family planning programs in the 1980s, in practice men were at best an afterthought; policymakers did not judge the participation of men in contraceptive use as necessary, possible, or worthwhile, and therefore little effort has ever been made to involve men.

Domestic Institutions in Family Planning

In Mexico City and Oaxaca in the last three decades, family planning campaigns were designed to accomplish two key goals: first, to foster the regime of "personal choice" regarding the timing and number of children a couple wanted, and hence usher in the advent of democratic decision making and citizenship in this realm of social life; and second, to analyze, regulate, and control populations. In part this emphasis on control reflects feminist currents internationally that began in the 1970s, when women activists asserted the need to gain control over their own bodies reproductively and otherwise.[1] Even more, use of the term *control* reflected efforts on the part of states and international multilateral organizations beginning in the 1960s to promote economic development in the southern hemisphere through disarming the "population bomb" by lowering birth rates around the globe.

The reemergence of feminist movements in Mexico in the 1970s contributed to focusing attention on several issues related to family planning, such as demands for the legalization of abortion and greater legal penalties for rape and violence against women. Formally and informally, the guiding assumption in family planning, domestic violence, and other campaigns developed by feminist activists in Mexico during this time was that women can be changed, but men are largely a lost cause and not worth as much effort to try to change.[2] Mexico in the 1980s witnessed the development of reproductive health as a key platform of women's overall struggles for equality. This was true both at the level of the federal government and in particular communities. For example, in a pioneering study, Carole Browner (1986) showed how the new government family planning policies had to contend with local conflicts in the early 1980s between men and women over the value of population growth versus the benefits of birth control in a Chinantec-Spanish-speaking township in rural Oaxaca.[3]

Needless to say, no organization of or for men that focuses on men and questions of reproduction, contraception, abortion, and sexual violence has ever existed in Mexico or any other country. The silence of men on these issues has indeed been deafening—except, of course, when men have developed and implemented programs that aim to make women exclusively responsible for contraception and related matters. The only groups of and for men concerned with reproductive health have concentrated on medical problems like AIDS and other sexually transmitted infections (STIS). There has never been a groundswell demand on the part of men for contraception for men. Nonetheless, from the international funding agencies to Mexican state-run health institutions in Mexico to local NGOS working on issues of sexual health and birth control, the institutional bias to ignore or even exclude men from these arenas has had indisputable and enduring consequences.

By examining the history of family planning in Mexico and especially the state of Oaxaca in the last several decades, we may gain insight as to how men have intentionally or otherwise been excluded from most governmental and nongovernmental initiatives with respect to reproductive health in general and birth control in particular. In this way the expectation that men will not easily or generally participate in family planning has become a self-fulfilling prophecy. That is, if it is true that men do not participate nearly as much as women in contraception in Mexico, this is neither a question of men per se nor one of Mexicans. These truths are a result of wider international trends that in turn reflect widespread prejudices and priorities of the most powerful movers and shakers over the past several decades with respect to the global efforts around family planning. The present chapter aims in part to contribute to an emerging literature on men, contraception, and sexuality.

A final caveat may be in order: this chapter does not focus on individuals or personal negotiations regarding birth control or sexuality. Their absence is not meant to imply that discussions, debates, and resolutions by couples in Oaxaca regarding these matters are irrelevant. Although the term *agency* is sometimes overused, especially when individuals and groups fail to achieve desired results or do not even try, health institutions and state agencies are never monolithic, as I show in a recent ethnographic study of sex, birth control, and AIDS in Oaxaca (Gutmann 2007). Nonetheless, here I have chosen to examine how and the extent to which individuals and couples in Mexico are constrained by technical limits imposed by governing bodies, governmental, religious, and civic.

The Oferta Sistemática (for Women Only)

A Mexican state-mandated contraceptive program, Oferta Sistemática, was recently established to increase the adoption and use of birth control by women. With the Oferta Sistemática (roughly, "the Standard Plan"), every time a woman of childbearing age came into contact for any reason with a doctor, nurse, or other healthcare worker, whether in a clinic or in her home, she was offered contraception. (All forms of birth control are free in public health centers in Mexico.) It is significant that men were not part of the Oferta Sistemática, unless they happened to accompany their spouses, which meant that men were not as a matter of course asked about what form of birth control they might employ unless they specifically sought information about contraception. In this way, the female contraceptive culture emerged and was reinforced at the institutional level, including the public health system, so that women were systematically confronted by health personnel about birth control in ways that few men experienced.[4]

Although healthcare practitioners insisted that promoting birth control among women simply reflected the realities of the situation in which most women expected and were expected to be solely responsible for contraception, such interactions in reproductive health clinics reveal a form of medical profiling in which doctors and nurses reveal their own prejudices and preferences for women to assume this obligation (see Briggs and Mantini-Briggs 2003). In the same way, *metas* (targets) set by federal agencies for the promotion in local clinics of various forms of contraception are aimed at recruiting women as the "new users."

In an effort to examine negotiations between women and men regarding contraception—what Carole Browner (2000) terms the "conjugal dynamic" —in 2001 I interviewed women in a family planning clinic in Oaxaca. I sat with one woman who told me her husband had just returned "for good" from the United States and the two had decided they needed reliable contraception. They might still have more children, so they were looking for temporary methods. She was in the clinic to get an intrauterine device (IUD) inserted. I said to her, "I am sure you aren't looking for your husband to get a vasectomy, because that is a permanent form of birth control, but have you thought about other methods for men instead of getting an IUD put in?" The woman looked at me as if I were confused or maybe a little feebleminded. "Like what?" she gently inquired.

Of course, I had little to say by way of response. Other than condoms— and discounting withdrawal and rhythm as reliable forms of long-term temporary contraception for most men and women—no other method was widely available on the market, in Oaxaca or any other part of the world. Again, few birth control options existed for men. Thus the issue is not *if* there are few options for men, why not focus on women's contraception, but rather *why* there are few options for men, and what impact this might have on gender relations overall and reproductive health of both women and men in particular.

Histories of Men—Such as They Are

Histories of family planning and reproductive health usually focus on women, while men are rarely addressed except with respect to AIDS and STIs. The account to follow is thus unorthodox history.

Occasionally men are mentioned in passing, almost as an afterthought, as if men might have something to do with reproduction, but the implicit assumption is that men probably have little to do with birth control because they are generally reluctant to share responsibility for preventing pregnancy from occurring during their few seconds of ejaculation. The absence of men from histories of family planning is customary in academic disciplines that have pioneered research in reproductive health, such as medical anthropology, public health, and demography,[5] and men are so remarkably missing from reports and teaching materials produced by governments, international health agencies, family planning associations, and other educators that we might almost consider this a conspiracy of silence with respect to men and reproductive health.

How things might have been different were men able to avail themselves of widely accessible, safe, and reliable forms of birth control is, of course, impossible to predict with any certainty. Nonetheless one could speculate that certain factors involved in the urbanization of Mexico's population might have mitigated the emergence of an ever-more-severe division of labor with respect to child rearing. In the cities, women and men discovered that fathers who had previously taken their children to the fields to work could not do so with most forms of urban employment. Thus with respect to both conception and time spent with children, especially young children, by dint of proletarianization, the conditions grew for men to become ever more alienated from their progeny.

International conferences in Cairo and Beijing in the mid-1990s formally addressed the problem of men not figuring significantly in family planning efforts internationally. These conferences and the general climate in global health policy at the time led to local efforts in Oaxaca and other parts of Mexico such as training doctors in the no-scalpel vasectomy technique that had been developed in China twenty years earlier. For various reasons I explore elsewhere (Gutmann 2007), male sterilization as a popular form of contraception never achieved widespread acceptance.

Thus, in this way and others, the overall impact of Cairo and Beijing as measured by local-level changes ten years after the conferences was still limited. In part, I believe, this was the result of local health practitioners not supporting men's involvement in reproductive health and sexuality agendas, as often as not because of a concern that doing so would divert attention from pressing issues of women's health and sexuality. Not coincidentally, local reticence was inextricable from broader discomfort found within the ranks of international agencies and state institutions regarding the inclusion of men in any arenas related to gender and development. Men were not trusted by many practitioners to be responsible partners in health, while others viewed men as a threat to already limited financial and other resources (see Chant and Gutmann 2000).

By way of background information, Oaxaca de Juárez is a metropolitan area of around one-half-million people located in a mountain region some three hundred miles south of the Mexican capital. Approximately half the population of the state, totaling over three and one-half million people, self-identifies as belonging to one or another indigenous group, the largest being Zapotec and Mixtec. According to nearly all indices, living standards in the state of Oaxaca, especially in the countryside, are among the lowest in Mexico.

As in other parts of Mexico, so-called modern forms of contraception became widely accessible Oaxaca in the 1970s. Devices and methods like the condom and IUD were available to middle-class women and men living in the cities before this time—in fact, the science to manufacture the birth control pill was developed in Mexico in the 1950s—but widespread access to, and use of, these forms of contraception did not occur until the Mexican federal government launched major campaigns for family planning in the 1970s (see Brambila 1998). Although the history of family planning in Oaxaca is similar to that of the rest of the country, because of the area's higher proportion of people living in rural areas, higher percentage of indigenous peoples, and especially insidious poverty, Oaxaca has perennially received less funding, less information about sexual health and contraception, and less availability of medical care in general.

The history of family planning in Oaxaca is replete with the language of *control de población* (population control), *control de natalidad* (birth rate control), and *control de fertilidad* (fertility rate control). The term *salud reproductiva* (reproductive health), coined in the United States in the 1980s, is today widely employed in Mexico and throughout the world. Reproductive health was meant to shift the focus from population control to efforts to improve women's health, contraception, maternal and child health, midwifery, sex education, and access to abortion, and to help prevent problems like sexual violence, infant mortality, and STIs. As used in public health, development, and academic studies, the expressions *reproductive health* and *reproductive rights* generally refer to the reproductive health and rights of women. The subject of men's reproductive health, if raised at all, usually refers to STIS and problems of male organs like the prostate. Indeed, the notion of *men's* reproductive health and rights seems to many an oxymoron. Raewyn Connell (2005, 1813) discusses the contradictory history of "men's relational interests in gender equality" policy, finding that early assumptions that men and women had the same interests in equality have yet to be confirmed in practice. She argues that simplistic approaches to equality and rights can inadvertently conceal real differences along gender lines with respect to influence and needs.

The history of family planning in Mexico thus shares much in common with the history of family planning in other parts of the world. Perhaps for this reason one remarkable feature of the history of family planning in Mexico is how quickly the country went from being a bastion of pronatal policies as late as the early 1970s to a country in which contraceptive methods were adopted in a matter of a few years by millions of women (and few men), which then led to a dramatic decline in the fertility rate (the ratio of live births in Mexico, expressed per 1,000 women in the population went from 6.7 in 1970 to 2.2 in 2003) and the rate of population growth.

Pronatalism had multiple roots and various justifications, while the impediments to widespread adoption of contraception were legion. The teachings, language, and regulations of Catholicism—for example, the sanctity of the seed—represented obvious obstacles to the use of modern forms of birth control by followers of the church's doctrinal rulings on preventing pregnancy. Others in Mexico who were intent on guarding the country from imperialist encroachment insisted that only foreign capitalists would benefit from fewer Mexican births, and on these grounds decried contraception as interference in the internal affairs of the country.

Pronatalism in Mexico and Oaxaca

Although it would change spectacularly in the early 1970s, throughout most of the twentieth century, pronatalism was the official state ideology and a principle cherished by a nation that had witnessed millions dying in the revolution from 1910 to 1921. Population growth was not only not a problem but was encouraged to repopulate the country as a whole, to spread needed workers to its more remote but economically strategic areas, and to vault Mexico into the ranks of more important regional powers. Children represented more hands in the countryside as well as social security during old age in the cities—the more children, the greater one's chances of survival later in life. The dominant cultural ethos held that "big families were not merely a reflection of antiquated or 'macho' values . . . but rather an adaptation to an economically extremely precarious situation in which the majority of the Mexican population found (and finds) itself" (Márquez 1984, 314).

Throughout the early 1960s, Mexico's economic growth was double its population growth. As long as the economy grew at a faster pace than the population, government and business leaders believed that there would be no problem sustaining the younger generations. On the contrary, a young workforce was needed to fill the factories and populate the underdeveloped cities and regions of the country. Not only was family planning unnecessary in the view of the authorities, but as the secretary of public health stated in 1962, birth control was antithetical to Mexican religious and social values. Nonetheless, despite this policy from above, the view from below was distinct. As in other countries, Mexico's mortality rate declined, and life expectancy grew over the course of the twentieth century, from a life expectancy of 24 in 1895, to 48 in 1950, to over 75 in 2006. A key component contributing to this rise was the declining rate of infant mortality, which consequently led to women and men no longer needing or seeking to have as many children to ensure that some would survive. Unlike in many other countries, however, fertility rates did not begin to decline in a commensurate fashion until the 1970s.

Worldwide debate unfolded in the 1960s regarding the population problem. Meanwhile, in Mexico, pronatalism reigned and naysaying academics and policymakers were largely ignored, as were the voices of international organizations trying to influence Mexico's family planning politics.[6] According to the Sanitary Code at this time, contraceptives were to be distributed only with a medical prescription. This proved to be far less of an obstacle for people in major urban centers who had the social connections and financial means to obtain contraceptives, whereas obtaining birth control was invariably more difficult for most citizens of limited social and economic capital. At this time the government restricted the manufacture of contraceptives and prohibited all advertising for family planning. During his presidential campaign in 1969, Luis Echeverría went so far as to state that "to govern is to populate" (*gobernar es poblar*). It was not until April 1972 that the government formally announced a wide-ranging family planning program for the entire country.

By 1976, even in rural areas where prevalence rates lagged significantly behind urban centers, 14 percent of married women of childbearing age reported using birth control. By 1981 this figure increased to 27 percent, and by 1987 it was 33 percent (see Potter 1999).

Culturalist explanations that insisted Mexican women would be reluctant to adopt birth control in large numbers were thus significantly flawed and proved unable to predict the sea change in women's contraceptive practices. Yet what authorities learned about women in the process of implementing family planning programs in Mexico was unfortunately seldom used when it came to involving men in these projects. To this day, analyses of monolithic and monochrome Mexican men and their machismo, sexual attitudes, proclivities, and practices have proved far more stubborn to dislodge. To the extent that male sexuality has been understood in Mexico in unitary and simplistic ways, public policy, including with respect to contraception, pregnancy, and child rearing, has shown little more imagination or ability to engage men in contraceptive projects. Reproductive health policies have consequently been designed so that women alone are held ultimately responsible for family planning. Mexican men's supposedly uniform negative attitudes with respect to birth control, child spacing, and decisions about the number of children a couple might desire were seldom challenged by state or nongovernmental authorities in the early years of the twenty-first century. This can partially be traced to the manner in which the first family planning campaigns were fashioned, often, as we shall see, under the aegis of liberal international multilateral agencies and foundations, which explicitly or implicitly excluded men from the process.

The 1973 About-Face

In April 1972, Mexico launched a new national family planning program with the slogans "Paternidad responsible" (Responsible parenthood) and "La familia pequeña vive mejor" (Small families live better). Over the next two years, the federal government activated a series of programs and policies aimed at kick-starting "population regulation." In February 1973, a new Sanitary Code abolished Article 24 of the Mexican Constitution, which had prohibited the advertising and sale of contraceptives.

The abrupt about-face in population policy led to a rapid and sharp decline in fertility rates in Mexico, a decisive refutation of the views of policy wonks who had predicted that Mexican women would not acquiesce to contraception for religious, moral, and practical reasons. The predictions of "those who thought that Mexico's high fertility was entrenched" were quickly dispelled (Alba and Potter 1986, 63).

What accounts for this spectacular turnaround is a key question in the history of population and family planning in Mexico and Oaxaca. Economic pressures were clearly central to Echeverría's decision, early in his presidency, to staunch population growth. Although Mexico still enjoyed a healthy economy, annual rates of economic growth had slowed by the early 1970s. Additionally, migration within Mexico from the impoverished countryside to the cities was increasing rapidly, and the appearance of overpopulation worried many officials. Academic demographers in league with interested foreign foundations and agencies at long last seemed to find a receptive audience in positions of power. Yet at the same time, population control became yet another vehicle for the ruling party, the PRI, to influence and control the lives of the Mexican citizenry, in this case, within a few years beginning in the 1970s, by seeking to manage the intimate realms of sexuality and contraception for tens of millions of women (McCoy 1974, 399). Throughout this reversal of policy, to be sure, the Mexican government did not want to appear to be responding to demands of the United States for Mexico to lower its birth rate. Nonetheless it was difficult for Mexican authorities to conceal that these new policies were in part very much the result of strong international coercion, especially from the United States and affiliated funding agencies like the World Bank.

International pressure on Mexico during the 1960s and 1970s was tied inextricably to the sordid history of imperialism and colonialism from the time of the eugenics movement in the 1920s through campaigns for sterilization in Latin America, and subsequent dire prognoses by the CIA among other agencies of the United States that argued for population control as a way to reduce revolutionary movements and protect strategic U.S. interests in the Southern Hemisphere.

How could contraceptive use have become so widespread in a relatively short time in a Catholic country? The short answer to this question is that Mexico has long had an inconsistent and flexible relationship with its particular brand of Catholicism. Although Catholicism in contemporary Mexico has played an enormous role in preventing the legalization of abortion, it has had little bearing on other issues relating to sexuality and reproduction, and indeed in 2007, abortions were legalized in Mexico City. Throughout most of the twentieth century, following the adoption of the 1917 Constitution, in which the church was prohibited from owning property and was brought under the strict supervision of the Mexican federal government, anticlericalism has existed side by side with obeisance to Rome. As state and church became ever-more-separate institutions, doctors came to substitute for priests as the ultimate authorities on family planning, in the formulation of the former director of Mexfam, the Mexican affiliate of the IPPF (International Planned Parenthood Federation; see López Juárez 2003).

Additionally, the lack of opposition to artificial birth control on the part of the church should also not be exaggerated. Despite pronouncements by church leaders, innumerable local priests certainly continued to counsel to their parishioners against the use of contraceptives. In practice this meant targeting women once again, both because far more women than men attended church regularly in Mexico and because in the Catholic Church, as well as in the Mexican health system, women were de facto considered most responsible for family planning and most responsive to injunctions from religious authority. The adoption of the birth control pill and other forms of contraception by millions of women in the 1970s and beyond, however, illustrates that although significant, these countervailing efforts were on the losing side of the debate. As Catholic strictures against artificial contraception became more anachronistic, undoubtedly some clergy turned a blind eye to such transgressions to ward off dwindling church attendance and membership.

From the outset, family planning campaigns in Mexico were aimed at women far more than at men. The conclusion most commentators have drawn regarding the surprising change in contraceptive practices and the subsequent decline in fertility in Mexico is that women proved far less religiously bound and more concerned with providing their fewer children with better educational opportunities and material privilege than some analysts had suspected possible. Women in Mexico quickly adopted the slogan "Smaller families live better" as soon as government health institutions presented them with the opportunity to do so.

If at all considered by planners, they considered men as neutral or begrudging partners in birth control. That is, although they (belatedly) acknowledged that women's desire to have fewer children would prevail over all sorts of other mitigating factors (like their Catholic prejudices), they also assumed that men still had to be thwarted from their preordained natural tendencies. Representing an emerging consensus in the Mexican government, Gilberto Loyo, former Secretario de Gobernación and longtime PRI spokesman on population matters, published a paper in 1967 in which he commented: "It can be said that to some degree in the rural areas and to a greater degree in lower class urban areas women—oppressed by the number of children they have, by their poverty, and by the irresponsibility of their husbands—attempt to control birth by inducing abortion, (many times with regrettable consequences) or by ineffective contraceptive means" (Loyo 1974, 187).[7] In this way, Mexican men were officially labeled "irresponsible" with respect to family planning. Planners identified men in the countryside and even more the poor men of the urban centers as bad influences and cultural barriers to containing Mexico's population explosion. Yet to the extent that irresponsibly spreading one's seed was considered natural to men in Mexico and elsewhere, culturalist assumptions about what curbing fertility rates might entail shaped the government's ensuing efforts; women were targeted for change, while men were all but ignored as long as they did not interfere with these efforts.

The key foreign institutions involved in population politics in Mexico in this period included USAID, the UN Fund for Population Activities (UNFPA), the IPPF, the World Bank, the Population Council, and the Rockefeller, Ford, Hewlett, Mellon, and MacArthur foundations. Family planning shifted from a more strictly medical matter to a global enterprise involving billions of dollars spent annually in services, fees, and products, and population policies became central to overall economic, political, and social programs throughout the underdeveloped world (see Caldwell and Caldwell 1986; Ford Foundation 1991).[8]

In Mexico and elsewhere, women were the key to future success in family planning, though invariably, in every country and every international agency on earth, the persons responsible for developing and implementing family planning policies and projects were overwhelmingly men from the ruling and professional classes. This meant that women had to be convinced not to view "modern contraceptive methods as potential threats to their health and even to life itself" (Alba and Potter 1986, 64) and to accept their responsibility as women to "protect themselves" by using birth control. Remarkably enough, in Mexico as throughout the world before the arrival of the birth control pill, men had been more active participants in preventing pregnancy. Indeed, they were often the key players in methods like withdrawal and condom use (Schneider and Schneider 1996). This pattern changed with the pill and other female forms of contraception that the international agencies promoted so heavily beginning in the 1960s, spawning in turn a female contraceptive culture and the effective marginalization of men from more significant involvement in birth control.

Men as targets of policies and programs were not explicitly brought into the family planning equation until the 1994 International Conference on Population and Development, in Cairo, and a year later at the Fourth World Women's Conference, in Beijing (see Chant and Gutmann 2000), though of course men all the while had been genuinely concerned with preventing pregnancies—as well as implicated in making babies.

Contraceptive Targets

In 1977, Conapo, Mexico's National Population Council, announced goals to reduce the rate of population growth in the country, so that by the year 2000 the rate would be 1.0 percent. A crucial component in reaching these goals was the contraceptive prevalence targets (*metas*) set by the council that same year. From that date until the present, every clinic and hospital in Mexico has been assigned specific numbers of women they must try to convince to accept one method of birth control or another. The targets were method specific, with the highest priority given to the IUD and female sterilization. As Potter (1999, 717) writes: "The critical statistic for public hospitals and maternity clinics was the percentage of mothers who accepted one of these methods immediately following delivery."

With the contraceptive target system, the Mexican government decided to intervene in the sex lives of its citizens. Sexual reproduction was medicalized, and institutionalized medicine became the regulator of fertility and normative reproductive practices. Although called targets, these goals were in effect quotas, as clinics suffered penalties, at least indirectly through loss of prestige and clout within the healthcare system, if they consistently fell short of the federally established goals. Conversely, clinics could expect extra resources if their numbers were significantly over target. The target-quota system of promoting contraception among women was of a piece with other nationally mandated healthcare programs such as the Oferta Sistemática, which compelled all medical personnel to encourage birth control use every time they meet with women for any other reason as well.

In all facets of family planning campaigns sponsored by federal and state governments in Mexico, a notable underlying theme is the promotion of modern methods of contraception in contrast to traditional methods like withdrawal, rhythm, and abstinence. The decline in fertility rates is obviously not a simple result of accessibility and adoption of birth control of any kind. Undoubtedly, millions of Mexicans decided they wanted fewer children. Often-cited reasons for wanting fewer children included having more money for their children's education and for their general well-being. At the same time, the ideology of "modern is better" pervaded discussions on birth spacing, number of children, and contraception.

Conclusion

The modern history of family planning, in Mexico and the rest of the world, is largely the history of women and birth control. It is also an institutional history, because international and national, governmental and nongovernmental, organizations have played pivotal roles in developing family planning campaigns and contraceptive products and promoting the use of one or another birth control method—among and for women. Mexico's particular history of benign pronatalism was followed by intensive and widespread efforts to lower population birth rates throughout the country in a short period of time. These efforts were generally highly successful, no doubt in part owing to the common desire of women (and men) for smaller families, as well as contingent factors such as the essential abstinence of the Catholic Church from attempting to derail the spread of contraceptives. Smaller families reflect the process whereby Mexican women (and men) selectively choose which church doctrines they will adhere to, and, to cite Gloria González-López (2005, 244), demonstrate that Mexican women in particular "are neither submissive nor passive, but are active individuals who mediate Catholic teachings on sexual morality based on their personal subjectivities."

In studying men's reproductive health and sexuality in Oaxaca, among other things I tried to determine the influence of negotiations in couples with respect to contraception. This method was inherently problematic because such negotiations take place over years if not decades, and more importantly, couples do not make such decisions in isolation from the larger contexts influenced by pharmaceutical companies, government health institutions, the Catholic Church, and other outside actors. The global political economy is central to every decision regarding birth control by couples in every home in Oaxaca, regardless of how personal and intimate the choice may seem to the men and women themselves.

Notes

My thanks to Carole Browner and Carolyn Sargent for the invitation to participate in this project, to the other members of the seminar, and to those who have taught me much about reproductive health and sexuality, especially Ana Amuchástegui, Stanley Brandes, Raewyn Connell, Soledad González, Marcia Inhorn, Ana Luisa Liguori, Richard Parker, and Mara Viveros.

1. See, for example, *Our Bodies, Ourselves*, published in 1973 by the Boston Women's Health Book Collective. English-language versions of this text were passed around among feminist activists and scholars in Mexico in the 1970s.

2. This point has also been made to me repeatedly by feminist activists from organizations helping battered women in Mexico City and Oaxaca. See, for instance, Gutmann 2007, chapter 8.

3. On the history of NGOs and reproductive health generally in Mexico, see González Montes 1999.

4. An earlier version of this essay that was written for the seminar "Reproduction, Globalization, and the State" was subsequently incorporated into my ethnography *Fixing Men: Sex, Birth Control, and AIDS in Mexico* (California, 2007), especially chapter 5.

5. Exceptions to this situation are Greene and Biddlecom 2000; Bledsoe, Lerner, and Guyer 2000; and Dudgeon and Inhorn 2003, 2004.

6. Including the International Planned Parenthood Federation (IPPF), the Ford Foundation, the Population Council, and the United Nations Population Fund (UNFPA).

7. Often translated as secretary of the interior, the Secretario de Gobernación represents the second most powerful national political office in Mexico.

8. Amuchástegui (2001) writes about the effect of scientific knowledge on sex experiences and about the history of sexuality in Mexico.

Antiviral but Pronatal? ARVs and Reproductive Health

The View from a South African Township

Globalization is an econo-technological institutional process with a pervasive, if irregular, impact. It has brought technological access to the forefront of political debates over global inequality. In high-income countries, treatment with antiretrovirals (ARVs) became widely available in 1996, and AIDS-related mortality dropped sharply. In contrast to conventional wisdom that such therapies would remain beyond the reach of most HIV-positive people in developing countries, improving access to ARVs has become officially a global priority. While this has yet to be realized in most African countries, South Africa has undertaken the largest public ARV treatment program in the world. At the same time, reproductive decision making is overlooked in Africa in the face of AIDS. Reproduction and AIDS are kept separate but are in fact linked through competing global programs.

Reproductive health and rights agendas have focused attention on important issues that were not emphasized in previous debates over population control—who controls fertility, reproductive decision making, the ethics of contraceptive methods, and the impact of gender relations in the household, clinic, and national policy environment. Reproductive health as a global agenda can provide an opportunity for including social issues under its vast umbrella. In other work, I have examined the possibilities of integrating AIDS into the normal interventions to promote reproductive health (Richey 2003, 2005, 2006, 2008). When global discourses are translated in local contexts of HIV/AIDS, reproductive health in many African communities might best be understood as remaining healthy enough to reproduce. South Africa has one of the highest rates of contraceptive use and the lowest fertility rates in

Africa, yet the gendered importance of childbearing persists perhaps both in spite of and because of the omnipresence of HIV/AIDS.

South African AIDS is exemplary of the embodiment of history, as portrayed by Fassin (2002, 2007). Yet contraceptive and ARV technologies are future-looking interventions in the ways that they are meant to prevent, to stave off an unwanted future. It is in clinical-level interactions that we see negotiations over possibilities that are inextricably bound to an embodied past. Therefore an exploration of AIDS and contraceptives in South Africa cannot take place outside the macro-context of race, political struggle, state building, and the economic realities of contemporary South Africa, best characterized by poverty, empowerment extremes,[1] and gross and gaping inequality, known as the "distributional regime" (Seekings and Nattrass 2006).

Reproductive decision making in the context of the AIDS clinic reignites classic debates over the rights of the individual versus the rights of the community, the meanings of motherhood and maternal identity, and the appropriate control of sexuality by the state vis-à-vis governance of the self (cf. Glenn, Chang, and Forcey 1994). The self on ARVs as linked to the geopolitical realm of AIDS treatment both globally and locally has been termed the "therapeutic citizen" (Nguyen 2005). Yet in the situation of reproductive decision making by HIV-positive women, the stakes are higher, the boundaries less discernible, and the meanings even more contingent owing to the urgency of the disease and the poignancy of the processes of giving life. To begin to understand this, we must find a way to gender the therapeutic citizen to reintegrate the biopolitical struggle of ARVs with the social issues percolating within the therapeutic state.

Methodology

This research is, in some respects, an anthropological examination of AIDS interventions from the standpoint of politics and policy. The empirical material for this chapter comes from fieldwork in the Western Cape Province of South Africa from June until December 2005. I became most interested in the participant observation work I was permitted to conduct at the Heshima Clinic for HIV/AIDS treatment on which most of this chapter will draw.[2] The clinic is my site of inquiry because of its unique position as a site of translation and struggle between high modernist discourses of medicine, neoliberalism, and development and national discourses of cultural, Africanist, traditional medicines (*sangomas*), economic apartheid, and global discourses of abjection (Ferguson 1999; Kristeva 1982). The clinic where I worked is hardly a neutral geographic site. Consisting of a smallish, well-kept cement building, four prefabricated "bungalow" annexes, an AIDS support group's fledgling vegetable garden, and parking space for about five cars within a high chain-link fence, the clinic is a highly politicized space. Patients, service providers, and researchers enter at their own, varied risk. Everyone in the township knows that Heshima used to be the mother-and-baby clinic and now it is the AIDS clinic, although the sign outside says something less descriptive. Within the chain-link fence, power is legitimately wielded by the state. The inhabitants are commissioned with the authorized use of medicine.

Furthermore, in the province that least frequently resembles an integrated picture of the New South Africa's "rainbow nation," the clinic is a space of legitimate socio-racial-culture contact, if not equal exchange. Doctors (and researchers) drive in from Cape Town's leafy suburbs; counselors and nurses come from other townships or racially mixed geographic spaces, and patient advocates come from the diverse localities around the clinic's township area. Patients come from the local township, from other townships, or from other poorer parts of the country. There is no residency requirement for ARV treatment, just a commitment to return to the clinic for the required regular follow-up visits. The clinic provides the rare opportunity to examine the mixes of different agendas that cut across lines of race, class, and South African history.

Therapeutic Citizenship

Drawing on concepts of biological citizenship (Petryna 2002; Rose and Novas 2005) that link biomedical science to the ways that claims are made by and against the state for biomedical resources and rights, therapeutic citizenship examines how citizens' identity with illness constitutes a "parallel and derivative citizenship" (Nguyen 2010, 145). Therapeutic citizenship is useful for placing personal negotiations of illness within an explicitly political and institutional framework. Linking moral obligations with economic imperatives in a way that emphasizes relationships and interactions, therapeutic citizenship provides us with a way of thinking about the individual and the collective and allows us to "bring the state back in" (see the classic Evans, Rueschemeyer, and Skocpol 1985). This therapeutic state, however, is neither the nation-state of international relations, nor the developmental state of liberal longings, nor the mezzo level of multilevel research (sitting conveniently below global and above local), but is a performative apparatus and an ethical project. As such, the states of this state are multiple and different. One particular area for provocative inquiry I take up here is how the therapeutic state constructs its citizens as gendered.

This chapter draws from Nguyen's (2005) discussion of the complex biopolitical assemblage of HIV/AIDS that has been able to stitch together apparently disparate phenomena such as condom demonstrations, CD4 counts, sexual empowerment, compliance with drug regimes, retroviral genotyping, and an ethic of sexual responsibility into a remarkably stable worldwide formation. Therapeutic citizenship is a biopolitical construct based on a system of claims and ethical projects that arise out of the conjugation of techniques used to govern populations and manage individual bodies. Therapeutic citizens operate within a therapeutic economy (the totality of therapeutic options in a given location and the rationale behind legitimate access to them), which may be structured by monetary exchange but is also embedded within "regimes of value" (moral economies, networks, patronage, etc.) (Nguyen 2005).

However, further work is needed to conceptualize the therapeutic citizen, specifically as it relates to a particularly gendered notion of citizenship. Nguyen himself described an "unexpected challenge" to his clinical work as a physician providing ARVs in the Ivory Coast: women who became healthier returned to sexual life and childbearing. This turned up in the clinic as an "adherence problem." Women would disappear from the clinics and come back nine months later with a baby. Nguyen explained that one of the nurses had summed up why the women felt they had to hide to reproduce: "It's not authorized to get pregnant when you are on treatment."[3] Can it be possible for women in a culture of nearly universal childbearing and high levels of reproductive desire to become authorized as therapeutic citizens? This chapter explores how we can gender the therapeutic citizen through an understanding of reproductive decision making by women on ARVs within a South African AIDS clinic.

Mapping the Local Terrain of a Township in Western Cape Province, South Africa

It would be naive to surmise that equitable systems for providing lifesaving drugs could exist outside their historical context of overlapping indices of inequality. Global political economy, race and ethnicity, gender, regionalism, religion, nationalism, and politics will all impact the way that the ubiquitous rollout of ARVs will take place in developing countries. Furthermore, gendered constructions of the therapeutic citizens of the ARV state will serve multiple, if perhaps predictable, agendas. For example, a doctor in the Western Cape stated that "men are more likely to take a macho denialist approach," but women "as caregivers are more immediately and forcefully concerned with their own health" (Casey 2005, 50).

My analysis draws on a South African case study from a vertically structured, multisited ethnography within two highly contentious policy realms: family planning and AIDS treatment. South Africa probably has more than five million people living with HIV/AIDS—the highest number of any country in the world.[4] South Africa also has had extremely high levels of contraceptive use, with 75 percent of women having ever used contraceptives, and 50 percent currently using a modern method, according to Demographic and Health Survey data from 1998.

The South African state-sponsored family planning program officially began in 1974, a time of rapid urbanization and forced resettlement of the Black population into "homelands," vast labor migration, rising levels of unemployment, and increasing militancy against the apartheid regime (Kaufman 2000, 105). While the program was officially nonracial, most research emphasized the provision of family planning with the state's desire to control the Black and Coloured population (Brown 1983, 1987; Chimere-Dan 1993; Klugman 1993, cited in Kaufman 2000). Still, ever-increasing numbers of Black women have been adopting contraception for as long as data have been available.

On AIDS issues and treatment, the national government has been notorious for its lack of leadership. President Mbeki questioned the link between HIV and AIDS, accused scientists of racism, and called ARVs poison while supporting regimens of African potatoes and garlic as good alternatives to ARVs for AIDS treatment (see Nattrass 200). Still, on November 19, 2003, the South African government published the *Comprehensive Plan on HIV/AIDS Care* to provide universal coverage of ARVs within five years. Policy progress is measured according to rollout rates. These rates represent the percent of people who progress to AIDS and get ARVs. By the end of 2005, national HAART coverage was approximately 25 percent (meaning that only one in four people who needed HAART was receiving it) (Nattrass 2006, 5). Significant differences still exist between the provinces. Some provinces have exceeded a 50 percent rollout, but there are huge variations among worst-performing provinces (Mpumalanga, Free State, and Limpopo), covering barely 20 percent of those who need care. Western Cape is, not surprisingly, doing the best in the treatment rollout, with total HAART coverage of over 55 percent at the end of 2005 (Nattrass 2006, 5) and even more coverage available today.[5]

ARV provision in the Western Cape takes the form of a highly verticalized intervention. The Western Cape Province more closely resembles Uganda in its political approach to AIDS than it does to the other provinces in South Africa. Public-private partnerships flourish, linking pharmaceutical companies, bilateral and multilateral donors (like USAID and the Global Fund), and the provincial government of the Western Cape.[6] One of the leading ARV doctors in the region compared the HAART rollout to a "military operation" (Naimak 2006, 13).

The Western Cape has a lower disease burden than other provinces in South Africa. Its HIV prevalence rate among antenatal clinic attendees was 15.4 percent, about half of the national average of 29.5 percent (Department of Health 2005). Western Cape is the best-endowed province in the country for doctors, specialists, and hospitals, with approximately 73 doctors per 100,000 people (Abdullah 2005, 246–47). Geographically manageable, two-thirds of the province's population resides in greater Cape Town. However, the poorest areas with the highest burdens of disease have the fewest facilities and the lowest number of doctors per inhabitant in the city (Department of Health 2004).[7] Furthermore, nearly three-fourths of the population is dependent on public health services (Department of Health 2004). The Western Cape also has the highest development index ratings in the country, alongside the highest Gini coefficient (a measure of income inequality): the area is both rich and plagued by inequality.

The level of inequality in South African society presents particular challenges for providing and receiving healthcare for AIDS. The founder of one of the province's largest ARV clinics and coauthor of the country's national ARV treatment guidelines concluded: "All programs are focused on the 'oppressed' and the 'innocent.' . . . All of our programs are focused on women and children. . . . Men are guilty. . . . Men are the perpetrators" (Casey 2005, 50). Relations of struggle and blame shape the way in which therapeutic citizenship must be understood.

Heshima Clinic

Heshima Clinic is located within the oldest township in the Western Cape, dating back to 1927. In many ways, Heshima Clinic is a best-case scenario for ARV treatment in South Africa. Unlike most of the Western Cape's HAART facilities, Heshima is an integrated clinic, where ARVs are distributed together with primary health services, including family planning, nutritional counseling, and limited psychological services. The clinic is well managed and mostly protected from huge NGOs and their accountability demands so that staff can conduct their clinic work with minimal disruption. The site is also groomed to demonstrate success in an ongoing subregional political feud in the health sector. According to the regional director responsible for the clinic, Heshima has an ideal staffing ratio, runs under shared leadership instead of a military model, and is an operational setting as opposed to one focused on research.

Before turning to descriptions of the clinical interactions, I give a rough outline of the treatment terrain from the patient's perspective. In doing so, I am charting the "usual" path of treatment flow as I saw it most often: this is neither the official protocol for how treatment should happen nor the path taken all of the time. Most often, ARV treatment should begin with a visit to the patient advocates for the first counseling session. Patient advocates are the lowest-paid, semiskilled youth counselors who go on home visits and are on call around the clock for ARV patients. Patient advocates provide meaningful links between the real people and their caregivers and are the only service providers who are required to be local—that is, to live in Heshima. After the session with the patient advocates, a patient should have two visits with the ARV adherence counselors. These are highly skilled counselors, one male and one female at Heshima Clinic, with experience in voluntary counseling and testing (VCT) for HIV. They are responsible for counseling patients into adherence and detecting any potential adherence problems before patients are permitted to begin ARV treatment. A visit to the nutritionist should also take place but often does not, and a visit with a psychologist may be prescribed for patients facing clinically manageable psychological problems.

On Thursdays, Heshima Clinic holds mandatory three-hour staff meetings for all its team members. Together they decide on ARV initiation. The terms for assessment are both medical and social. Patients must have a treatment buddy—a sort of enforced, minimal biosociality (Rabinow 1999a,

411). They must have been to the requisite counseling sessions, have a contact person (if they lack a proper address in the catchment area), and show no significant signs of drinking or drug problems or severe mental illness. Once selected, a patient must perform responsibly as a therapeutic citizen by stating that he or she will use a condom, plan pregnancies with the doctor, try to receive appropriate government disability grants, eat well, refrain from traditional medicines, inform the clinic before traveling, especially before returning to the Eastern Cape,[8] and adhere to medication.

Border Defense of the Therapeutic State

ARV treatment presents interwoven relationships of treating the self and the mother—representing a new twist on the historical feminist debates between the self, the fetus, and the maternal relationship. Exposure to pregnancy necessarily risks exposure to HIV, as procreation involves unprotected sexual intercourse. As we will see from discussions of the clinic interactions, there is an implicit separation between procreative sexual relations and all other types of sexual behavior. Procreative sexual relations are governed by appropriate consultative processes between the therapeutic citizen and her physician, and all other sexual behavior falls under the strict control of the condom. Yet this separation between the mother and the sexually active woman not only is illogical, it represents a fundamental difficulty of gendering the therapeutic citizen. Treatment counselors tell women that they must use a condom every time they have sex to protect themselves from reinfection with a resistant virus and to protect their partners. At the same time, the counselors advise women on ARVs to plan pregnancies with their physicians.

At the Heshima Clinic, approximately fifteen people on average are considered for placement on ARVs each week. There are more women than men.[9] Most of the women are mothers; some are pregnant. In the province, at least one-third of all HIV tests are done on pregnant women under the Prevention of Mother-to-Child Transmission of HIV (PMTCT) program, and the other two-thirds of those testing for HIV also include mostly women.[10] Although the "typical" ARV patient is a woman of childbearing age, few studies have been done so far on family planning for women living with AIDS in the Third World. The existing ones emphasize the need to link contraceptive and AIDS interventions into a convenient service for women (de Bruyn 2004, 2005; Preble, Huber, and Piwoz 2003; Best 2004). However, family planning practices are also used as meaningful performances of therapeutic citizenship, as I will demonstrate from the ARV team meetings at Heshima Clinic.

As mentioned earlier, once a week the entire ARV team meets to discuss the patients who are being worked up for treatment. The team sits around a long table with copies of the patients' case summaries. The dialogue on each case begins with a review of the medical report from the physician responsible for the patient, followed by a review of the report written by the social worker; however, the social worker's report is often missing. Then the patient advocate gives an oral summary of the home visit and personal situation, and the adherence counselors describe their sessions with the patient. If the patient has seen the psychologist or nutritionist and further comments are available, they are presented as well.

Together with other relevant social criteria for ARV readiness, such as alcohol abuse or difficulty disclosing to a treatment buddy, contraceptive status is assessed for almost all of the women who seek treatment. This assessment is not a simple matter of ensuring that women on ARVs do not reproduce, although that may be the outcome. It involves a complex negotiation of reproductive management for the patient's own good. How this good is determined involves investigation, speculation, and, to some degree, the participation of the women themselves.

The biomedical report is the first determinant of whether a therapeutic citizen is potentially able to become pregnant. Some women who are very sick are not considered "at risk" of pregnancy. One example is the case of Xoliswa, a potential patient for starting ARVs. Because she was so ill, the team agreed that she had to be sent to a hospice center for constant care while beginning the treatment regime.[11] Still, her doctor noted at her case discussion that the team will "rediscuss family planning when she's better."[12] The doctor recognized that the goal of ARVs is to bring Xoliswa back to life, and in doing so, she will be likely to return to reproduction.

Social issues, or the situations and relationships that must be negotiated as part of living with AIDS and in which ARV treatment plays only one part, have a significant effect on how a woman can be a therapeutic citizen. One example comes from Phumla, a twenty-four-year-old unemployed mother of two children, ages five and seven. The family slept on the floor of a one-room shack owned by Phumla's friend and her friend's boyfriend. When the team was considering her for treatment, the discussion turned to her support structure. The patient advocate reported that Phumla's sister had refused to be her treatment buddy but had found a friend to help out. Phumla had had no regular sexual partner since she was diagnosed as HIV positive six months earlier. Phumla said that she wanted another child sometime in the future but was currently taking the contraceptive injection. Having successfully performed as a therapeutic citizen thus far, Phumla was allowed to begin ARV treatment. However, the social issues of sexual and reproductive desire, gender relations, familial instability, and poverty persist as limitations on Phumla's therapeutic citizenship.

Another example comes from Faith, a potential ARV patient who sparked a debate among the team members as physicians tried to negotiate their role in her social issues and her family planning. Faith and her family were victims of recurrent seasonal fires attributable to cheap cookers that regularly raze sections of the local informal housing settlements to the ground. She had two children who stayed with their grandmother in a different township. When the team met to discuss her case, Faith had been living for months in a tent, pitched in another informal settlement far from her home, and was complaining about a lack of food. However, Faith traveled to the Heshima Clinic for care because she said that she wanted to return and was ready to start ARVs. Her compliance with the TB treatment was reported in her file as "excellent." The program head then asked the physician: "So are you going to put her on family planning or not?" The doctor responded, "It's up to them. If we are forcing them, they are not compliant." A different doctor supported the first one: "They didn't understand that condoms are not as effective as the injection. What happens if they fall pregnant? How bad is it going to be?" The program head ended the discussion: "We should be thinking about family planning in a broader context of family planning, not just contraception."[13]

Implicit here is that the physician must take into account the social issues of Faith's life when formulating her treatment regime—including a contraceptive component. However, the doctors' discussion of responsibility for contraceptive choices and how these choices relate to compliance is informative. As both of the previous examples demonstrate, ARV compliance must be negotiated within fundamental poverty constraints (where will you sleep, where can you get money, what do you eat) that are likely to be exacerbated by having more children. Yet women are entitled to make their own reproductive choices, and these choices may contravene such planning for many reasons. Providers are relying on patient advocates' descriptions of spaces (geographic, racial, sexual, and economic) that they do not inhabit. This translation dance is not always successful. For example, one young woman's name was on the pharmacy list for having neglected to pick up her prescribed medicines; according to her patient advocate, she was unwilling to start ARVs because she did not want to use the contraceptive injection.

When a female patient begins her ARV regimen, doctors must try to estimate the probability that the woman will become pregnant while on the medication. The potential for drug interactions with the pregnancy is just one factor that must be considered, alongside all possible side effects, effectiveness, and desirability of the pregnancy. Additionally, the macro-constraints of cost and availability and the disparity between regional health systems must also be considered for patients at Heshima Clinic. The following example illustrates the particular difficulties of prescribing an appropriate drug for treatment with the first-line regimen. The most desirable drug, Efavirenz, is not recommended for use during pregnancy because of its link to birth defects. Instead doctors must prescribe Nevirapine for women who are likely to experience intended or unplanned pregnancy. However, for maintaining a woman's health, Nevirapine needs more consistent monitoring and follow-up than does Efavirenz.[14] In an interview, one physician stated that because this sort of intensive monitoring rarely happens, even in the best situations in South Africa, her clinic is usually "anti-Nevirapine." Instead, her clinic usually makes all women get a contraceptive injection and use Efavirenz.[15] This is an attempt to ensure that women get the best possible ARV treatment without risking birth defects in the case of a pregnancy. However, the issue of pregnancy is not the only determinant in the clinic; the disparity between regional health systems also plays a role. Because Nevirapine is cheaper, less-wealthy clinics and regions are more likely to use it for their first-line ARV regimen for women. At Heshima, where many patients come from the Eastern Cape and can be expected at some point to return, doctors might actually be doing female patients a disservice by prescribing a better Efavirenz regime, because a woman might have to switch to Nevirapine if she chose to return home.

The team struggled with these issues in the case of Catherine, a forty-year-old mother of five children. Catherine was married to an HIV-positive man and depended on his government disability grant for support. She lived in a room that sheltered seven families. When the team discussed Catherine's case at the meeting for ARV initiation, it was observed that she had completed counseling to start ARVs months earlier but had disappeared when the time had come to actually pick up the medicine from the pharmacy and begin taking the pills. Catherine had said that because of disclosure issues with the six other families who lived with her, she did not want to start the drugs. It was also noted that although her living situation had not changed, she had recently become so sick that she was ready to start the ARVs. Although Catherine's file noted that she had been taking the contraceptive injection, after looking at her chart, the doctor reported that there was no evidence that she was actually using any method of contraception. Thus, because the likelihood of pregnancy seemed high, she was started on the ARV regimen that includes Nevirapine, just in case she fell pregnant.

Discourses of liberal individualism, choice making, and reproductive rights frame the policies and practices at Heshima Clinic. Yet a recent patient was noted to have "just started on contraception two weeks before because [the clinical staff] forced her."[16] Others are described as "being on family planning specifically for the ARVs." Together with the social issues, women on ARVs must consider both the possibility of an AIDS-infected baby and the potential for birth defects attributable to the mother's treatment regime. ARV treatment complicates the negotiating logics, already difficult to disentangle from poverty and fertility desires, for realizing reproductive choice.

Clinical-level data remind us that it is worth explicit research consideration that women with AIDS do get pregnant, whether they are on treatment or not. As PMTCT expands into HAART in developing countries, we need more studies on how mothers and their children negotiate AIDS care. ARVs and contraceptives are not channeled through the consistent imposition of biopolitical discipline relying on medical authoritarianism, as one might expect given South Africa's political, racial, and economic history. Instead, we see complex negotiations between "ought" and "can," "possibility" and "probability," ethics and protocols. All of which are conducted on the basis of highly imperfect information, requiring multiple layers of translation within a context of complicated and sometimes competing agendas. Women and their providers are pragmatically negotiating a messy terrain of social issues and complicated biosociality in which the fact that women are regularly overvictimized does not mean that they adequately control their sexual or reproductive lives. It is in these interactions where women do have input into the decisions made about their health—even in a formal, medical setting—where the possibility of performing as a gendered therapeutic citizen becomes important.

Gendering the Therapeutic Citizen: Future Directions

Therapeutic citizenship exists as "a form of stateless citizenship whereby claims are made on a global order on the basis of one's biomedical condition, and responsibilities worked out in the context of local moral economies" (Nguyen 2005, 142). Paul Roux, a well-known Cape Townian physician, described his treatment experiences with mothers on ARVs. These women have high rates of pregnancy when they feel that they have become healthy again. A practitioner and pragmatist, he explained: "You can't expect to restore someone to personhood and not allow them to procreate."[17] How, then, will it become possible for women to be full therapeutic citizens whose gendered claims are taken seriously within both the global order and the local moral economy?

Do therapeutic citizens have more rights on the basis of their illness, or do they live under the constraint and surveillance of semiauthoritarian technologies? The global trend toward highly verticalized interventions into public clinics by SWAT teams armed with pills reaffirms the place of the state in developing countries at the same time that public health is put under stress by these very interventions. Evidence from fieldwork in the Western Cape suggests that matters of clinical concern over reproductive health and AIDS care come at the interface of social issues and ARV technologies. We cannot simply use existing knowledge about ARV treatment regimes wedded with models of reproductive desires and contraceptive use. Therefore the performance aspect of the therapeutic citizen becomes invaluable, as does the translation effort of the patient advocate, who is situated in a no-man's-land of the biopolitical state—neither fully citizen nor sovereign.

Therapeutic citizens, we might be led to believe, do not reproduce. But as the case study here demonstrates, women on ARVs do reproduce, demanding a reconsideration of therapeutic citizenship. Thus the potentially reproductive therapeutic citizen destabilizes an entire Eurocentric hegemonic tradition in which being a citizen—or being a state—is masculine and reliant on a rights-seeking individual. While it may be the case that biological citizenship is both individualizing and collectivizing (Rose and Novas 2005, 441), negotiating pregnancy and ARVs brings different relational subjectivities that are neither individual nor collective. Do women who are already therapeutic citizens and biomedical beings and have become accustomed to routine monitoring, biosocial audits, and complex negotiations between people and pills attribute different meanings to reproductive decision making? Is it reasonable to expect that women on ARVs take a far more active role in evaluating, planning, and controlling their procreation than women who are not undergoing AIDS treatment? How can we meaningfully integrate social issues into our understandings as more than just justifications for "noncompliance"?

The conceptual difficulty of gendering the therapeutic citizen promises further knowledge on both therapy and citizenship. Perhaps this speaks to the limits of HIV/AIDS in people's lives: the disease is not determining in ways that are clear, unilateral, functional, or consistent. If women with AIDS reproduce in ways that bear a striking resemblance to the reproductive practices of women without AIDS, why should this be so surprising? Women on ARVs who want to become pregnant while remaining good therapeutic citizens must exercise a vast and steadfast discipline of the self and the sexual other, and they must additionally master the performance and pragmatism of dealing effectively with the concurrent potentiality of life and death.

Notes

1. I refer to the contemporary debates surrounding "Black economic empowerment"; see Ponte, Roberts, and van Sittert 2007.
2. Heshima is a pseudonym. I am grateful to the Metropole Region of the Western Cape for research clearance for this project and to Elizabeth Seabe for research assistance.
3. From a talk by Vinh-Kim Nguyen at Copenhagen University, May 18, 2006.
4. The HIV prevalence statistics are notoriously ideologically biased; reputable statistics from different sources vary by more than a million people in their estimates of the number of South Africans living with HIV.
5. This represents the number of people on HAART in both public- and private-sector provision as a percentage of the number of people needing HAART estimated by the ASSA2003 demographic model.
6. The provincial government entered into partnerships with at least six other NGOs or research-based initiatives for AIDS treatment in public facilities in the Western Cape (Naimak 2006, 7).
7. See Chopra and Saunders 2004 for a discussion of the public health disparities between communities within the Western Cape.
8. The population movements between Eastern and Western Cape are a persistent challenge for the health sector, as most patients, even long-term residents of the township,

can be expected to return home for traditional ceremonies, important holidays, and family affairs. These events are blamed for much of the clients' nonadherence.

9. Physicians interviewed in Cape Town estimated that between 70 and 80 percent of their ARV patients were women, because men do not come forward to receive treatment (Casey 2005, 48).

10. Fareed Abdullah, public lecture, University of Cape Town, September 23, 2005.

11. The clinic has a cooperative relationship with one hospice organization that will admit patients who are very ill and starting treatment in case they become sicker while suffering from immune reconstitution syndrome.

12. Field notes, September 9, 2005.

13. Field notes, October 20, 2005.

14. Efavirenz and Nevirapine are types of medicine called non-nucleoside reverse transcriptase inhibitors (NNRTI). NNRTIs block reverse transcriptase, a protein that HIV needs to make more copies of itself.

15. The injection is favored for its effectiveness and because its provider-dependency makes for easier monitoring by the clinic staff.

16. Field notes, October 20, 2005.

17. Paul Roux, presentation at the PATA Conference, Cape Town, November 29, 2005.

Birth in the Age of AIDS

Local Responses to Global Policies and Technologies in South India

The HIV/AIDS pandemic, along with biomedical treatments and global health programs to prevent mother-to-child transmission of HIV, is transforming birth experiences of women throughout the world. But these global trends of disease, medicine, and health policy interact with social and cultural contexts in distinctive ways, creating locally specific responses to reproduction in the age of AIDS (Whiteford and Manderson 2000). Based on ethnographic research on women, HIV/AIDS, and reproduction in Tamil Nadu, India, conducted for one month in 2002–3 and six months in 2004, this chapter examines the social processes through which pregnant women discover their HIV-positive status and the ensuing birthing experiences of those women. This is a historically and regionally specific case study of the impact of the intersection of international global health policy, state policy, and local practice on the reproductive lives of HIV-positive women in Tamil Nadu at the beginning of the new millennium (Ginsburg and Rapp 1995).

Through an examination of these intersections, I demonstrate how the social practice of medicine is linked to the social practice of kinship and marriage for women with HIV who seek reproductive healthcare in Tamil Nadu. This is evident both in the context of receiving an HIV-positive diagnosis and in the context of birth itself. Furthermore, while pointing to obstacles that women living with HIV faced in accessing basic obstetric care, I illustrate pragmatic strategies that these women employ as they navigate the institutions of both medicine and family (Lock and Kaufert 1998).

Setting the Scene

Of the fifty HIV-positive women whom I interviewed, twelve knew they were HIV positive before or during a pregnancy, and all twelve decided to continue with the pregnancy and delivery (Van Hollen 2007). These women came primarily from the lower socioeconomic sector of society. The average total annual household income reported was US$864. The average level of education of all twelve women was the sixth standard (sixth grade). All twelve of these women came from lower-caste communities. Six identified themselves as Hindu, and the other six reported that they had been born into Hindu families but had converted to Christianity. Their average age was twenty-eight. All had been married at some point; some were in their second marriages after having become AIDS widows at a young age.

The births of all twelve women were hospital births, which took place in Chennai (formerly Madras, the capital of Tamil Nadu) and in Namakkal District (a largely rural district in Tamil Nadu and home to India's largest trucking center in the town of Namakkal). All but one had given birth to their babies while knowing their HIV status since 2000. The year 2000 was a watershed year for mother-to-child transmission programs in India, since it was in 2000 that the Indian government's National AIDS Control Organization (NACO), in collaboration with UNICEF, piloted its Prevention of Parent to Child Transmission (PPTCT) program. In 2004 the PPTCT program was officially administered in select government maternity hospitals throughout Tamil Nadu to provide free counseling and HIV testing to pregnant women and to provide single-dose Nevirapine treatment (an antiretroviral therapy) to HIV-positive mothers and their newborns at birth, which can reduce HIV transmission rates from 25–30 percent to 8–10 percent.[1] This chapter focuses on three case studies of women from Namakkal District who gave birth in 2000, 2002, and 2004. These cases allow us to see both continuity and change through time in this district, a district that has gained international notoriety for having one of the highest HIV-prevalence rates in India, a fact that is attributed to the centrality of the trucking industry (TNSACS 2004; Jain 2002, 72).

I begin with an analysis of the narrative of a woman from Namakkal District whom I call Saraswati,[2] not because her story is representative of all the birth experiences but because it includes many of the key themes that emerge in other women's stories: the lack of informed consent along with the duplicity and pragmatism of both medical personnel and family members in the process of HIV testing, and the stigma and discrimination against HIV-positive women in maternity hospitals coupled with private acts of resistance against such discrimination.

Saraswati Gives Birth: 2000

Saraswati was twenty-four when I met her, and she had a four-year-old son who was HIV negative. When she was seventeen, she married a lorry driver. She became a widow at twenty-one when her son was one year old. She recounted the experiences of her pregnancy and birth of her son in 2000:[3]

> I first learned of my HIV status when I was five months pregnant when I went for my first prenatal checkup with a private doctor. Since my husband was a "lorry driver," they did an HIV test without saying anything and without asking my permission. And then they told me that I was "positive." . . . My parents and my mother's younger brother were the only ones who knew about my status at first.

In Tamil Nadu, women like Saraswati often do not get any prenatal care until well into their pregnancy. Thus they discover their HIV status at a late stage in their pregnancy, often precluding the possibility of abortion (Van Hollen 2007). Saraswati's HIV test was carried out without informed consent. My research suggests that lack of informed consent was not uncommon in private prenatal care. In Saraswati's situation, her status was disclosed to her, but I heard of several cases in which the private medical institutions simply referred patients elsewhere without disclosing their HIV status. Some women living with HIV told me that private medical practitioners do not require informed consent because they consider HIV testing to be like other routine tests. Others told me that the staff in some private hospitals fear that a patient may refuse to get tested given the option, and that since hospital personnel will not treat anyone who is HIV positive owing to their fears of HIV transmission during medical treatment, they simply test without informed consent so that they can refer any HIV-positive patient to private or public hospitals that are known to accept HIV patients. Public maternity hospitals with PPTCT programs are required to obtain informed consent for HIV testing. However, based on my observations of pretest counseling and testing in four government PPTCT centers in 2004 and on my discussions with women who had attended such centers, it is clear that the degree of informed consent carried out in such facilities is uneven (Van Hollen 2007).

Saraswati continued her account:

> My husband was on the road for his work when I found out about the HIV. I realized at that point that my husband must have had HIV even before we were married because before our marriage he was taking medicines from Majeed's clinic in Kerala.[4] When I had asked him about those medicines at the time of our marriage, he had told me that it was for some other minor illness. After I learned about my HIV status, I told my parents about the Majeed medicines, and my parents and I decided that if my husband had been keeping this a secret, he would not agree to get tested now. So when he came back home, we took him to the hospital and got him tested on some other pretense without his knowledge. He wouldn't have agreed otherwise. We didn't tell him that I had tested HIV positive. My doctor had cheated me, so I cheated my husband [she says, laughing].

This passage points to the multiple levels of duplicity that emerge in response to an HIV-positive diagnosis and affect marital relationships and broader kin and community relationships, as well as the doctor-patient relationship. The secrecy surrounding testing and the disclosure of an HIV diagnosis is a result of the stigma of HIV within medical settings and within the confines of the family; at times members of these two arenas are adversaries, while at other times they are collaborators in schemes of deceit. The kinship and marriage fault lines along which such schemes were played out are by no means predictable.

Most of the HIV-positive women whom I met believed that their husbands were aware of their HIV-positive status before the women themselves were tested but that their husbands had kept their HIV status secret to avoid blame and conflict within the family. Many, in fact, told me that they believed their husbands had known of their HIV status even before marriage. Yet it was increasingly women's HIV status that became known to other family members first, since women were now being tested for HIV during their pregnancy. As a result, women were being blamed for bringing HIV into the family.

In part due to the recognition of the unequal attribution of blame that could result from prenatal HIV testing, counselors in the government's PPTCT program were advised to urge women to convince their husbands to be tested at the same time that the women themselves would be tested. Governmental and nongovernmental organizations involved in international HIV/AIDS prevention work, such as the WHO, UNAIDS, UNICEF, USAID, and the CDC also advocate partner testing in their guidelines for pretest counseling during pregnancy.[5] But the Indian government has taken this emphasis one step farther than these other organizations by actually calling its program the Prevention of *Parent*-to-Child Transmission, rather than using the global health policy appellation of the Prevention of *Mother*-to-Child Transmission (PMTCT; italics mine). The government of India chose to substitute *parent* for *mother* to increase the husbands' involvement in the program (including HIV testing), to decrease the stigmatization of HIV-positive women, and to acknowledge and raise awareness about the fact that husbands have been primarily responsible for infecting their wives. This is one example of the ways in which global policies are mediated through national state policy. The tendency to place HIV testing and counseling squarely within a set of kinship and marriage relationships is not only a policy move on the part of the government but also reflects the social and cultural understanding of HIV/AIDS and reproduction for the women, families, and medical personnel.

It is clear from Saraswati's comments quoted earlier that the medical personnel colluded with Saraswati and her parents to test her husband without his knowledge. This demonstrates that a concern with protecting themselves from HIV in the medical setting is not the only factor leading medical staff to bypass informed consent. Another reason for bypassing informed consent is that HIV is not viewed as a private, individual issue so much as it is seen as a social issue, and particularly a family issue, that may warrant the abnegation of individual rights. The Indian government's policy at that time did require written informed consent for HIV testing, but this was clearly not always enacted in practice. In the WHO, UNAIDS, UNICEF, USAID, and CDC joint guidelines for pretest counseling during pregnancy in "resource-poor" contexts, written informed consent was and continues to be considered imperative. Meanwhile, however, CDC recommendations within the United States have recently shifted to an "opt-out screening" approach in which "patients should be informed orally or in writing that HIV testing will be performed unless they decline" (CDC 2006, 10).

Saraswati's account also demonstrates that stigma within medical settings resulting from fears of transmission through medical interventions was clearly intense in 2000:

> After I tested HIV positive, my doctor told me that she could not attend to my delivery. I saw two or three other doctors who also told me very openly that they would not attend my delivery. I didn't receive any medical care during my pregnancy at all after that. I wasn't even given iron tablets. Those doctors told me that I should have my delivery in a public hospital in Erode where HIV patients are cared for. I went to that hospital in Erode, and the doctor there said that he would care for me during my delivery.

Saraswati went on to describe the events of the birth:

> Ten days before my due date, I went to that hospital in Erode and checked in. But . . . when I showed the nurses my papers with my HIV-positive test results, one nurse said, "You people from Namakkal, you have no other work but to come to our hospital for all these kinds of things. We can't treat you!" and told me to go back to Namakkal. Then the doctor . . . came and scolded those nurses and said to me, "See, the staff here won't cooperate, so it's better if you go to Namakkal." He gave me the name of a private doctor in Namakkal.

Her birth story continued:

> When I reached that private doctor in Namakkal, he said that he could care for me, but he said that it might be hard to save me or my baby, and he asked us to have 20,000 rupees ready. The doctor said that since I was HIV positive, I might die having a normal delivery, so I would have to have a cesarean. He also said that a cesarean might help protect the baby.

The explanations given for conducting a cesarean are confusing here. Cesarean section is recommended to prevent HIV transmission from mother to child, although it was not typically done for that reason in the public hospitals in Tamil Nadu that have PPTCT programs, since the procedure was considered to be too costly to carry out for all HIV-positive mothers. But for this private practitioner, cost would not be an obstacle, since he was charging Saraswati 20,000 rupees for the procedure. This represented approximately three and a half months of her husband's total income at the time, and like the vast majority of Indians, she did not have access to any kind of health insurance to defray her medical costs. What is confusing is that Saraswati also said that the doctor claimed that the cesarean was necessary to save her own life. It is not clear whether she misunderstood him, or he incorrectly believed this, or there was some medical reason for this, or this was purely driven by a profit motive.

Saraswati went on:

> After the delivery . . . the nurses refused to change the "glucose drips" for me because they said that they had developed a high fever since they had touched me the day before. So I said, "Instead of letting it go dry, I will just pull the needle out of my hand myself." I started crying, and my mother started wailing. Then the doctor heard this and came in, and the doctor changed the "bottle" himself.

What is interesting to note here are the different representations of the nurses versus the doctors. In this section, as well as the earlier section when Saraswati was in the hospital in Erode, it is clear that she feels that it is the nurses who are the prime perpetrators of discriminatory practices, whereas the doctors—both male and female—are represented as much more caring and as stepping in to do the work of the nurses when the nurses refuse. This difference is probably a reflection of doctors' better education and training in the treatment and care of HIV/AIDS patients compared to nurses and other supporting staff at that time, resulting in fewer fears about HIV transmission among doctors than among other medical personnel.

When I asked Saraswati if she or the baby received any treatment to prevent the transmission of HIV, she said that she didn't think so, that she was never informed about anything like that, and that she did not remember having any tablets or injections for that during delivery. She did, however, remember the doctor's advice about caring for her newborn.

> After the baby was born, the doctor told me that I should wash my hands carefully every time before I touched my baby, that I should not breast-feed the baby, and that I should not lie near my baby, since my breath shouldn't touch the baby. When people saw me treating my baby this way, everyone came to know about my status. My son was very active, and the older women in the village would say, "Even when you haven't given mother's milk, your son is so active. Imagine how healthy and active he

would be if you would breast-feed!" When these older women said that, my grandmother told them why I was not breast-feeding, and in that way the whole village came to know about my HIV status.

Although the earlier passage suggested that the doctors were more knowledgeable about the modes of HIV transmission, here we see that this knowledge may have been uneven in 2000, since the doctor needlessly told Saraswati to avoid touching or breathing close to her baby, yet also advised against breast-feeding, which can be a mode of mother-to-child transmission. We also see in this section how HIV-positive women in Tamil Nadu may be criticized by their community for not breast-feeding their newborns (due to a strong cultural value placed on breast-feeding), and how this public critique may lead to unintended disclosure of their HIV-positive status, often resulting in community-wide stigma.

Jayanthi Gives Birth: 2002

Two years later, Jayanthi gave birth knowing that she was HIV positive. Jayanthi had discovered her HIV status during the eighth month of her pregnancy with her second child. She had been married at the age of twenty and became a widow at twenty-four, three days before the birth of her second child.

As with Saraswati, Jayanthi's account of the process of discovering her HIV-positive status reveals the kind of behind-the-scenes strategies of both family members and medical personnel. In her case, her husband had fallen very ill during her pregnancy, and Jayanthi's own father had taken her husband to the hospital for an HIV test, whereupon they discovered that her husband was HIV positive. Neither her husband nor her father had informed Jayanthi that they were going for the test or that her husband was HIV positive. But they did inform the doctors at the hospital where Jayanthi was going for her prenatal care. Jayanthi's husband and her father asked the doctor to inform Jayanthi of her husband's status via the prenatal counselor. We see from this example that doctors and other personnel working in the health service sector are often expected to play important roles as mediators for families.

The United States mandates confidentiality of a patient's HIV status, reflecting a perception of HIV as a private, individualized disease. Among the communities in Tamil Nadu where I conducted this research, knowledge of someone's HIV status was perceived as a family affair, as something to be either disclosed or kept secret from particular relatives, and sometimes from spouses, and medical personnel participated as brokers in the flow of this knowledge among kin. The largest public hospital for HIV/AIDS treatment used a computer program to track down family relations to get them tested. Thus community practice and state practices parallel one another but diverge from the policies for medical practice in the United States and policy guidelines within global health policy that mandate patient confidentiality.

Jayanthi then recounted the events of her birth:

> After discovering that I was HIV positive, while I was still pregnant my doctor gave me a tablet and told me to take the tablet as soon as I began to have my pains. My pains came in the night, but I did not want to take that tablet because I was afraid that it would harm my baby. . . . I went to the Taluk hospital [public secondary care] in the night. . . . I did not go to the same hospital that I went to for my checkups so that the staff would not know that I had HIV. But the next day, one of my cousins came and told the nurses at that hospital that I had HIV. . . . They asked me to leave and go to the GH [Government Hospital for tertiary care] where they had treatment for HIV-positive mothers. But I refused to go. . . . Then all of the nurses went home and left me. I gave birth to my baby like that, alone, without any nurses there to help. I had terrible pain. I didn't receive any treatment. Not a single drop of medicine. Not a single injection.

Jayanthi's distrust of the medical system had led her to throw out the Zidovudine antiretroviral tablet, which her doctor had given her to prevent HIV transmission.[6] Her suspicions also motivated her to try surreptitiously to get care from another hospital without informing them of her HIV status, since based on the experience of her close friend, she was afraid that she would not get care at the hospital if they knew she was HIV positive. It is not surprising that women like Jayanthi will act pragmatically to fool the medical institutions if they feel that doing so is the only way to receive treatment.

Without interfering cousins such as Jayanthi's, it is also possible that such pragmatic efforts for survival could contribute to the spread of HIV in medical settings that are not set up to practice universal precautions for each and every normal delivery. Discriminatory processes within the hospitals lead to these kinds of strategies of secret resistance, which can fuel the spread of HIV and also helps explain why hospitals may not subscribe to informed consent for HIV testing. This creates a vicious cycle, detrimental to both HIV prevention and care.

Saraswati's grandmother had outed Saraswati's HIV status to the village in her attempt to defray the harsh criticisms about Saraswati's decision not to breast-feed. And Jayanthi's cousin had gone out of her way to come to the hospital in the middle of the night to disclose Jayanthi's status to the hospital staff, thereby making this known to the village community. Saraswati's mother and father had cooked up a scheme to force her husband to be tested to reveal his HIV status, whereas Jayanthi's father had acted in concert with her husband to keep Jayanthi from knowing that her husband was being tested and, initially, from knowing her husband's HIV-positive status. These cases demonstrate that in Tamil Nadu the social experience of HIV/AIDS runs along the grooves of kinship and marriage relationships that serve at times to protect the dignity and health of these women and other times to expose them to public indignities and prevent them from gaining access to knowledge and care needed to protect their health and the health of their future children. Clearly, as Carsten notes, kinship is not "intrinsically desirable," as anthropological analyses tend to assume (Carsten 2000, 28); it "can take both benevolent and destructive forms" (Carsten 2004, 9).

Vijaya Gives Birth: 2004

HIV/AIDS can disrupt and wreak havoc on kinship and marital relationships at the same time that kinship norms provide a framework for the social responses to HIV/AIDS. HIV/AIDS is thus reproducing and transforming kinship and marriage in Tamil Nadu, just as new reproductive technologies have been reported to do elsewhere (Strathern 1995; Franklin and Ragoné 1998; Becker 2000; Inhorn and van Balen 2002). This is starkly apparent in the growing numbers of young AIDS widows and the strategies that they and their families employ to respond to these premature disruptions of family life, strategies that sometimes involve the creation of "practical kinship" (Das 1995). Vijaya became an AIDS widow in 2000 when her first child was four years old. But she did not learn about her own status until four years later in 2004, when she was in the ninth month of her second pregnancy after having gotten married again, this time to the older brother of her deceased husband. Although they understood that Vijaya could have gotten HIV from her first husband, neither she nor her parents realized that she could transmit it to her second husband or a future child. "If I had known," she said, "I would have never agreed to remarry."

Vijaya's experience of learning about her HIV status did not involve the same kind of duplicity that characterized the stories of Saraswati and Jayanthi. Vijaya learned that she was HIV positive on her first prenatal checkup in a Taluk hospital in Namakkal District in the ninth month of her pregnancy. This was a hospital that had a PPTCT program in 2004. She received pretest counseling, gave informed consent for the testing, and received posttest counseling.

Vijaya was open about her HIV status with her husband and said that he was supportive of her, perhaps because of the role played by his own brother, perhaps because of a change in attitudes about HIV/AIDS as we move from Saraswati's experience in 2000 to Vijaya's in 2004. Yet Vijaya was far from public with her status, suggesting that the disease was still highly stigmatized.

Vijaya described the day of her birth:

> I went to the Taluk hospital when I started having labor pains. But the doctors and nurses would not see the delivery there. They referred me to GH. People from HUNS helped me go to GH. They got me admitted without telling the staff about my HIV status. It was only once I had been admitted into the hospital that we revealed my status.

From Vijaya's account, it is clear that even in 2004, women living with HIV in Namakkal District, one of the highest HIV-prevalence areas in India, still faced great obstacles trying to access basic maternity care at the time of delivery. The particular hospital that first refused to admit her when she was in labor was officially a PPTCT hospital. Furthermore, just as Jayanthi had attempted to access obstetric care while keeping her HIV status under the radar in 2002, women were still resorting to this tactic in 2004 even in a government hospital with a PPTCT program.

What is significantly different, however, is that Vijaya now had the backing of HUNS (HIV Ullor Nalla Sangam)—a nongovernmental network of HIV-positive people—to help her navigate the obstacles of the medical system. Among other advocacy activities, HUNS was providing access to legal aid for people living with HIV/AIDS and facing all forms of discrimination, including discrimination in medical settings. Once she was admitted into GH with the help of HUNS, there was no refusing Vijaya her treatment, and she and her newborn received Nevirapine to help prevent the transmission of HIV to her child.

Although others might view her experience as a circuitous path to obstetric care, riddled with obstacles, when I asked Vijaya how she felt about her birth experience, she replied, "I was completely satisfied with all the treatment and care I received from both the Taluk Hospital and GH." Vijaya's satisfaction with her medical care must be placed within the historical context of Saraswati's and Jayanthi's birth stories. From this perspective, we can appreciate that Vijaya's birth was a victory for poor women living with HIV, but a victory that still required a struggle. As I reflect on accounts like Vijaya's, it sometimes seems as though women the world over are reduced to feeling grateful for whatever medical care they are dealt, just because it is provided and their babies survive.

Conclusion

Each of these three births took place after the government's PPTCT project had been initiated (either in its pilot phase or its subsequent programmatic phase) and after treatment to prevent mother-to-child transmission of HIV had been made available in some private hospitals. Yet the mere fact that such treatments and programs exist tells us little about the lived experiences of pregnancy and childbirth for women living with HIV. My analysis of the births of Saraswati, Jayanthi, and Vijaya reveals that even though programs to prevent mother-to-child transmission were formally available, these three women all faced difficulties in obtaining obstetric care owing to ongoing stigma and discrimination in medical settings.

Furthermore, the practice of medical care for mother-to-child HIV prevention programs is not universally implemented in the same way across the globe but is shaped by local social organization and cultural understandings of HIV and birth. Local understandings and practices at times inform the state's interpretation of global health policy, as we see in the state's choice of nomenclature of the PPTCT program and the state's more family-centered interpretation of patient confidentiality. When we examine the social uses and practice of medicine in Tamil Nadu, it is apparent that HIV testing and care, particularly in the context of reproduction, are viewed not as matters pertaining exclusively to the patient as an individual but as events that involve broad networks of kinship and marriage. In Tamil Nadu an HIV diagnosis in the context of reproduction demands a careful and strategic but varied selection of alliances along kinship and marital lines that informs how knowledge flows and how care is or is not provided.

My study of three women's HIV experiences also demonstrates how medical personnel in Tamil Nadu are drawn into these family alliances and how the *practices* of medical care for HIV/AIDS—including the absence of uniformly applied informed consent for HIV testing and confidentiality—are responses to local sociocultural contexts. Medical personnel may become coconspirators trying to keep an HIV diagnosis hidden from some family members, or trying to expose an HIV status to other family members. Family members may in turn inform medical personnel of someone's HIV status even when a patient is trying to keep that information away from the doctors and nurses. For the three women in this study, there were instances where the medical personnel's links to, and participation in, kinship and community networks were beneficial to them, and other times when these connections worked against their own interests. Above all, what these three case studies reveal is that whether women living with HIV are confronting stigma and discrimination in medical institutions or within their extended kin and community networks, their vulnerable situation itself demands that they engage in complex, pragmatic, and often creative strategies just to obtain basic obstetric services.

Notes

My research was supported by the Fulbright Foundation and the University of Notre Dame's Institute for Scholarship in the Liberal Arts. I am grateful to all the women who participated and to those who facilitated this research: P. Kousalya (PWN+), Dr. P. Kuganantham (UNICEF), Jeypaul (HUNS), and R. Meenakski (SPMD). Thanks also to the following research assistants and translators: S. Padma, Punitha, Jasmine Obeyesekere, Sharon Watson, Rajeswari Prabhakaran, Dr. Dasaratan, and Sheela Chavan.
1. From Libman 2004. See also "Second Phase of Anti-retroviral Programme Begins—Tamilnadu, India," posted on the AIDS-INDIA Listserv, March 1, 2005. The article originally appeared in the *Hindu* newspaper on February 28, 2005.
2. All names of research participants are pseudonyms.
3. All the interviews in this paper have been translated from the original Tamil. Words in quotation marks indicate that the original was in English.
4. See Van Hollen 2005 for a discussion of Majeed's claims to a cure for HIV/AIDS.
5. See the Women, Children, and HIV website at http://www.womenchildrenhiv.org.
6. While Nevirapine was provided in the official PPTCT program, Zidovudine was provided during the pilot phase.

Competing Globalizing Influences on Local Muslim Women's Reproductive Health and Human Rights in Sudan

Women's Rights, International Feminism, and Islamism

Articulating the centuries-long processes of globalization has received increasing attention in anthropology, from Eric Wolf's analysis of Europe and the "people without history" (1982) to Arjun Appadurai (1990) and the global cultural economy, with numerous ethnographic studies in the postcolonial frame. The task of observing and analyzing the concrete local realities that manifest the process of globalization is extraordinarily challenging. As globalization has unfolded, the spread of ideas, ideologies, images, institutional structures, and the state has required that additional weight be given to forces that are exerting contradictory pressures on people's lives, decisions, and cultural practices. Anthropologists' ethnographic studies of the incorporation of global influences on local practices have identified varying responses to different elements, from resistance to syncretistic inclusions to enthusiastic adoptions of new opportunities or cultural change.

During the past thirty years, in my study of Sudanese health issues— which has focused especially on female genital cutting (FGC, or FGM, female genital mutilation)—I have used theoretical concepts of feminist anthropology, political economy, and globalization to link the local experience of reproductive health to the expansion of capitalism and the dynamics of challenges to patriarchal relations (Gruenbaum 2001, 2005). But in fieldwork in Sudan in 2004, I found that the competing force of political Islam, or Islamism, has become increasingly more powerful and influential. Its influence goes beyond resistance to the external power of Western capitalism to become a competing form of globalization, delegitimizing local cultural authority to insert a form of globalization, one that is much harder to resist.

In this chapter, I examine the forces of change affecting the cultural contexts of female genital cutting (for definitions and description, see the appendix at the end of the chapter), sexuality, and reproductive decisions in several areas of Sudan. I consider the feminist, public health, and human rights movements that are strongly influenced by Western and capitalist processes of globalization, and I address the competing globalizing influences of Islamism, specifically its Wahhabist tenor.

Feminist Activism against Female Genital Cutting

I have often pondered the Egyptian physician-activist Nawal El Saadawi's pithy salvo at the foreign anti-FGC campaigners, criticizing their ultimately unhelpful "them-helping-us" rhetoric, which amounts to "colonialism in disguise" (El Saadawi 1980). To women of the regions where forms of female genital cutting are practiced, the Western feminists who displayed ethnocentric polemics to denounce such harmful traditional practices were attacking the right of African and Middle Eastern women to determine the targets and timing of their own struggles. Such outsiders essentialized African and Middle Eastern women's lives, making the condition of their genitals the most salient feature, for which insensitivity mainstream Western feminism has been duly criticized (see James and Robertson 2002).

While several researchers have presented cultural contextualization and nuanced understandings of the harmful traditional practices of female genital cutting (Assaad 1980; Boddy 1982, 1989, 1998; Gruenbaum 1982, 1996, 2001; Hayes 1975; Morsy 1991, 1993), much recent work has focused on change and efforts to end the practices (Abusharaf 2000, 2006; Shell-Duncan and Hernlund 2000). The rhetoric of "eradication"—a term that robs social actors of their agency—reflects globalizing influences of Western feminism, public health, and human rights movements, all of which seek to free women and girls from traditional practices that harm their health and rights. And yet the local energy for change provided by African and Middle Eastern women in their own postcolonial struggle to define and assert their rights and improve their lives refutes any stale notion of women's passivity. As Gwendolyn Mikell points out, African and Middle Eastern women have faced a challenge in attempting to simultaneously affirm their identities in a context of global oppression while "transforming societal notions of gender and familial roles" (1997, 1). Mikell argues that African feminism is shaped by resistance to Western hegemony as well as being rooted in cultural legacies of Africa (4), both of which are profoundly evident in the debates over female genital cutting, as the work of Ahmadu (2000), Abusharaf (1998, 2000, 2001), Mikell (1997), and others demonstrates. Writers who have taken strong stands against the practices with what I would argue is insufficient attention to the contexts of women's lives—for example, Lightfoot-Klein (1989), Hosken (1980, 1982), Walker (1992), Walker and Parmar (1993), and Daly (1978)—contribute to the climate of ethnocentric Western hegemony, whether it is feminist or not, provoking resentment and even backlash. Stanlie James and Claire Robertson (2002) provide a spirited review of the ways in which the anti-FGC polemics of the U.S. writers, in particular, have damaged the sense of respect for transnational sisterhood on this issue. Robertson characterizes such Western representations of FGC as "reducing all of Africa to one uncivilized place; reducing African women to the status of their genitals, presumed to be infibulated, and Africans to being sadistic torturers or victims; and reducing all FGC to its worst form, infibulation" (James and Robertson 2002, 60).

It is incumbent on national activists in countries affected by FGC to engage in their own liberation process—and indeed, African and Middle Eastern women in their homelands and in the global North have long since taken the lead in this effort, as the work of scholars and organizations such as RAINBO and the Inter-African Committee against Harmful Traditional Practices (IAC) has shown (Abdalla 1982; Abusharaf 1998, 2000, 2001; Dorkenoo 1994; El Dareer 1982; Toubia 1985, 1993, 1994).

Leaders of the Sudanese women's movement have a long history of activism and a lengthy agenda of social practices and economic conditions that need to change for the betterment of the lives of women and girls (Abusharaf 2001, 117–19; Hale 1996, 2005). As Hale has pointed out, local issues of women's culture, with their generative and transformative potential, have been pushed aside to some extent by the privileging of the transnational over the local. Hale argues that transnational institutions, such as the Sudanese Women's Union (linked to the Sudanese Communist Party and related international institutions), as well as the National Islamic Front and other Islamist groups, have both looked for new solutions outside women's traditional local culture (2005).

In the process, many Sudanese traditions have been suppressed, either as not modern or as non-Islamic, respectively, depending on which of the competing globalizing processes has gained the upper hand. Insofar as female genital cutting practices are addressed, then, even indigenous leadership may end up circumventing some Sudanese women's "process of liberation" to achieve more urgent results. But insofar as local Sudanese leaders have contributed to and welcomed the international conventions and declarations, efforts at cultural changes necessary to implement the agreements about women's and children's rights are simultaneously liberating and globalizing.

Opposing Change

Opponents of feminist agendas in Middle Eastern countries frequently accuse activists of pro-Western or anti-Islamic views. Indeed, although there were indigenous efforts to modify or end FGC historically (see Abusharaf 2001), the best-known anticircumcision campaigns in Sudan and other African countries were colonial, taken up in the spirit of "civilizing" the subject countries (Boddy 2007). In Sudan, for example, when modern midwifery training was introduced in the 1920s, students were educated not to circumcise. A law in Sudan against unlawful circumcision formally banned infibulation in 1946, a decade before independence. Although key Sudanese religious and medical leaders supported the law, its enforcement provoked protests by religious and other leaders who saw it as a British colonial imposition (Abusharaf 2001, 119; Boddy 2007; Gruenbaum 2001, 206–7; Toubia and Rahman 2000). The law, which was preserved for another four decades after independence, went unenforced until it was deleted from the criminal code under Islamist revisions in the 1990s (Malik 2004). Activists' calls for new legislation to reinstate the prohibition and extend it to ban all forms of FGC have met with distinct reluctance from political leaders.

Islamist Global Influences on Female Genital
Cutting and Reproductive Health in Sudan

Despite the recent peace accords in the civil war between southern Sudanese forces and the central government—which many had hoped would usher in an era of secular multicultural tolerance throughout the country—the government of Sudan continues to pursue an Islamist political structure for northern Sudan. Moreover, appeals to Islamic nationalism have been used widely by Islamists, and they are often successful at persuading Sudanese Muslims—who want to be loyal to Islam and do the right thing—to suppress elements of culture that more learned religious leaders declare to be un-Islamic. In this context, the growth of several Islamist and Wahhabist organizations such as the Ansar al-Sunna ("followers of the traditions of the Prophet") has made human rights and feminist agendas, as well as deeply rooted Nile Valley cultural traditions that were syncretized into Islam (e.g., zar spirit possession, river rituals, some wedding rituals, etc.), targets of attack. Public opinion is responsive when policies and political views appeal to Islamic orthodoxy, which affects reproductive health in the areas of FGC reform, early marriage, family planning, restrictions on women's activities, and sexuality.

There is support among Sudanese religious scholars and imams for the rejection of female circumcision as not Islamic in origin and not required by Islam, and such religious leaders are being encouraged to articulate and spread this message by international organizations like UNICEF and CARE, as well as Sudanese associations such as the Sufist Council. Others continue to use Islam and the sayings of Mohammed to justify the preservation of FGC practices, arguing that it is ennobling for Muslims to do the mild form mentioned by the Prophet in the Hadith. Indeed, the conservative Sudanese Muslim and professor of gynecology Dr. Sittalbanat advocates the practice as Islamic. Dr. Sittalbanat has developed a technique for removal of just a thin membrane from the clitoris, a technique that she calls "*sharia* circumcision." This new term is powerful: unlike the *sunna* circumcision terminology, *sharia* implies that the procedure cannot be made illegal, since it is protected or even required by religious law.

Although movement activists want a new law, none wanted another law that bans only the very severe form of circumcision known as pharaonic, which includes both clitoridectomy and infibulation, preferring to have no specific law than one that allows exceptions. Despite the dramatic harm reduction involved in doing the lesser form (Shell-Duncan 2001), any law that allowed "the mild type" (one of the rather ironic terminologies in use to avoid the association with religion implied by the term *sunna*) would undermine any enforcement. People could simply label whatever they do as sunna, a problem that was identified more than twenty years ago (Gruenbaum 1982). Testimony in hypothetical court cases would be problematic. One cannot rely on self-report as to the type of FGC—which is also a limitation of surveys or interviews both because of people's desire to sound pious (sunna) and because of the uncertainty many women have about exactly what was done to them—and physical examination of scarred vulvas is socially un-acceptable and unenforceable.

Sudanese movement activists no longer use the Arabic term *sunna* because it falsely confers religious legitimacy on the practices. The Arabic word *khifad*, often translated as "reduction," is also out of favor because the term echoes the verb in the controversial "weak" Hadith of the Prophet that is used for the claim that FGC is sunna. Sudanese activists now favor the neutral term *khitan* (cutting) so as to include all forms of FGC without religious connotations.[1] Reformers have also endeavored to establish a positive term for the uncircumcised state—*salmah*—so they can talk about what they favor in positive terms; *salmah* connotes a positive state of purity and well-being without being cut.

Local Discourse for Change

Although efforts against FGC have been conducted for decades, convincing people to abandon the practices made only slow progress for most of the twentieth century. In the northern two-thirds of the country, prevalence of some form has remained fairly steady at around 90 percent. But today many observers are convinced—though concrete data are scarce—that the incidence of new cutting (as a percentage of the girls at risk) is beginning to decline in some contexts and that the less-severe types of cutting (clitoridectomy and excision, WHO's Types I and II) are gaining in popularity. The activists, physicians, and others I interviewed in Khartoum and Omdurman consider this to be a strong trend among the urban middle class in particular. However, traditionally uncircumcised southern Sudanese who have settled in the north—displaced by the civil war that ended in 2004—are said to have begun to adopt the customs of the north. Among these internally displaced migrants, FGC is believed to be gaining adherents. Western ethnic groups displaced by the conflict in Darfur, some of whom have not practiced severe infibulations, may face a similar future as they are forced to settle among people with different customs.

What struck me about the dialogues in both rural and urban settings in 2004 was that the discourse was shifting from justification of circumcision based on honor, morals, marriageability, and the belief that it was religiously permitted or encouraged to a discourse of doubt and questioning. While there may yet be a majority of hard-core defenders of the practice among women, I encountered more openness among many of the younger generation who were willing to consider whether it would be better to change. For them, all the considerations—health, rights, and religion—were salient. But to judge from discussions in the seven rural communities where I worked in 2004, the main deterrents to rapid change seemed to be the risk that a daughter would be unmarriageable (due to shame or preferences of potential husbands) and the social pressure and peer pressure of shame and mockery of others. The strongest argument that seemed capable of driving the hesitant to consider change was the idea that Islam prohibits infibulation.

Elsewhere I have discussed the process of change for the two communities of my longitudinal ethnographic study and observations from short-term research in five other communities (e.g., Gruenbaum 2005). The following short summary highlights the local dynamics and the global influences affecting female genital cutting especially.

In Garia Wahid, a community I have studied since 1976 (Gruenbaum 1982, 1991, 1996, 2001), a noncircumcising, subordinate ethnic group, the Zabarma, had initially resisted the adoption of FGC despite their linguistic and some social acculturation to the dominant group, the Kenana Arabs. During the 1970s, the subordinate Zabarma, originally from West Africa, had lived in a separate village, preserving their language and female segregation customs, experiencing only limited contact with women of neighboring groups, leaving the women relatively free of social pressure to acculturate to the dominant groups' FGC practices. After many of them relocated to a planned village for tenants on the new Rahad Irrigated Scheme in 1978, they were exposed to new influences from the dominant Arabic-speaking group. In my subsequent research I found that although initially reluctant to alter their traditions, there had been several significant changes, including sending some girls to school and responding to the peer pressure to adopt circumcision. By 2004, I learned, most of the Zabarma mothers reportedly opted for a compromise sunna form for their daughters, to avoid fights among the girls. They described it as only a partial clitoridectomy, rather than the pharaonic form—just enough to avoid social problems.

The Kenana Arabs had not changed their practices in 2004. Although still doing infibulation, their attitudes toward pharaonic circumcision had begun to shift. They had greater awareness of the social movement against it, and many women and men expressed cautious support for change. Midwives say they won't do infibulation anymore, but "only the sunna," anticipating a change in Ministry of Health administrative policies that would punish midwives who practice FGC,[2] and both men and women were aware of this. But although the Ministry of Health, like the doctors' professional group the Sudan Medical Association, has adopted an eradication policy to eliminate all forms, some practitioners and clients believe sunna may be allowed.

The rural ideas about this were reinforced by the views of other midwives and the trainees I interviewed, including the former traditional birth attendant now undergoing formal training—I sought her out for an interview at the midwifery school in Fau—and the other trainees doing practical internships in Garia Wahid. All are thoroughly indoctrinated with the new anti-infibulation message. The director of the midwifery school said all graduates are required to take a solemn oath not to infibulate, and violators would be sanctioned with removal of their equipment, suspension of their right to practice, and recall for additional training.

In the 1970s, the elderly grandmothers were the strongest and most respected defenders of FGC. Their generation relied on folk remedies and traditional birth attendants who rarely traveled to cities. The younger generation of grandmothers today has experienced more travel, trade, government services, media, a multicultural community, and the education and labor migration of some of their children. For them, FGC is not so strongly tied to morality—horrified visceral reactions about shame are not as common—and they are listening to both the health messages and the idea that the practice may not be required in Islam. Moreover, although the older women still largely support FGC, the younger adults could openly discuss the possibility of change in their presence without censure. Nevertheless, marriageability of daughters continues to be a major concern, and the young mothers of the Kenana still want to do the sunna form so that their daughters will be accepted.

The Gezira, an irrigated area in the country's central region, has been the recipient of decades of development, including schools and other social services. It is not surprising that the progress against FGC has been stronger there, but it has not been rapid. The community of Abdal Galil, where I worked since the 1970s, was exposed to the anticircumcision movement earlier than was the Rahad area. But except for a few families who had quietly switched to sunna, the community had largely resisted change until about 1994 or 1995, several years after the trained midwife had adopted an intention to give up pharaonic infibulation. Around 1989 she became convinced that infibulation was not Islamic, but it was not until several years later that her client families were willing to accept this new opinion, which was being heard from educators and the media. Since the mid-1990s, most young girls have been spared infibulation, although clitoridectomy or partial clitoridectomy was still being practiced, as I witnessed in 2004.

Like the larger cities, Abdal Galil and other parts of the Gezira are changing FGC practices more rapidly than other rural areas because of greater access to education, urban migration, rural electrification, and the media. Radio and television programs discuss health issues and offer religious perspectives against FGC. It is my impression that it has become rare for adult women not to have heard the arguments against pharaonic circumcision, and they have heard it from religious shaykhs on the radio or television as well as health educators and their own healthcare providers at the community's health center. Some of the younger mothers I spoke with had begun to discuss the idea that if infibulation is not necessary, perhaps clitoridectomy is not necessary, either. Giving up infibulation had been a major transition: the scar tissue barrier to penetration was not there anymore for their daughters. If girls could be expected to stay moral without that, they reasoned, perhaps the removal of the clitoris was similarly unnecessary. Again, this was discussed in the presence of grandmothers who still wanted to see the girls infibulated.

What may have helped the discourse in Abdal Galil was the experiences of early adopters of change—families who quietly took their daughters to urban midwives or doctors who did less damage. The fear of daughters' unmarriageability or intense shame did not materialize for the innovators, emboldening others to modify the severity, if not abandon the practices altogether.

Globalization and Islamism: Other Reproductive Health Issues

The public health and human rights agendas of international organizations and nongovernmental organizations (e.g., UNICEF and CARE) have included several additional initiatives that impact reproductive health. Although population control is considered a politically inappropriate goal today, the provision of family planning methods has been embraced as a positive goal by such organizations as well as by the Sudanese feminist movement. In the seven rural communities and the urban environments where I worked in 2004, I saw examples of those who strongly favored family planning. The ideology of "be fruitful and multiply" and being willing to welcome "as many children as God gives" as a religious dictum had begun to be modified in some contexts. (I collected no systematic data on this topic, but questions about preferred age of marriage and ideal family size were a regular part of the discussions in my participant observations.)

Urban, middle-class, educated women with whom I discussed the preferred family size frequently said two, three, or four children, preferably gender balanced, and they emphasized their desire to ensure that their children were well taken care of and well educated. For some of the rural women, too, the desired family size seemed to be somewhat smaller than two decades ago. Nevertheless, some reproduction continued to be vital to one's well-being and marital success, and infertility was a serious dilemma for those affected by it.

In several rural conversations, though, the Cairo Conference (the United Nations International Conference on Population and Development in 1994) was brought up by people who believed the ideas about population and family planning were Western and anti-Islam. Those who expressed these views, most of them men, were very much in favor of rejecting the Western ideas about limiting family size and favored having as many children as possible. For them, the story of the polygynous man (who had had several wives over a long period of life) who had fifty-four children (or fifty-four sons, in another version) was a sort of folk hero, doing great things for his country by providing so many good farmers and leaders, and so forth. My questions about how they would overcome limitations of land and opportunity if many people had such high reproduction were usually scoffed at, quoting scripture about God's encouragement to reproduce and voicing trust in God to provide for their well-being. "Sudan has oil!" was another idea—many expect that all of them will somehow benefit from that.

The interest in smaller families is for child spacing, health, and increasingly economic considerations as development leads to more expenses, especially for urban children and those who attend school. One doctor I interviewed in the rural hospital in Um Sayyala, in fact, implored me to help him find a way to get a supply of contraceptives for his patients, since so many wanted them but found them too expensive.

On the face of it, this appears to be a challenge to the Islamic discourse, particularly in light of some religious teachers' advocacy for early marriage and reproduction. At the same time as education, development, human rights organizations, and others are pushing for later marriage for girls, religious leaders of several sects are encouraging marriage at early ages for both young men and young women. For example, in the late 1980s and early 1990s, the government of Sudan offered incentives to promote marriages of young people who could not otherwise have afforded to marry. The government provided couples with free registration, bus rides to large wedding celebrations for dozens of couples to celebrate their marriages simultaneously, and plots of land to build their houses. Some religious shaykhs, too, promoted early marriages. In the early years of the new century, large, simplified group wedding celebrations were sponsored by the late Shaykh al-Borai in North Kordofan, who provided beds, other furnishings, and a small sum of money for each marrying couple. Such measures arose in response to the escalating costs of marriage evident in the 1970s and 1980s because of Sudanese labor migration to the Gulf and inflation in costs, in some cases due to extravagance. Young people in one of the villages where I had worked were remaining unmarried through much of their twenties at that time, and people saw this as a problem. With the encouragement of shaykhs, some of whom pointed to the prophet Mohammed's marriage to Aisha as an example of the desirability of early marriage, parents are feeling justified and proud of marrying their daughters young, at the same time as countervailing encouragements are making it possible for more girls to get places in school and gain opportunities for jobs. Since my information on this is qualitative, I cannot determine whether there are demographic trends associated with these factors, but I am convinced that this is an important area for further research.

Sexuality has also been addressed in religious discourse. Elsewhere I have explored the issue of sexuality and sexual pleasure as they relate to the FGC issue in Sudan (Gruenbaum 2006), suggesting that one of the reasons many women cling to their belief in the importance of infibulation is that they consider a tight vaginal opening essential to their husband's sexual satisfaction.

An idea that has been circulating recently in Sudan is that for Muslims, their religion grants both husbands and wives the right to sexual pleasure. This idea, based on interpretation of scripture, is being articulated by certain of the religious leaders who are engaged in the movement to stop female circumcision as un-Islamic. The idea that cutting the clitoris might interfere with sexual pleasure thereby becomes not a question of women's human rights, Western decadence in relation to sex, or health but a question of theology. For these teachers, Islam supports female sexual pleasure and opposes all forms of female circumcision.

Women's Empowerment and Religious Authority

Elsewhere I explain that the efforts of the anti-FGC movement to create shortcuts to women's empowerment entail two sorts of difficulties. First, women and their communities do not always put stopping FGC or any other externally defined goal at the top of their lists. The TOSTAN organization's approach, used with such apparent success in Senegal, provides resources to enable local communities to define their own priorities; they have found that once the leadership skills and organizational capacities are better developed and the most pressing priorities are addressed, the additional goal of ending FGC usually does emerge as educators teach community groups about human rights. Reformers must be prepared with resources, patience, and participatory models for this strategy to work.

The international women's movement has sought greater empowerment for women. Is this, therefore, an international, globalizing, feminist agenda? Or does the fact that so many national and local institutions embrace the empowerment goal suggest that it resonates with the local struggles? Are reformers prepared to accept the priorities set by empowered women and communities, even if doing so means they are slow to accept changes to their FGC practices?

Since Sudanese and other Muslims who circumcise women have often assumed there is a religious justification or at least permission for FGC, using progressive Muslim teachers to denounce the association of FGC with Islam is certainly powerful. Several organizations rely heavily on the participation of religious shaykhs, side by side with political leaders and health providers, to educate and persuade communities to consider change (I describe this process in more detail in Gruenbaum 2005).

But as useful as religious arguments may be at the local level, elements of global forces influence the ways in which religious movements articulate their teachings, command loyalties, and transform cultural practices. The impact of conservative Islamist groups like the Ansar Sunna in eastern Sudan can alter the cultural practices and use Islam to stop infibulation but preserve the so-called sunna form of FGC. Such interpretations of Islam bear marks of the international Wahhabist movement—a globalizing force in its own right.

Conclusion

Reproductive health issues in Sudan must be understood in terms of the dynamics of diverse cultural roots; the impact of colonial and postcolonial political economy; and contemporary globalizing factors with media, labor migration, education, and healthcare. But the women of Sudan are also being buffeted by clashing global ideologies. On the one hand, the globalizing impacts of Western capitalism and the state may deliver messages about globalizing value systems of human rights, women's and girls' rights, and health promotion while transforming traditional productive systems into capitalist economic structures. The competing globalizing efforts of political Islam, on the other hand, seek to uproot traditions and replace them with supposedly authentic Islam, guiding both community values and the laws of the state.

As I have argued elsewhere, conservative forces opposed to ending FGC or other changes in reproductive health in Sudan often blame the Western feminist agenda, but they do so to discredit Sudanese leaders. But Sudanese reformers claim ownership of their values, promoting women's rights and choosing their directions for the future based on their own discussions about how best to improve the lives of women and girls and protect the dignity and self-respect of women and the health and well-being of children.

Appendix: Female Genital Cutting in Sudan

The most common Sudanese form of FGC is the World Health Organization's Type III, consisting of the removal of the prepuce, clitoris, labia minora, and most of the labia majora, followed by infibulation, or stitching closed, of the labia across the urethral and vaginal openings, leaving a single tiny opening for urination and future menstrual flow. Usually performed before girls reach the age of seven, this procedure, once healed, leaves a smooth surface of skin and scar tissue that later presents a barrier to intercourse, which many people hope will help prevent premarital sex or pregnancy. At the time of marriage and first intercourse, the opening must be stretched, torn, or surgically opened.

Although there are no recent or accurate figures on the types of cutting practiced, the consensus among activists today is that a growing percentage of people in Sudan have begun to practice a less severe form of cutting, the World Health Organization's Type I, removing all or part of the prepuce and clitoris but avoiding infibulation. Another percentage has abandoned the practices entirely, particularly among the urban, educated classes.

Notes

This chapter is based on the paper prepared for the workshop "Reproduction, Globalization, and the State" at the Rockefeller Foundation Bellagio Study and Conference Center, Bellagio, Italy, June 1–7, 2006. The research was supported by a sabbatical leave and travel support from California State University, Fresno, as well as research consultancies with UNICEF Sudan and CARE Sudan. I am grateful to the Institute for Women, Gender, and Development Studies at Ahfad University, Omdurman, Sudan, for affiliation and facilitation of my research in Sudan in 2004. All views expressed are my own and do not reflect the opinions of the institutions with whom I have worked. Portions of this paper were presented at the Society for Applied Anthropology and Society for Medical Anthropology joint meetings in Dallas, Texas, April 2004, and at the Sudan Studies Association in Santa Clara, California, May 2004. Special thanks to Samira Amin Ahmed, Balghis Badri, and Samia El Nagar.

1. The prophet Mohammed is said to have allowed reduction but not destruction of the female genitals, based on an oft-cited Hadith, or saying, to a midwife during his lifetime: "Reduce, but do not destroy." The authenticity, as well as the interpretation of the intention, is much debated. For a fuller discussion of religion and female genital cutting, see Gruenbaum 2001, 60–66.

2. The majority of communities continue to be served by traditional birth attendants with no formal training, and the Ministry of Health has had little or no control over their practices heretofore. In several states, however, the government health officials, assisted by international NGOs, are now recruiting traditional birth attendants for either intensive short-term training to upgrade their skills or full training for a year or more in one of the professional schools of midwifery.

PART II

Biotechnology, Biocommerce, and Body Commodification

Part II explores state-sponsored guidelines and laws defining and regulating reproductive technologies and their local interpretations and (re)inventions. Global advances in reproductive technologies and state responses to them in the form of legal and ethical guidelines are transforming widely shared notions of kinship at the local level. These reassessments of how to define family bonds are informed by social and culturally specific constructs of the person, kinship, and descent. Each of the three chapters in part II explores local interpretations of how authentic children are to be produced and accounted for and how recent advances in reproductive technologies have challenged conventional understandings of what constitutes an appropriate family.

In "Reproductive Viability and the State: Embryonic Stem Cell Research in India," Aditya Bharadwaj explores how infertile couples seeking to ameliorate the associated stigma may become complicit, albeit poorly informed agents, in the search by India's biotechnology industry to obtain legal embryos for stem cell research. Bharadwaj shows that informed consent is not a major concern for many of the doctors who aid infertile couples with in vitro fertilization (IVF) treatment. This in part is because under Indian governmental guidelines, embryos cannot be harvested solely for research purposes, so doctors encourage infertile couples to donate their extra, unneeded embryos produced through IVF as a "gift" to science. Bharadwaj shows how Indian infertility specialists, infertile patients, and their government coproduce a set of practices that strengthen the Indian biotechnology industry and better position the country as a biotech superpower.

Marcia C. Inhorn's "Globalization and Gametes: Islam, Assisted Reproductive Technologies, and the Middle Eastern State" reveals a different side of infertile couples' IVF experiences. Whereas Indian practices are shaped in part by state guidelines, in Muslim countries, IVF falls within the domain of family law governed by religious law (*sharia*). Inhorn examines the implications of differences between more restrictive Sunni—and more flexible Shia interpretations of sharia—for the IVF experiences of couples living in various Middle Eastern countries. Her chapter reveals how religious law is being (re)interpreted, and in some cases circumvented, by infertile couples despite explicit religious sanctions. It also highlights some of the ambiguities surrounding the kinship of children conceived through IVF.

In "Law, Technology, and Gender Relations: Following the Path of DNA Paternity Tests in Brazil," Claudia Fonseca explores how a different reproductive technology, DNA paternity testing, has, in paradoxical ways, also challenged and complicated conventional notions of kinship in Brazil. Historically, birth certificates were the main means to validate the social ties between parents and children. But in the 1990s, as part of a larger social justice movement, it was decreed that children had the right to learn the biological identity of their parents through DNA testing. While it was anticipated that the tests would be mainly used in child support claims by unmarried mothers and their children, they became unexpectedly popular among married men seeking to prove they were *not* the fathers of their female partners' children. Like the other chapters in part II, Fonseca's illustrates the larger point that global reproductive technologies are inevitably transformed by the particular cultural contexts in which they are deployed and the local strategic interpretations that accompany them.

These three chapters demonstrate some of the unintended consequences and social maneuvering that follow state imposition of formal legislation or guidelines to regulate reproductive technologies. With the ongoing global dissemination of information and technologies in the domain of reproduction, states and their structures, whether secular or religious, must confront a multitude of complex questions regarding the definition of legally and socially acceptable reproductive interventions—questions that also challenge individuals and families in distinct ways in different types of social formations.

Reproductive Viability and the State

Embryonic Stem Cell Research in India

In the middle of the twentieth century, two new functions of the state were added to the classic role of national security, namely, science and development. Ashis Nandy argues, "In the name of science and development one can today demand enormous sacrifices from, and inflict immense sufferings on, the ordinary citizen. That these are often willingly borne by the citizen is itself a part of the syndrome" (Nandy 1996, 1). Nandy's argument gains even more salience in the context of the burgeoning spread of neoliberal governance around the globe. The rise of biotechnology of embryonic stem cells (ESC) in India is partly contained in this new emerging global order. In this chapter, I situate the stigmatized bodies of Indian women and men seeking assisted conception within the broader political and scientific calculus of the Indian state. The conjoining of the global spread of neoliberal reasoning with the reasoning of the contemporary Indian state is central to framing policies that make Indian women and men "bioavailable" (L. Cohen 2005; Bharadwaj 2008) as suppliers of raw materials, such as eggs, sperm, and embryos, for stem cell research.[1]

The chapter opens an ethnographic register to explore how three constituents—the Indian state, in vitro fertilization (IVF) clinics, and "infertile" citizens—interact and have "co-produced" (Jasanoff 2004) the burgeoning research in embryonic stem cells. To co-produce is to be mindful that "the ways in which we know and represent the world are inseparable from the ways in which we choose to live in it" (Jasanoff 2004). The representation and experience of ESC research in India are informed by very different constituent realities, priorities, and points of departure. The state and medical establishments view ESC as the "next big thing to hit India after the country's software revolution" (Thorold 2001). The experience of certain citizens is more circumscribed: it is curtailed by a reality that has less to do with the science of ESC and more with rapidly evolving state policies and private-sector healthcare that frame citizens as raw materials, test sites, and eventual profit. Nevertheless, state policy, medical commercial priorities, and the infertile citizenry's social suffering conflate to co-produce both the ongoing growth in ESC research and the future (profitable) promise of therapeutic applications.

Two sets of citizens are prominent in this analysis. The first set comprises infertile individuals who are promised "free IVF for spare embryo" deals in the predominantly private-sector fertility clinics. The second set comprises fertility treatment seekers who are based in a public-sector IVF facility and agree to voluntarily give up embryos for research or adoption. While none of these individuals have ever actually given up embryos for research, they remain open to the possibility despite, or perhaps because of, the profound social suffering, stigma, and ostracism surrounding their infertility. It is tempting but simplistic to argue that the Indian state and the medical establishment are coercing these categories of individuals into giving up "spare" embryos.

Although exploitation is unquestionably one of the many factors at play, I focus more on understanding the structural shifts authored by the Indian state and how they implicate the reproductive lives of infertile citizens. I attempt to understand how "embryo surplus" infertility treatment seekers are enrolled in the scripting of a new kind of ethical governance. Their insertion into the bureaucratic calculus of the Indian state is important, as this further fuels the participation of the Indian biotechnology sector in a global economy where ethics, morality, science, and commerce are becoming increasingly intertwined. I conclude that certain categories of Indian citizens—predicated on ideas such as autonomy, consent, and choice—are more valuable than ever to the state as potential commodities. The real bone of contention here is not individuals giving away their embryos or exchanging them for free IVF but rather how the institutions of the state and biomedicine are stage-managing the creation of ethical conditions and spaces with economic as opposed to moral concerns in mind.

The Research

This chapter derives from a larger ethnographic research endeavor examining cultural complexities inherent in the production of embryonic stem cells in India. The research examines and problematizes the supply chain of human embryos from the point of conception in IVF laboratories to their eventual ongoing manipulation in public- and private-sector research facilities. I draw on ethnographic observations and forty semistructured, open-ended interviews with infertile patients undergoing fertility treatment such as IVF in two infertility clinics in New Delhi. One is located in an upscale South Delhi private hospital that caters predominantly to a middle-class and upper-middle-class urban clientele, and the second is publicly funded and based in New Delhi's army research and referral hospital. The bulk of IVF treatment seekers in the army facility are soldiers of the Indian army with rural, working-class backgrounds. This class contrast gives a rare comparative advantage to the research, given that assisted reproductive technologies in India—as elsewhere—are predominantly urban and middle-class phenomena.

The chapter also draws on interviews with clinicians and scientists in Delhi and Mumbai. I analyzed the treatment seekers' accounts for their views on giving and receiving gamete donation as well as sharing of spare embryos for research. I also questioned clinicians and scientists on the nature of their everyday practice, the ethics of procuring human embryos for research, and the nature and value of informed consent.

Infertile Bodies and Fertile Embryos in the Neoliberal Mode of Production

In India today, women's reproductive potential has come to be viewed as both a scourge—most graphically illustrated in aggressive and gendered nature of population control policies pursued by the state (cf. Van Hollen 2003)—and a boon in the shape of reproducers of the Indian state and economy. In great measure, India owes its rise to the army of its young workforce and a reserve pool of a staggering five hundred million people under the age of nineteen. In this respect, by fulfilling their traditional fecundity obligations within and outside the parameters set by the state, Indian women make their reproductive labor viable in the neoliberal mode of production. Women and their reproductive potential have remained at the heart of family planning policies in India, where the two-child norm has been promoted as the developmental ideal for much of the nation's postcolonial history. However, in the new century, infertile women and their technologically induced oocytes and embryos are rapidly becoming state subjects in need of regulated development, production, and local and global circulation. This is most graphically illustrated in the proposed ethical guidelines on infertility management and embryonic procurement sponsored by the Indian Council for Medical Research (ICMR 2006). Moves to monitor and regulate the steady growth in the number of IVF clinics, as well as egg and sperm donation in private-sector practices, has created a "furor" in the Indian medical community (Express Healthcare Management 2000), with the main bone of contention within the ICMR guidelines being the proposed prohibition of intrafamilial gamete donation. The medical community has reportedly taken strong exception to the state-sponsored ban on sperm donation by a relative or known friend of the wife or the husband, fearing that this would trigger paid donation and trade in semen.

However, should the guidelines become law, the consequences of such moves may in fact affect family-founding strategies employed within the clinical space, where tactical alliances are forged between select family members, infertile couples, and their clinicians to keep donor gamete IVF secret and on occasion as close to the agnatic blood relative as possible (Bharadwaj 2003, 2008). The question that arises is why the Indian state is inserting the market, and contractual commercial transactions, into a domestic moral economy of exchange and kin relations. These transactions are not mere examples of intrafamilial sharing, gift giving, and altruistic exchange but rather a context-sensitive and contingent way of making sense of reproductive disruption and family-forming strategies (Bharadwaj 2009). In many instances, intrafamilial arrangements are modern ways of doing tradition (Bharadwaj 2006), negotiating with patriarchal, gendered, and religious injunctions while conforming to the pronatalist imperative (more on this in the next section). For example, the ancient practice of levirate is still reenacted in IVF clinics where the sperm of a male agnatic relative is used to induce conception (Bharadwaj 2006). The practice of adoption, in the majority of cases, is similarly confined to the wider familial unit for deeply held cultural reasons (Bharadwaj 2003, 2008).

The neoliberal state in India is, however, seeking to outlaw these practices for reasons far more complex than mere social reform and protection of women from the excessive demands made by the patriarchal ideological order. On the contrary, the new laws hold the potential to create a body of medicalized childless citizens that can be garnered for extracting embryos and gametes to fuel the burgeoning rise in stem cell creation.[2] By putting in place strict procedures for informed consent, instituting a National Ethics

Committee, and ensuring the provenance of any potential stem lines accruing from human embryos, the Indian state is seeking to regulate ethical sources for procuring raw materials that resonate with the prevailing global standards and respond to international calls for better state control and regulation (Mudur 2001). These ethical sources, it appears, are imagined as fully informed, rational, and autonomous consumers seemingly liberated by the market from the fetters of outmoded and traditional reliance on familial support for "assisting life." These autonomous citizens can now be enjoined to sacrifice their biogenetic spare embryos with an encrypted provenance in the service of a booming "neoIndia" in much the same way as clinical trial subjects are considered the gold standard for ethically informed patients in contemporary India (cf. Sunder Rajan 2008; Bharadwaj 2008).

Spare Embryos: Consent, Choice, and Circulation

Unassisted infertile bodies compromise reproductive viability. Infertility or reproductive disruption on a similar scale is a profoundly disabling condition, especially in the context of classic patriarchy as found in the patriarchal belt extending from North Africa and the Middle East to southern and eastern Asia (Inhorn 1996; Inhorn and Bharadwaj 2007). The virulent stigma attached to reproductive disruption in India is therefore better understood when seen as shaped by pronatalist imperatives (Bharadwaj 2005). By pronatalist imperative, I mean patriarchal strictures that mandate reproduction, privileging and conflating motherhood with womanhood and fatherhood with manhood. Unlike fertility—where Rapp and Ginsburg (1995) argue that the notion of stratified reproduction helps clarify how "some reproductive futures are valued while others are despised"—in India, where the patriarchal normative and ideological order has for centuries had a vested interest in the reproductive futures of its populations, infertility poses a different set of questions (Bhattacharji 1990; Bharadwaj 2005). Thus, as in the past, in India today very often only one kind of reproductive future is despised, namely, a future obstructed by infertility (Patel 1994; Riesman 2000).

However, India in the recent past has been described as a nation with an embryo surplus (Jayaraman 2001). It is argued that a rich and steady supply of spare human embryos is emerging from the many state-of-the-art IVF clinics in the country. What is less well understood, however, are the exact modalities of procuring embryos for research, the process and nature of informed consent obtained, and the view of women and men who donate, gift, or give their biogenetic capital and how they view their contribution in the larger national and international context.

In my fieldwork in a privately owned stem cell research facility in Mumbai, it became clear that the spare embryos that were sourced from within their in-house IVF practice served as ancillaries to the larger stem cell research program. The admission was frank, candid, and the scientist in question (hereafter Dr. A) saw nothing remotely problematic about such practice. After all, he contended, there was a "well-informed" process of "informed consent" in place, and besides, the infertile treatment seekers were more interested in a quick pregnancy than in larger philosophical issues surrounding the potentiality of human embryos. This was to be later corroborated by yet another fertility expert in Mumbai (hereafter Dr. B). When probed further for clarification, Dr. A admitted that the notion of informed consent, which he regarded as "standard clinical practice," could, in the final analysis, actually be rendered deeply problematic depending on how facts were thought about and explained by individual clinicians. He followed this contention with a dramatic admission:

> I can sit here all day explaining to a couple how good it is to donate embryos for research or equally convince them otherwise if they at first instance appear to be hesitant or unsure and give me the slightest impression they shouldn't even think about donating. Either way it's up to me how I play it. I can convince a person either way.

In this statement, we see the jagged contours of the informed consent process and its constructed nature. A longer conversation with Dr. A exposed more specific details (*E* refers to the ethnographer):

DR. A: I think this holds true even in the Western countries. I mean, although we say things like informed consent, ultimately I think you—you [clinician] are a part of the decision making.

E: Hmm, true, yes.

DR. A: It happens.

E: Yeah.

DR. A: Even—even though you want to be completely out [of the consent-giving process], it's not possible to be completely out, because the couples often ask you, "Well, what would you do?"

E: Yes.

DR. A: Letting them know it's immaterial what I do because I'm not in a sim—similar situation.

E: Yes.

DR. A: Somebody who would suggest, it's completely out of the picture. I don't know because I cannot put my mind-set into yours. I cannot think because what you are thinking now is in that frame of mind. I cannot put—I can only tell you the pros and cons, explaining the picture you know, what it is . . .

And I—I choose the couple to whom I talk. Even if I have a couple who I think don't come from that background, education-wise, to understand the stem cells, I don't talk about it. I freeze it today. Because what happens is maybe they didn't look at me with a true understanding, they—is he going to use them in any case if I say yes or no? How do I guarantee this process.

Because they are the ones, who—you know, or some couples are so stressed, so stressed, I don't talk to them either. Because they're so stressed that in case of that treatment fails then has he [clinician] used the good embryos for them running stem or giving me the bad embryos? Or you know, has he compromised my treatment? So I talk to couples who I think would understand this, and they should have the minimum.

Dr. B went even further to expose the problematic aspects of the so-called informed and consented donation of embryos. He began by offering conventional accounts about profound social stigma and ostracism faced by infertile couples and how the bulk of the pressure remains on women regardless of the exact reason for reproductive disruption. "If a woman with blocked tubes comes to you," he said, "You can only do an IVF for her, there is no other option."

The least expensive form of IVF in India costs about $1,500 per cycle, and in Dr. B's estimation, more than 50 percent of infertile middle-class patients struggle to cope with this price tag. He then told me about the number of desperate patients he sees in his clinic, asking for help and threatening suicide. The social stigma and ostracism associated with infertility in India is well documented (Riesman 2000; Bharadwaj 2011), and if it were not for this research, Dr. B's assertions could easily be critiqued as sensationalist and overtly exaggerated. However, it was his subsequent assertion that disclosed even more disturbing aspects of informed consent in Indian fertility clinics in the age of stem cell research.

If I go and tell one thousand infertile patients who need IVF and can't otherwise afford it that I'll give them free IVF, they'll say yes. If I tell them half of their embryos I am going to use for stem cells, do you think they'll say no? They will jump at the chance and sign any piece of paper. Somebody comes to me and says, "I need materials for stem cell research and I will fund IVF cycles in return," what do you think I will do, say no? Here patients are prepared to sign blank forms, forget informed consent.

Dr. B was espousing an ethic that saw no harm in using embryos for research as long as everyone involved benefited; for him there were only winners and no losers in this game. This mockery of an informed consent process is likely to generate a type of embryonic stem cell research that preys on profound social suffering. Over the past ten years, I have interviewed numerous infertile Indian women who fear abandonment and are desperately trying to salvage failing marriages and manage social ostracism, stigma, and social exclusion. Even within the conjugal context, couples struggle with extremes of emotional, physical, and financial depredation inflicted by invasive and expensive assisted reproductive technologies. Though purportedly rational consumers of conception technologies, their consent to comply with the treatment regime is almost always a feature of their delegitimated social location.

Altruistic Giving: Potential Embryo Donors Speak

The treatment seekers in this research understand the work ethic of free IVF for spare embryos slightly differently. While none of them had given up embryos for research, several did have embryos frozen, and I asked them to deliberate on the possibility of giving away their embryos. Although none had been offered free IVF in exchange for embryos, they responded to questions about the possibility of giving away gametes and embryos altruistically. The responses that emerged remained centrally focused on the contention that "so long as our treatment is not compromised, we don't mind giving away whatever they need." Dr. A had remarked earlier in the research that his patients who signed over their spare embryos did express concerns about the quality of embryos he used for their IVF cycles. He recalled assuring couples that only the best embryos were used for their treatment and the "less-than-perfect" embryos were spared for cell extraction. Dr. A's colleague and one of the senior scientists in the stem cell team had similarly observed, in response to a question about the proposed ICMR ban on generation of embryos for research, that the quality of embryos affected the quality of derived cells. Thus he thought that a better method ought to be conceived of, one that would allow access to higher-quality embryos for routine IVF cycles. There is, however, no way of ascertaining what quality controls and methods are put in place to make the selection process transparent.

Initial analysis of the patient data also indicates that despite the continuing concern for their own treatment and the propensity to link embryo donation to successful conception, most women were genuinely interested in helping other couples. The primary response of couples in this regard centered on the notion that if a situation were to arise that necessitated donating embryos, "it was better to give it to someone who was suffering needlessly the pains of infertility or science." As one middle-class woman in Delhi contended:

> You don't mind what happens to your embryo once you've been through such suffering. You start to see life differently. If it helps science and other people, they can do what they want with my embryos. Probably I wouldn't be saying this if I were not going through this.

This woman was anxious for a quick resolution and repeated that she was unable to think beyond her immediate suffering. Her response in this regard was informed by the ongoing emotional and domestic upheaval in her life and the feelings of altruism, sympathy, and a need for healing that she craved in her own pursuit of conception.

When asked to think through whether such disposal of "spare" embryos ought to be a voluntary donation or a paid commercial transaction, the overwhelming majority supported the idea of free giving, seeing it as a noble act and offering help to someone in need. For instance, the wife of an army soldier responded:

> If this brings some happiness in someone's life, then we shouldn't hesitate and help in whichever way. It is such merit to help someone in need.

This woman could not separate helping another person in need from research on embryos for possible future commercial exploitation. Unlike the anthropologist posing these questions, she was less skeptical, and her predominant refrain remained as follows:

If it is for research, humanity benefits; there is suffering in the world, so if a tiny bit from us [i.e., embryos] can contribute towards alleviating such misery, then why not?

Her husband smiled and nodded in agreement, and so did many others. These routine expressions of gratitude may derive from a variety of sources: army discipline, religious ideals, or deep appreciation of access to technologies of procreation inaccessible to them in the private sector. These individuals and couples were very happy to share, donate, and give, as long as there was some mechanism for setting up a meaningful dialogue with the clinic. Equally, it became clear that as long as infertility remains a deeply stigmatized condition and source of much symbolic and real violence in the lives of women, embryo donors will remain a vulnerable, exploitable source. Indeed, many of the so-called donors would willingly part with embryos for much less than a free IVF cycle.

Spare embryos therefore remain tainted entities from the point of conception, as their surrender for research or adoption by another infertile couple is inextricably bound up with the helplessness permeating the local moral worlds of the infertile in India. Their consent is informed by a very different social reality that is never addressed in the clinic but nevertheless is often exploited: subtle moral pressure for extracting spare embryos. Even altruistic sharing or giving of embryos is shaped by the social suffering wrought by infertility rather than informed consent in service of a rational science. The question remains: can spare IVF embryos in India ever represent a morally sound foundation for an ethical global biotech future?

Conclusion

The poor in a neoliberal world inhabit biologies that are routinely construed as waste (Scheper-Hughes 2000) and gain meaning only when recycled in a tangible, meaningful, and above all profitable sense (cf. Bharadwaj 2008). Thompson argues that in the "biomedical mode of reproduction," waste is seldom a political or logistical problem but rather an ethical one of how to designate life material (embryos) as refuse (Thompson 2005, 264). In the neoliberal mode of production, this problem is frequently addressed by resorting to recycling socially and ethically defined surplus that cannot otherwise be gainfully accumulated (see Bharadwaj 2008).

This is partly in line with larger developments in the field of biotechnology, where a discernible "shift from kind to brand" is very much in evidence (Haraway 1997, in Franklin 2003). Dealing with the emergent dimension of innovation and market strategy in the business of stem cell manufacture, Sarah Franklin (2003) has recently described the ways in which concerns about public opinion are literally being built into new life-forms. The Indian state has thus far remained relatively indifferent to the need to establish policy surrounding embryonic bioproducts like stem cells.

However, the concerns that the Indian state is seeking to build into stem cell research by enacting regulations and installing ethical protocols will emerge in distant global spaces. The Indian state and its future biotech investments are locatable in a moral geography where local and global ethical sensibilities have become curiously joined. The need to embed embryonic stem cell science in India within the purview of legal and ethical scrutiny can be situated within the larger concern for managing the increasingly collapsing domains of local and global publics. The biosociality (Rabinow 1996) of Indian publics is as yet unexpressed (Bharadwaj 2008), but preemptive moves influenced in large part by Euro-American ethical and governance protocols appear to have been embraced by the Indian state, despite the relatively apolitical nature of embryo research there. It is easy to conceive of this show of solidarity as yet another instance of the global shaping the local, but in fact, the concerns that drive these moves in locales like India are more pragmatic. In India, strategies to ensure the provenance and strictest ethical scrutiny of embryonic entities do not appear to be a local cultural response to existential questions but rather are a strategic investment in future global markets, potential scientific collaborators, probable international lay consumers of embryonic entities, and their ethical and moral thresholds (Bharadwaj 2009).

The conception story of embryonic stem cell biotechnology in India therefore emerges in a context of vast risk for human exploitation. It may not seem to be as brutalizing as the trade in human organs in India and elsewhere (Das 2000; L. Cohen 1999, 2000), yet the very creation of an entity labeled "spare embryo" raises problematic moral and ethical issues. While the state, scientists, and clinicians may take cover in the safety of procedures of informed consent, expressions of informed choice create little more than sanitized paper trails that mask profound social suffering. The resultant provenance of an embryonic stem line remains similarly tainted but obfuscated. Couples in this research who invoked the vocabulary of altruism and greater good drew heavily on their continuing struggle with infertility, the social suffering it produced, and an innocent (perhaps even naive) hope that their charitable act might benefit someone, somewhere, struggling with the debilitating social, economic, and personal consequences of infertility (cf. Bharadwaj 2009).

In this context, the role played by the Indian state becomes significant. As discussed earlier, the recent Indian Council for Medical Research draft guidelines on stem cell research and regulation—in line with Euro-American legal thinking—expressly forbid the generation of embryos for the sole purpose of obtaining stem cells. This leaves only one potential exploitable source—the infertile IVF treatment seeker—and the generation of spare embryos. While the Indian state does offer donors a promissory note of future benefit accruing from their embryonic contributions, all potential biotech futures that their infertile bodies make imaginable remain out of bounds for the "informed" donors as they sign away access to future breakthroughs in exchange for free IVF. Alternatively, they voluntarily surrender embryos but remain unaware of their future rights. The contract between the consenting citizen and the state is bypassed.

As Scheper-Hughes succinctly argues, the neoliberal defense of the individual right to sell might well be problematic, since in all contracts there are notable exclusions (Scheper-Hughes 2000, citing Das 2000, 197). In this respect, future prospecting remains the sole domain of the corporate and pharmaceutical players that underwrite IVF with one eye on the generation and procurement of spare embryos and the other on the potentially profitable futures these spare embryos could help create. Whether citizens now enrolled by the Indian state as an ancillary to the production of profitable therapeutic futures remain a notable exclusion in the contract or a benign reality will become apparent as these futures come to fruition. For now, embryo donors remain excluded from future benefit sharing within the private sector, especially since the suggested government guidelines for stem cell research are yet to become enforceable law.

In the final analysis, reproductive disruption in India is made viable as much through the science of conception and embryonic stem cell generation as by governance and regulatory modalities of the Indian state. In a post–Cold War global order, the calculus that drives ethical and legal convergence between nation-states in search of a morally and ethically unproblematic production and circulation of biogenetic entities can no longer be articulated in nationalistic, local, or regional terms. The neoliberal ethic operates on a global scale where shared morality and ethics become necessary conditions for the international circulation and accumulation of capital. As Sunder Rajan argues, "Many of the tactical and strategic articulations of the Indian state tend not to be 'resistance' to global orders of techno-scientific capitalism, even while they might rescript hegemonic imaginaries in ways not imagined" (2006, 83) or—as this research suggests—now becoming imaginable.

Notes

This chapter is a condensed version of some of the main themes in the monograph *Local Cells, Global Science: The Rise of Embryonic Stem Cell Research in India* (2008). I am grateful to the editors, Carole Browner and Carolyn Sargent, for their generous feedback and support, and to the Bellagio conference delegates, whose comments and suggestions made a profound difference to the analysis.

1. The development of stem cell research in India has been part of a larger policy pursued by the Indian state since 1985, when the government began investing in the creation of a centralized department of biotechnology (DBT) as the nodal agency for policy, promotion of R&D, international cooperation, and manufacturing activities. To date, close to US$500 million has been invested in this venture. Now, with the establishment of Reliance Life Sciences, an Indian private biotech company, both public- and private-sector research institutions are forging ahead with transnational collaborations. Both centers have met the U.S. administration's criteria for derivation of human embryonic stem cell lines.

2. India has begun putting systems in place to meet the Good Manufacturing Practice, or GMP (Financial Express 2005), as well as ethical protocols that require informed-consent embryo donations as a basic admissible standard. At a press conference in November 2005, India's union science and technology minister described how the Indian government not only sought to strengthen stem cell research in the country by extending accreditation to companies to do research, but also required these companies to follow the GMP's international guidelines so that their products could be marketed globally (Financial Express 2005).

Globalization and Gametes

Islam, Assisted Reproductive Technologies, and the Middle Eastern State

In the new millennium, the Middle Eastern assisted reproductive technology (ART) industry is flourishing, with hundreds of in vitro fertilization (IVF) clinics in countries ranging from the small Arab Gulf states to the larger but less prosperous nations of North Africa (Inhorn 2003; Serour and Dickens 2001). This development of a mostly private Middle Eastern ART industry is not surprising: Islam encourages the use of science and medicine as solutions to human suffering and is a religion that can be described as "pronatalist," encouraging the growth of an Islamic "multitude" (Inhorn 1994; Musallam 1986).

Yet relatively little is known about Islam and technoscience, if technoscience is defined broadly as the interconnectedness between science and technology through "epistemological, institutional, and cultural discursive practices" (Lotfalian 2004, 1). As Lotfalian notes in his recent monograph *Islam, Technoscientific Identities, and the Culture of Curiosity*, a glaring lacuna exists in the literature on science and technology in cross-cultural perspective, particularly from the Islamic world (6). This dearth of relevant scholarship clearly applies to the cross-cultural study of ARTs and third-party donation. For example, in the seminal volume *Third Party Assisted Conception across Cultures: Social, Legal, and Ethical Perspectives* (Blyth and Landau 2004), not a single Muslim society is represented among the thirteen country case studies.

Clearly the time has come to examine the globalization of ARTs to diverse contexts in the Muslim world, particularly given the rapid development and evolution of these technologies over time. As I argue in this chapter, assisted reproduction in the Muslim Middle East bespeaks a complex global assemblage (Ong and Collier 2005) of technologies, gametes, legislation, religion, money, and ideas involving the pursuit of conception. That infertile Muslim couples are willing to participate in this world bespeaks the love, commitment, and ardent desire for children that characterize most ART-seeking couples in the Middle East, qualities that are rarely emphasized in the Western media discourses about purported Middle Eastern violence, religious fanaticism, and the cruelty of Muslim men to women. As I have argued elsewhere (Inhorn 2007), the love between infertile couples is fueling the ART industry in the Middle East. It is also causing some Muslim couples to venture across deepening Sunni-Shia religious and political divides in search of human gametes (i.e., donor sperm, oocytes, and embryos), even at a historical moment when tensions between these two Muslim communities are at an all-time high (Nasr 2006).

As we will see, practices of assisted conception are now tied to varying Sunni and Shia religious attitudes toward gamete donation, codified in authoritative Islamic fatwa declarations and sanctioned by Middle Eastern states to varying degrees. In general, Middle Eastern states have imposed little governmental oversight on the IVF industry. This relaxed regulatory environment stands in stark opposition to many highly regulated Western European nations (Franklin 1997; Jones 2008; Storrow 2006) but is similar to the United States, where there is little if any explicit governmental regulation and an IVF industry that is largely free market regulated and profit driven (Spar 2006). However, this is where a U.S.-Middle East comparison ends: namely, despite minimum government standards and intervention, the Middle East is characterized by a strong and effective religious regulatory environment, in which various practices of assisted conception are allowed or disallowed in the absence of explicit state mandates, laws, or professional codes. Indeed, the very strength of the religious regulatory environment— and the internalization of these regulatory guidelines by IVF practitioners and patients—has effectively allowed the Middle Eastern nation-state to turn its regulatory attention elsewhere (for better or for worse, as we shall see). Furthermore, religious regulation of ART has led in recent years to two clear patterns of ART practice, which follow the growing Sunni-Shia sectarian divide in this part of the world. Namely, all Sunni-dominant countries in the Middle East ban third-party gamete donation, while at least two Shia-majority nations now practice gamete donation.

This chapter focuses on two nations of each type—Egypt and the United Arab Emirates, both Sunni-dominant countries, and Iran and Lebanon, both Shia-dominant countries—where I have conducted extensive field research on ARTs with hundreds of Muslim couples.[1] The interaction between religion and the state will be highlighted for each country. To do so requires examining fatwas, or non-legally binding but authoritative Islamic religious decrees, as well as the subsequent ethical and legal rulings that are being issued by some Middle Eastern states to enforce or, in some cases, overturn these fatwa rulings (Moosa 2003; Tremayne 2006, 2009). Understanding the rapidly evolving religion-state nexus surrounding ARTs in the Muslim world is imperative. Perhaps unlike any other major region of the world, Islamically imposed religious restrictions guide clinical practice throughout the Middle Eastern region, with relatively little state legislation or intervention. Religious mandates affect not only what clinics are able to offer to patients but also what patients are able to accept as morally permissible in their personal treatment quests.

Indeed, a key question is how the religion-state nexus actually plays out in everyday practice—in the actual "making of Muslim babies" within Middle Eastern IVF centers (Inhorn 2006a). The Harvard medical anthropologist Arthur Kleinman (1995, 45) has coined the term "local moral worlds" to describe "the commitments of social participants in a local world about what is at stake in everyday experience." In the Middle East, understanding local moral worlds involves asking what Muslim ART seekers think about IVF and specifically donor technologies. How do disparate Sunni-Shia stances toward gamete donation influence the local moral worlds of infertile Muslim couples desperate to produce a child? When faced with the need for donor gametes to overcome infertility, what do Muslim IVF patients, whether Sunni or Shia, actually do? Understanding local moral attitudes toward science, technology, medicine, and religion in the Middle East requires ethnographic engagement with reproductive actors themselves, including those who seek human gametes across national and sectarian divides.

ARTs in Sunni Islam

It is important to begin in the Sunni Muslim world, where the earliest fatwas on ART practice emerged and the first clinics opened in the Sunni strongholds of Egypt, Saudi Arabia, and Jordan. The Grand Shaikh of Egypt's famed religious university, Al-Azhar, issued the first fatwa on medically assisted reproduction on March 23, 1980. This initial fatwa—issued only two years after Louise Brown's birth in England, but a full six years before the opening of Egypt's first IVF center—has proved to be truly authoritative and enduring in all its main points. In fact, the basic tenets of the original Al-Azhar fatwa on IVF have been upheld by other fatwas issued since 1980 and have achieved wide acceptance throughout the Sunni Muslim world.

The Sunni Islamic position on assisted reproduction clearly permits IVF, using eggs from the wife with the sperm of her husband and the transfer of the fertilized embryos back to the uterus of the same wife. However, since marriage is a contract between the wife and husband during the span of their marriage, no third party should intrude into the marital functions of sex and procreation. This means that a third-party donor is *not* acceptable, whether he or she is providing sperm, eggs, embryos, or a uterus (as in surrogacy). As noted by the Islamic legal scholar Ebrahim Moosa (2003, 23):

> In terms of ethics, Muslim authorities consider the transmission of reproductive material between persons who are not legally married to be a major violation of Islamic law. This sensitivity stems from the fact that Islamic law has a strict taboo on sexual relations outside wedlock (*zina*). The taboo is designed to protect paternity (i.e., family), which is designated as one of the five goals of Islamic law, the others being the protection of religion, life, property, and reason.

As a result, at the ninth Islamic law and medicine conference, held under the auspices of the Kuwait-based Islamic Organization for Medical Sciences (IOMS) in Casablanca, Morocco, in 1997, a landmark five-point declaration included recommendations to prevent human cloning and to prohibit all situations in which a third party invades a marital relationship through donation of reproductive material (Moosa 2003). Such a ban on third-party gamete donation is effectively in place in the Sunni world, which represents approximately 90 percent of the world's 1.4 billion Muslims (Inhorn 2003, 2005; Meirow and Schenker 1997; Serour 1996; Serour and Dickens 2001).

But to what degree are these Sunni fatwa declarations actually followed by physicians in the Muslim world? A 1997 global survey of sperm donation among assisted reproductive technology centers in sixty-two countries provides some indication of the degree of convergence between official discourse and actual practice (Meirow and Schenker 1997). In all of the Sunni-dominant Muslim countries surveyed—including the Middle Eastern countries of Egypt, Kuwait, Jordan, Morocco, Qatar, and Turkey, as well as a number of non–Middle Eastern Muslim countries including Indonesia, Malaysia, and Pakistan—sperm donation in IVF and all other forms of gamete donation were strictly prohibited. As the authors of this global survey note, "In many Islamic countries, where the laws of Islam are the laws of the state, donation of sperm was not practiced. AID (artificial insemination, donor) is considered adultery and leads to confusion regarding the lines of genealogy, whose purity is of prime importance in Islam" (Meirow and Schenker 1997).

The statement "the laws of Islam are the laws of the state" warrants further investigation, for it is not accurate, technically speaking. Islamic law, called *sharia*, governs family law (i.e., personal status law) in most Middle Eastern societies. However, separate civil legal codes, often imposed during periods of French and British colonial rule, govern most other areas of law throughout the region.[2] ARTs come under the aegis of Islamic family law, given that they are used to produce offspring for infertile couples. The association of ARTs with Islamic sharia has given religion outstanding power to dictate the scope and contours of clinical practice in the Muslim world, effectively weakening state intervention or civil law in this area.

Egypt is a case in point. Over the past twenty years, Egypt has supported a thriving IVF sector with approximately fifty IVF clinics. Five of these clinics are located in government hospitals and receive some state funding to offset expenses for the infertile poor (Prof. Mohamed Yehia, personal communication, July 29, 2007). However, as in most Middle Eastern countries, Egypt's IVF sector is highly privatized and exists beyond the official gaze of the state. Opening an IVF clinic requires licensure by the Egyptian Ministry of Health, based on guidelines set forth by the Egyptian Medical Syndicate. However, the Egyptian Medical Syndicate has based its bioethical guidelines for clinic operation on the early fatwa issued by Al-Azhar, as well as the subsequent recommendations of the 1991, 1997, and 2000 conferences on ARTs organized by Al-Azhar's International Islamic Center for Population Studies and Research and endorsed by the Al-Azhar clergy (Prof. Gamal I. Serour, personal communication, July 30, 2007).

Professor Gamal Serour, director of the center at Al-Azhar, laments the comparable lack of Egyptian state involvement in this process. "Unfortunately, there have not been any attempts to legislate IVF in Egypt," he writes. "The state controls the practice of IVF through licensing these centers. Centers have to abide by the guidelines laid [out] by the medical syndicate concerning premises, personnel, equipment, facilities, sterilization, etc. Every center must obtain approval of the medical syndicate followed by a license from Ministry of Health (MOH) before they start their programs." However, he adds, the "regulations environment in Egypt is poor. It stops at the phase of issuing a license. There is no regulatory body that supervises or inspects the work done; neither is there an obligatory registry for compiling data. Of course, inspection occurs whenever a catastrophe occurs" (personal communication, July 30, 2007). Concurring completely with this assessment, Mohamed Yehia, one of Serour's IVF colleagues at neighboring Ain Shams University in Cairo, describes the regulatory environment in Egypt as "very loose and mainly governed by the doctor-patient relationship" (personal communication, July 29, 2007).

The fact that, in practice, doctors and clinics operate with little government interference does not mean that "anything goes" in either Egypt or other Sunni Muslim countries. Indeed, what is quite remarkable is the degree to which the fatwa banning third-party donation is morally internalized and hence followed by both practitioners and patients in the Sunni Muslim world. Sunni Muslim physicians in the Middle East appear loath to offer gamete donation to their patients. According to them, clinics in the Sunni-dominant countries simply do not use donor technologies, which violate the sharia guidelines. Instead, if couples with recalcitrant infertility ask about gamete donation, they are either discouraged by their physicians from pursuing it further or are referred out of the country, primarily to Europe.

Indeed, most Sunni Muslim IVF patients would never dream of "doing donor" and desire their clinical care from a Sunni Muslim IVF physician who shares this conviction. In the hundreds of interviews that I have conducted with Sunni IVF patients in disparate Middle Eastern settings, the vast majority agree completely with the religious prohibitions on gamete donation, arguing that gamete donation (1) is tantamount to adultery, by virtue of introducing a third party into the sacred dyad of husband and wife; (2) creates the potential for future half-sibling incest, if the offspring of the same anonymous donor meet and marry; and (3) confuses kinship, paternity, descent, and inheritance in the emphatically patrilineal societies of the Muslim Middle East. According to them, preserving the "origins" of each child—meaning its relationship to a known biological mother and father—is considered not only an ideal in Islam but a moral imperative. The problem with third-party donation, therefore, is that it destroys a child's *nasab*, or lineage, an act that is considered immoral in addition to being psychologically devastating.

Sunni Muslim IVF patients use the term "mixture of relations" to describe this untoward outcome. Such a mixture of relations, or the literal confusion of lines of descent introduced by third-party donation, is described as being very "dangerous," "forbidden," "against nature," "against God"—in a word, *haram*, or morally unacceptable. It is argued that donation, by allowing a "stranger to enter the family," confuses lines of descent in the patrilineal societies of the Muslim Middle East. For Muslim men in particular, ensuring paternity and the purity of lineage through known fathers is of paramount concern. Thus a donor child could only be viewed as an *ibn haram*, literally "son of sin." The child will be deemed illegitimate and stigmatized even in the eyes of its own parents, who will therefore lack the appropriate parental sentiments (Inhorn 2006b).

This firm conviction that parenthood of a "donor child" is an impossibility is clearly linked to the legal and cultural prohibitions against adoption throughout the Sunni Muslim world (Inhorn 1996; Sonbol 1995; Zuhur 1992). The original Al-Azhar fatwa prohibiting third-party gamete donation also prohibits adoption of orphans, considering both acts unallowable. As a result, few Sunni Muslim IVF patients will contemplate adopting an orphan, stating with conviction that it is "against the religion." According to Arab men, an adopted child, like a donor child, "won't be my son" (Inhorn 2006b).

Given this local moral world, most Sunni IVF patients are extremely concerned about making their test-tube babies in a morally correct fashion. To that end, seeking out a trustworthy Sunni Muslim IVF practitioner is a concern for many patients. In the United Arab Emirates (UAE), the global hub of Middle Eastern transnationalism (i.e., less than one-quarter of the total population of four million are Emirati nationals), a controversial draft law to govern Emirati IVF centers included a clause stating that to be licensed by the Ministry of Health, every IVF center must have at least two Muslim practitioners, one an IVF specialist and one a laboratory technician. Attempting to reflect the UAE's multicultural population, two government ministers present at the legislative hearing argued that "science and medicine have no religion" and that "the UAE constitution does not discriminate against any citizen on religious grounds." Nonetheless the majority of those present at the hearing on July 3, 2007, voted to include the controversial Muslim practitioner clause in the draft law (Salama 2007). Ultimately, however, the requirement of a Muslim IVF practitioner did not pass into UAE law, when it was implemented in January 2010.

Having said all of this, it is extremely important to point out how things have changed for Shia Muslims since the beginning of the new millennium. Shia is the minority branch of Islam centered in Iran and found in parts of Iraq, Lebanon, Syria, Bahrain, Saudi Arabia, Afghanistan, Pakistan, and India. It has been much in the news lately because of the U.S.-led war in Iraq, the summer 2006 war between Lebanon's Hizbullah and Israel, and the current tensions between the United States and Iran.

Until recently, most Shia religious authorities have supported the majority Sunni view: namely, they agree that third-party donation should be strictly prohibited. However, in the late 1990s, the Supreme Leader of the Islamic Republic of Iran, Ayatollah Ali Hussein Khamanei, the hand-picked successor to Iran's Ayatollah Khomeini, issued a fatwa effectively permitting donor technologies to be used under certain conditions (Abbasi-Shavazi et al. 2008; Clarke 2006, 2007, 2009; Tremayne 2006, 2009). With regard to both egg and sperm donation, Ayatollah Khamanei stated that *both* the donor and the infertile parents must abide by the religious codes regarding parenting. However, the donor child can only inherit from the sperm or egg donor, as the infertile parents are considered to be like "adoptive" parents.

However, the situation for Shia Muslims is actually much more complicated than this. Because the Shia favor a form of individual religious reasoning known as *ijtihad*, various Shia religious authorities have come to their own conclusions about sperm and egg donation. There are major disagreements about

> whether gamete donation without bodily contact truly constitutes zina, or adultery;
>
> whether donation is permissible at all if the donors are anonymous;
>
> whether the husband of an infertile woman needs to do a temporary *mut'a* marriage with the egg donor, then release her from the marriage immediately after the embryo transfer, to avoid zina, or adultery (such mut'a marriages are condoned in Shia but condemned in Sunni Islam); and
>
> whether a Shia Muslim woman married to an infertile man can do a mut'a marriage with a sperm donor (an illegal state of polyandry), or

whether she should temporarily divorce her infertile husband and remarry him after accepting sperm from a donor.

In theory, only widowed or otherwise single women—who are not currently married—should be able to accept donor sperm, to avoid the implications of zina, or adultery. However, in all the Muslim countries, single motherhood of a donor child is unlikely to be socially acceptable.

Indeed, in a most interesting legislative turn of events, the Iranian state has issued a law making sperm donation officially illegal—thereby effectively overruling Ayatollah Khamanei's fatwa-based permission of sperm donation. Namely, a law on embryo donation passed in 2003 in the Iranian parliament (*majlis*) and approved by the Guardian Council (a religious watchdog body that endorses every bill before it becomes law) has restricted gamete donation to married persons. Although the law is brief (less than one page), it states clearly and succinctly who can and cannot donate and receive gametes. Egg donation is allowed, as long as the husband marries the egg donor temporarily—ensuring that all three parties are married. Sperm donation, on the other hand, is legally forbidden, because a sperm donor cannot temporarily marry an already married woman whose husband is infertile. Quite interestingly, however, embryo donation—which involves both sperm and egg from another couple—*is* allowed to overcome both male and female infertility. Because an embryo comes from a married couple and is given to another married couple, it is considered *halal*, or religiously permissible (Tremayne 2006, 2009).

The social and biological implications of embryo donation are quite interesting. For Iranian couples unable to produce a child because of male infertility, embryo donation allows them to bypass the problem of the husband's weak (or absent) sperm. However, embryo donation does *not* allow a presumably fertile wife of an infertile husband to contribute her own ova, in effect severing her biological ties to the donor child. Furthermore, and most strikingly, embryos donated from another married couple involve *both* egg and sperm donation. Although direct sperm donation via the injection of another man's sperm in the wife's womb is bypassed, embryo donation still disrupts male paternity and involves the acceptance by an already married woman of another man's (and woman's) gametes. Moreover, a woman's acceptance of another couple's embryo is effectively like gestational surrogacy, which is strictly prohibited in Sunni Islam. Nonetheless, cases of surrogate motherhood are occurring in Iran, despite the lack of firm legislation regarding this practice (Garmaroudi, n.d.; Tremayne 2009). Some Iranian clergy and physicians are presently advocating for future laws permitting all forms of donation as well as surrogacy. Once passed into law, gamete donation and surrogacy will be difficult to stop. Meanwhile, some IVF physicians in Tehran—as well as in the Shia-dominant country of Lebanon, which is closely following the Iranian lead—are using the legal and regulatory vacuum and original "permissive" fatwa of Ayatollah Khamenei to practice all forms of gamete donation among their desperate infertile patients.

Lebanon, the Middle East's most religiously diverse country, has attempted to legislate against third-party gamete donation and to limit ART access to married couples. However, (1) because of the strong Shia Muslim presence in that country, (2) the inability to achieve consensus among Lebanon's seventeen other confessional communities, and (3) the effective breakdown of the Lebanese state in recent years, the legislative process has been suspended indefinitely. Indeed, with its long history of sectarianism and religious infighting, Lebanon represents a case par excellence of religious rule at a time when the state—and its corresponding legislative and regulatory structures—is in chaos.

In the midst of this governmental vacuum, ART decisions are left largely to the better judgment of IVF doctors and their patients, based on their own understandings of the religious rulings, as well as personal moral convictions, which are often deeply internalized. Those married infertile Shia couples who are *truly* concerned about carrying out third-party donation according to either religious or legal guidelines may find it difficult to move forward, particularly when it comes to sperm donation. Yet, having said that, in Lebanon as in Iran, at least some Shia couples *are* beginning to receive donor gametes, as well as donating their gametes to other infertile couples. Since the new millennium, donor gametes and embryos are now being donated and procured by infertile couples in IVF clinics in Shia-majority Iran and Lebanon, the only two countries in the Muslim world where third-party donation is being practiced today. For infertile Shia couples who accept the idea of donation, the introduction of donor technologies has been described as a "marriage savior," helping to avoid the "marital and psychological disputes" that may arise if the couple's case is otherwise untreatable.

Who are the sources of these donor gametes? In the Lebanese IVF clinics in which I worked, some of the donors were other IVF patients (mostly Shia Muslims who accept the idea of donation), some were friends or relatives (including egg-donor sisters), and some were anonymous donors who provided their ova for a fee. In at least one clinic catering to a largely conservative Shia clientele, some of these donors were young, non-Muslim, American women, who travel from the Midwest to Lebanon for extra payment to anonymously donate their eggs to infertile Lebanese couples. Ironically, those most likely to receive these "American eggs" are conservative Shia couples, who accept the idea of donation because they follow the teachings of Ayatollah Khamanei in Iran. In Lebanon, such couples are generally members of, or sympathizers with, Lebanon's Hizbullah political party, which is officially described by the U.S. administration as a terrorist organization.

Furthermore, in multisectarian Lebanon, the recipients of these donor eggs are not necessarily only Shia Muslim couples. Some Sunni Muslim patients from Lebanon and from other Middle Eastern Muslim countries such as Egypt and Syria are quietly slipping across transnational borders to "save their marriages" through the use of donor gametes, thereby secretly going against the dictates of Sunni Muslim orthodoxy. That such reproductive tourism is done in secrecy—usually under the guise of a "holiday in Beirut"—is quite important, given the moral condemnation of gamete donation in the Sunni Muslim countries. Although such Sunni Muslim gamete seekers may have made peace with their own moral decisions to use donor technologies, they often remain extremely concerned about maintaining anonymity and confidentiality to avoid moral censure of themselves and their future donor offspring.

Not surprisingly, several of the Arab patients I met who were pursuing donor gametes in Lebanon were extremely concerned about achieving phenotypic similarity with their donor offspring. They did not want "black" children, nor did they necessarily want "white," Euro-American-looking children. They wanted children who looked "Middle Eastern" like themselves—hence their journeys to Lebanon for that purpose. As I learned on a visit to Iran in 2006, scores of Sunni Muslim Gulf Arabs from countries such as Saudi Arabia and Kuwait are traveling to Tehran in pursuit of gametes that have been donated by Shia Muslim Iranians in clinics there. Given that most Gulf Arabs could afford to travel outside the Middle East, Persian-Arabic phenotypic similarity may be an important factor in the pursuit of Iranian gametes, a fascinating topic for future research.

Conclusion

In short, the arrival of donor technologies in both Lebanon and Iran—the only two Middle Eastern countries where these services are offered today—has led to a brave new world of reproductive possibility never imagined when these technologies were first introduced there more than twenty years ago. These technologies have engendered significant medical transnationalism and reproductive tourism; mixing of gametes across national, ethnic, racial, and religious lines; and the birth of thousands of IVF and now donor babies to devout infertile Muslim couples. For their part, at least some infertile Muslim couples, both Shia and Sunni, have begun to reconsider traditional notions of biological kinship, even if "social parenthood" of a donor child is still not widely embraced in the Middle Eastern region (Inhorn 2006b). Nonetheless, because donor technologies are now available in the Shia world, the power of the Sunni Muslim ban on third-party donation is being weakened across the region, with some infertile Sunni Muslim couples reconsidering their own anti-donation moral stances. As a result of these social processes, Shia gametes are finding their way into Sunni bodies despite the regional antagonisms between these two religious sects. Indeed, in the new millennium, the case of assisted conception and gamete donation provides compelling material for the study of Islamic technoscience in practice—a study that is ripe for anthropological investigation as these technologies make their way to diverse Muslim societies around the globe.

Notes

My field research has been generously supported by multiple grants from the National Science Foundation and the U.S. Department of Education's Fulbright-Hays Faculty Research Abroad program. I am also grateful to all the Middle Eastern IVF patients and staff who have made my research possible over the years. *Alf alf shukran!*

1. Since 1988, I have undertaken long-term field research in four Middle Eastern societies —Egypt (1988–89, 1996), Lebanon (2003), "Arab Detroit" (2003–5, 2007–9), and United Arab Emirates (2007)—with additional research-related trips to Syria (2002–3), Cyprus (2003), Lebanon (2006), Iran (2006), Egypt (2007), and Qatar (2007). I have conducted in-depth ethnographic interviews with nearly six hundred patient couples and numerous IVF physicians and clinic staff members, the vast majority of whom are Muslim. For a more comprehensive discussion of my research methods and fieldwork experiences, see Inhorn 2004.

2. The notable exceptions are Iran, Sudan, and Somalia, where Islamic law has been imposed on all citizens (including non-Muslims) in matters other than family law.

Law, Technology, and Gender Relations

Following the Path of DNA Paternity Tests in Brazil

During the 1990s, a seemingly insignificant technological procedure—the DNA paternity test—went, in Brazil, from novelty to
routine. At the time, the country was experiencing the effervescence of
social movements bent on promoting the democratic principles of the
new 1988 constitution. Along with the idea of "justice for all" came the
notion that, since all citizens had a right to paternal identity, the DNA
exam—then going for the prohibitive price of US$450 a case—should be
financed by the state.

By 2001, when I began my study in different judicial spaces of Porto
Alegre (capital city of the state of Rio Grande do Sul), the various
strands of popular appeal, legal aid, and burgeoning labs had pulled
together to produce nearly a thousand paternity suits a month entering
the court system in my state alone, corresponding to approximately
7 percent of the region's annual number of births. The hypothesis that
originally inspired this phase of my research was that nowhere else in
the world did one witness so dramatic a surge in the public airing of
paternal doubts. Viewing the situation as the historically situated local
assemblage of a global form (Ong and Collier 2005), I set out to investigate the various influences—local as well as transnational—that might
explain Brazil's singular reaction to this bit of modern technology. The
exercise proved most interesting. On the one hand, the scrutiny of DNA
tests served to highlight Brazil's specific mix of democracy, free trade,
and gender relations. On the other, particular attention to transnational
connections ended up putting in question the very premise of Brazil's
singularity.

To explore the problem posed here, I have found it necessary to use a variety of research techniques. In the first part of the chapter, which centers on the role of congressmen and judicial administrators in the formulation of government policy, I have relied largely on documental sources, many of which were gleaned from public-service sites on the Internet. To address the attitudes of men and women who bring their complaints to court—the theme of the chapter's second half—I carried out ethnographic fieldwork between 2002 and 2003 in different instances of the Rio Grande do Sul (Brazil's southernmost state) judicial system. At the office of free legal aid (hereafter referred to as *defensoria*) where people initiate their suits, I took advantage of the routinely long wait in line to locate and converse with those seeking a paternity test. I was able to observe the ensuing sessions in Conciliatory Court, where judges, allotted fifteen minutes per case, attempted (usually in vain) to bring the litigants to a consensual accord. I also spent time at the public laboratory, where, from eight to twelve every morning, an average of thirty-five couples and their offspring were scheduled to draw blood for the exam. At the lab, besides conversing with people as they awaited their turn, I was able to establish quantitative data on the monthly average of tests, the percentage of negative results, and the geographic provenance of clients. Finally, I was given access to legal dossiers at Family Court, where I could take stock of the written pleas used by plaintiffs and defendants as they disputed paternal identity. The picture that emerges from the nearly one hundred individual cases I was thus able to piece together serves as complement to the analysis of the norm-making instances at the legislative and judiciary levels.

Science and Social Justice

Given the intellectual history of Brazil's elite, wherein positivism weds science to progress (Holston and Caldeira 2005), it comes as no surprise that broad sectors of the population quickly embraced DNA tests as a tool for social welfare. At the turn of the millennium, newscasters were commonly airing unusual situations in which the DNA test thus proved useful. In one such case, they reported on young Indian girls who were supposedly forced into prostitution in brothels bordering on cattle farms in the remote western pampas. Discovering who had fathered their numerous children not only would be a way of procuring child support—possibly from well-off ranchers —but, when the girls were underage, would also permit the identification and prosecution of child abusers. Another sort of scandal that occupied a great deal of media space concerned babies stolen from maternity wards. The most famous story involved Doña Vilma, a white, middle-class house-wife who had thus acquired at least two of her five children, tranquilly raising them to adolescence. A chance photo of her youngest, a teenage boy, made available on the Internet, had sparked the suspicions of the child's biological family, struck by the strong physical resemblance with family members. But it was the DNA test that finally restored the young man to his rightful parents and put the mother who raised him behind bars.

While such sensational cases cemented the association, in viewers' minds, between the paternity test and just solutions to serious conflicts, lawmakers, in congressional debates, were voicing hopes that the test might bring the benefits of modern society to more Brazilians. There had been much to-do during the late 1990s about "delayed birth registration," involving 25 percent of the country's children who, especially in the poor, inaccessible north-eastern regions, would often go years without a birth certificate. With no ready data on "fatherless children" (those who have a birth certificate, but with no register of paternal identity), congressmen consistently confused this category with that of delayed registration. It was as though the cam-paigns that extended registration at birth to more and more of Brazil's children were somehow linked to the search for fathers.[1] The implicit mes-sage was that both these problems were fated to disappear, thanks to the modernizing project of nationhood. Of still more central concern: in public debate, it was understood that holding men responsible for the children they had engendered would bring an end to a good part of the population's poverty. And Brazil's high percentage of female-headed households was fre-quently cited to justify the need for free access to paternity tests.

As DNA paternity tests were gradually included in the list of citizens' rights, it fell to federal congressmen—deputies and senators elected at the state level—to guarantee free access to those who couldn't afford the com-mercial price. In December 2001, the congress passed a bill (Federal Law 10.317) including DNA paternity tests in a law, half a century old, on state-financed legal aid. However, between 1995 and the approval of the 2001 law, there had been no fewer than twenty congressional proposals to facilitate access to the DNA paternity tests. The list of authors included partisans from leftist as well as conservative parties, representatives from the country's northern hinterlands as well as from its most metropolitan neighborhoods, feminists as well as supporters of the traditional family. From the look of things, the DNA paternity test was deemed a popular issue with the electorate, guaranteed to bring in precious votes.

It is important to consider this expansion of services within the context of a worldwide concern with using the judiciary to promote social justice (Santos 2000). As Brazil emerged from a military dictatorship (1964–85), the judiciary, long considered a white elephant of inefficiency, was catapulted into the role of spearheading the country's democratic renewal. In these circumstances, access to justice—thoroughly embedded in the spirit of the new 1988 constitution—signaled a desire to speed the benefits of democracy and spread the services of the modern nation-state to even the poorest elements of society. Among other measures, defensorias were opened in each state, aspiring not only to provide free judicial aid but also to protect basic rights (Schuch 2009). As many analysts observing similar processes in other parts of the globe have since pointed out, this multiplication of judicial services has not necessarily resulted in a less cumbersome system. The judicialization of social life has, however, involved an ever-increasing number of citizens who now look to the courts to settle even minimal details of their daily interactions (Nader 2002; Ewick and Silbey 1998; Debert, Gregori, and Piscitelli 2006).

What interests us here is how, in Brazil, the DNA paternity test became a symbol of this access to justice. Especially after the 2001 bill was passed, the office of free legal aid in many states took up the refrain that linked the DNA paternity test to social justice. For example, in 2002, the defensoria in Rio Grande do Sul put out a flier aimed at promoting the test in rural areas and cities far from the state capital. The release opens with a statement on "every citizen's right to recognized filiation," which now, thanks to the state government, was to be guaranteed by the office of free legal aid, and in record time (the two-year waiting period was allegedly cut to ninety days). Mixing references to the 1990 Children's Code as well as to the "personal drama of hundreds of state citizens" who did not have money to pay for the test in a private lab, the document's final paragraph outlines the modern (i.e., American) democratic ideals propelling this cause:

> In the United States, more than 95 percent of the paternity tests are done solely with DNA. In fact, this is the natural way, often impeded by economic disparities between societies that prevent the [enactment] of equal rights for all. In our state, access to the test has become a democratic

right. This is a question of science and law marching together, available to all [citizens], whatever their social class.[2]

It would appear that underlying the defensoria's enthusiasm for paternity tests lies the belief that certain disputes do not require elaborate judgments; rather, they involve cut-and-dried issues that are quickly settled once one has correctly identified the scientific evidence (Geertz 1983). Injustice here occurs when the facts are falsified or defective and when they are slow or, worse, not accessible. According to this philosophy, similar to one that, in the United States, has moved paternity suits out of family courts and into bureaucratic administration (Crowley 2001), the facts speak for themselves. "Marching together with science," legal agents are able to spend less time on each case, doubling their production rates, with the added advantage of being certain that justice, sheltered from fallible human judgment, has been done.

The Mixed Message of the Law

Considering the various and at times contradictory undertones that support the publicly funded DNA test, it should be no surprise that laws concerning a child's paternal identity also deliver an ambiguous message. On the one hand, evidence supports the optimists who view present pro-paternity policies as the culminating point of a century-long trend introducing cosmopolitan values into Brazilian family law. Discrimination against out-of-wedlock children fathered by married men dwindled after the 1977 divorce law. This law provided that the filial bond was irrevocable and such children could aspire to the same inheritance rights as legitimate offspring. It was, however, only in 1988, with Brazil's most recent national constitution, that the principle of equality between all children became imperative. Today it is irrelevant under what conditions a couple conceived their baby; the child will have full rights, equal to those of any "legitimate" offspring born to his mother or father. Furthermore, as of 1992, the so-called Paternity Law (n. 8560) specifically promotes the paternity of children born out of wedlock, decreeing public assistance for investigation in cases of reluctant fathers and prohibiting any discriminatory mention (i.e., "illegitimate") on a child's birth certificate.

Nonetheless there is a more somber side to present-day paternity laws—at least in Brazil—that few observers have noted. Despite legal advances compelling *un*married men to register their "fatherless children," the law, over the past hundred years, has progressively broadened the right of *married* men to *refute* their paternal status. According to the 1916 Brazilian Civil Code, a married man was automatically the father of his wife's baby if the child was born at least 180 days after their marriage or within 300 days of their legal separation. His only hope to deny paternity was to provide proof of total sexual impotence or of prolonged conjugal separation—and even in such cases, he had a two-month window after the child's birth to press suit (article 348 of the 1916 Civil Code).

In 1943 the law increased a man's possibilities to refute paternal status by creating the following addendum to article 348: "No one can disclaim the status registered on a child's birth certificate *unless by proving error or false registry.*" It is significant that Brazil's 2002 Civil Code maintains this loophole at the same time that it eliminates traditional restrictions. Today a married man may contest his paternal status without having to demonstrate impotence and without worrying about date limits. A married man may press suit to deny paternal status of children that are full-grown: his right to do so does not expire, ever.[3]

It is thus interesting to note that at the same time that there has been an ostensible move toward promoting legal paternity, especially of children born out of wedlock, more and more loopholes have been created that endanger the status of children who were heretofore considered legitimate. Optimists may opine that fatherhood has never before been more certain, and that men have never been held more legally responsible for their children than they are at this moment in history. As I will attempt to demonstrate, it would be equally accurate to suggest that, seen from another angle, paternity has never before been so uncertain, nor have men been so hopeful about escaping paternal responsibility.

Law as Practice

Policymakers in Brazil tend to project DNA paternity tests as a useful technology for ordering social life (J. C. Scott 1998)—for inducing the country's citizens to register their children and establish responsible households. Those people who frequent the court system may, on the other hand, have their own objectives for seeking a test. My field data suggest that working-class Brazilians have been quick to pick up on DNA technology and are responding en masse to the call for access to justice. However, as they go about settling interpersonal disputes, their individual use of the law does not always correspond to the expectations of the country's administrators.

The Dance of Documents

I had been listening to a custody dispute when a *defensor* called me over. "Come listen to this case! Now we're getting into *maternity* investigations!" The details I then heard from an extremely affable pair of young adults cooing over their blond, blue-eyed child did not exactly correspond to the defensor's description, but they did present an interesting case. The lanky youth in his early twenties, I discovered, was Abel[4]—a man who worked odd jobs and whose joy in life was taking care of small farms on the edge of town. The young woman, contrary to my original impression, turned out to be his younger sister. The man's four-month-old son had been incorrectly registered in the name of another father. Abel described how he had first brought his girlfriend home to live with him and his parents, and later moved with her into a rented house. Less than a year after moving in with Abel, the young woman, who was now four months pregnant, moved out, returning to her previous companion, who subsequently registered her baby as though he were the father. "He knew good and well the child wasn't his, but he registered it just the same!" At present the young woman had once again run away, but not without first dropping the baby off with its "true" father's family. Hugging her nephew possessively, Abel's sister explained: "We're all crazy about him. We just have to make sure that no one tries to steal him away." The judge said there would not be a problem: "All we have to do is run a DNA test, proving that Abel is the father, and they'll automatically cancel the other birth certificate."

How is it, one wonders, that this dance of documents, the false registry of one father and the legal switch of names, can be considered "no problem"? According to Holston and Caldeira, "Illegality and improvisation have always been the conditions under which the urban poor have created their spaces in Brazilian (and most Third World) cities" (2005, 394). These authors are not alone in suggesting that a highly idealized legal framework, typical of the Brazilian elite's modernist pretensions, propelled the Brazilian working classes toward the margins as opposed to bringing them into the disciplined sphere of the state.[5] In other words, facing official demands that had little to do with their everyday existence, people found ways of skirting the law or adjusting it to their own needs. Although Holston and Caldeira hold that this situation has changed with the social movements and redemo-cratization of the 1980s and 1990s, my examination of legal practices suggests that the distance between officialdom and the working classes continues to be routine.

Thus it is widely recognized that a stepfather who wants to cut the red tape implied in legal adoption might readily take out a birth certificate on his new mate's children as though he were their biological father. Stepfather adoption is certainly the most common "ideological falsification" I encoun-tered in my files. However, it is not entirely unusual to encounter *mothers'* names that have been altered; for example, when a woman registers her grandchild as though she were its biological mother. Legal operators dealing with pension benefits are well aware of this strategy.

These cases not only reveal how working-class people bend state bu-reaucracy to their own ends but also bespeak something of the eminently social bias that has traditionally guided the definition of kin. As the Brazilian saying goes: "Pai é quem criou" (father is whoever raises the child). Accord-ingly, until recent times, people seem to have used a child's birth certificate as a way of officializing an already existent social relation as opposed to simply registering a biological fact.

No Shrinking Violets Here

Lorraine, a solidly built black teenager, readily accepted my invitation to hold the boisterous two-year-old in her arms as she sat down to converse with the defensor. "Everyone falls in love with Toninho," she sympathized. "We're all crazy about him." Behind her, a lean young man with dreadlocks, some ten years her senior, beamed his approval. At first glance, I once again erroneously took this group to be a congenial nuclear family—a couple and their son—but in their chatty asides to me, I realized that I was looking at three generations of an extended family. Lorraine, escorted by her maternal uncle, had brought along her little nephew Toninho, "just for fun," while her own month-old baby stayed home with his grandmother. As with many of the families I have contacted, this situation once again illustrated the diffi-culty of assessing which children go with which adults.

Lorraine had indeed come in for a paternity test. She told her story in a matter-of-fact way without anger or embarrassment. The baby's father was her neighbor, seventeen years old, like herself. She made a concession to dominant morality and the endless campaigns against teenage pregnancy when referring to her age: "I'm very young to be a mother don't you think?" However, there was nothing in her demeanor that might be termed *traditional feminine modesty*. She didn't pretend, as did women in generations past, that she was seduced with promises of marriage (Caulfield 2000). On the contrary, she readily admitted she got pregnant after a one-night stand, and after I suggested that the boy, as her neighbor, had long had his eye on her, Lorraine retorted: "It's more like I had my eye on him!"

Lorraine's forthright manner was common among the women whom I encountered (or whose pleas I read) during my research (Fonseca 2003). Although they generally rebuffed accusations of promiscuity, claiming fidelity at the time of conception to one sexual partner, these women did not seem particularly apologetic about having pre- or extramarital affairs. While there may have been a time when unwed mothers sought, above all, the reparation of their damaged reputations through marriage, today's moral climate is quite different. During the past decades, we have witnessed the steady erosion of civil-law marriage. People today are marrying later and having children earlier than ten years ago. Divorce and separation are extremely common. Twenty-five percent of the population comprises couples who, living in common-law unions, simply don't bother getting married. Of course, part of this trend away from legal marriage may be due to economic hardship.[6] But a good part is no doubt due to present-day attitudes that have practically ended the moral distinction between married couples and common-law unions and have removed much of the discrimination against unwed mothers and divorcees.

To some extent, one could suggest that DNA technology has allowed the law to keep abreast of the changing sexual mores. Although there is strong evidence that working-class morality never fully corresponded to bourgeois ideals, family courts have historically imposed elitist standards: judging seduced maidens in terms of their virginal attitudes, married women in terms of their domestic-bound virtue, and divorced mothers in terms of their chastity (Fonseca 1997). Even in recent court files, men who could afford a lawyer seldom failed to include insinuations regarding the woman's loose sexual behavior in their pleas against fatherhood. That the couple had first met in a bar and had slept together on the first date, and so on—all might count as evidence of her supposedly loose morals. In classical fashion, the mere possibility of multiple sexual partners was understood to exonerate any and all from paternal responsibility.

However, over the past ten years, there has been a gradual change in the courtroom atmosphere, led not by lawyers but by those judging the cases. Today judges seem utterly uninterested in the woman's sexual behavior. It is no longer of the slightest relevance if she slept with one man or many. Such considerations might be relevant in a custody dispute, in which the court checks on the adequate material and moral conditions in which a child is raised. Paternity investigations involving a putatively simple biological fact are quite another matter. In other words, although DNA cannot be credited with having caused women's liberation, it has permitted legal operators to sidestep moralistic censorship of what in other times would have counted as loose female behavior.

Men in Growing Doubt

Nonetheless, before crowing too much victory, we should consider another facet of the test. While lawmakers were presenting the DNA paternity test as a way for consolidating nuclear families, other, more popular uses began to appear in the mass media. Television showmen would delight their spectators by luring into the studios real-life couples ready to air conjugal disputes in exchange for a free test. In a circuslike atmosphere, men would rant on about their former spouse's promiscuity while the women would indignantly protest their innocence. Newspapers published headlines describing how DNA testing settled the reluctant paternity of Pelé and Mick Jagger, while simultaneously reporting on how other famous figures were proved innocent by the DNA test when wrongly accused of fathering a child. Tuning in to the local radio stations, one could hear songs with lyrics such as "Não precisa fazer teste de DNA, a criança é a cara de você" (No need to do a DNA test, the kid's your spitting image). Of course, such songs might also inspire men to pay closer attention to physical resemblances and entertain the idea of a test if appearances were not up to expectations.

Little by little, as I advanced deeper into fieldwork in Rio Grande do Sul's court system, I began to see that, almost echoing the media hype, in many cases it was not the women but the men who were seeking to judicially clarify their paternity. Rarely would a man question the paternity of his live-in mate's child; however, once he was separated from, or had never taken up residence with, his child's mother, the DNA test seemed to represent a last hope for exempting him of responsibility. Of course, I found the classical cases of young Romeos or married men who under no circumstances would have voluntarily owned up to their brief amorous adventures. But I also found what seemed to be an ever-increasing number of ex-boyfriends, common-law husbands, and even divorcés—men who in previous times might well have tranquilly accepted their paternal status—who, prodded on by the possibilities of this new technology, now wanted "absolute proof" before legally assuming so serious a role (Fonseca 2009).

This attitude is well illustrated by Jair, a young man I observed in a preliminary court session. Confronted with his former live-in girlfriend and her babe-in-arms, he was asked by the judge: "Are you the father of this child?" His response came without hesitation: "Not yet." In other words, like so many of the young and not-so-young men I encountered, he was inclined to recognize his paternal identity (quite different, of course, from paternal responsibilities) only after "clearing up a certain doubt" through the use of a DNA paternity test.

How, one might ask, do women, heretofore the major source of truth as to their child's paternity, feel about the routinization of the DNA tests? Such feelings, scantily expressed in the legal briefs, were easier to read during interviews at the public laboratory. Young, unmarried girls, like Lorraine, who admit to a fleeting liaison, appear almost grateful that their former mates are willing to come in for a test. They hope to thus transform an informal acceptance into a binding obligation. However, women such as a certain Lucirene, who had lived with her former companion for five years before he took off with another woman, clearly see the test as an affront: "He knows good and well he's the father of our little boy. He's asking for a test just to make trouble." On another visit to the lab, I encountered a couple and their infant son awaiting a test. Here it was the seventeen-year-old girl's mother who, once out of hearing range of her grandchild's father, took me into her confidence: "Sure he's here to do the test. He says he wants her and the baby to move in with him. But my daughter says it's over. She's suffered too much humiliation. Having to do the test was the last straw." Many women we spoke to expressed variants of this emotion: what men took as their right and court clerks as routine, women saw as an accusation not against their sexual morality but against their honesty. The doubt in everyone's mind can, after all, persist only on the premise that these women are liars.

Altogether, my fieldwork experience, centered on people's use of law in Brazil, led me to believe that the association between DNA paternity tests and justice is more complicated than it originally appears. The agency of men and women taking their complaints to court reveals notions of filiation, family, and gender relations far different from those imagined by policy-makers. Ironically, rather than encouraging the conventional conjugal family, the technology appears to have undone, at least in certain cases, the classical legal and social package that took marriage and filiation as an indivisible whole. While they appear less and less inclined to submit their private conjugal relations to state approval, people are appealing more than ever to state services to define parent-child ties.

Global Route or Local Detour?

How might we explain the response of Brazilians to this new form of technology, the DNA paternity test? Just how distinctive is the Brazilian case? Are we dealing with a global form that follows the same route all over or a local detour created by the specificity of Brazilian circumstances and culture?

My first impression, that Brazilian, or at least Latin, men are particularly susceptible to jealous suspicions, was quickly put to rest by further research. In the United States, Canada, England, and Australia, a good part of the online literature I encountered on DNA tests concerns the subject of paternity fraud—men who are "unfairly" obliged to support children with whom they have no biological tie.[7] *Nonpaternity* appears to be the analytical term used by (again, mostly Anglo-Saxon) researchers who delight in transcultural comparisons in which the actual nonpaternity of suspicious fathers supposedly ranges from 25 to 40 percent (K. Anderson 2006). It is just such a perspective that led an enthusiastic Canadian scholar to suggest that, in the name of justice and to prevent fraud against misattributed fathers, "at the very least" paternity testing should take place systematically at the time of divorce. "For the sake of the children's well-being, more attention should be paid to the systematic testing for non-paternity, perhaps at birth" (Millar 2001, 73).[8] Similarities with the Anglo-Saxon world belie any tendency to attribute the test's popularity in Brazil to some sort of Latin American machismo.

On the other hand, as I extended my comparative inquiry beyond the Anglo-Saxon world, taking in the great variety of national responses to DNA technology, the idea of some sort of technological determinism, nudging us back toward a transculturally uniform image of men and their paternal doubts, appeared no more convincing. France, for example, has passed a law making the use of extrajudicial tests (including those provided through postal and Internet services) punishable by up to one year in prison and a €14,000 fine. Needless to say, in countries where people must procure a court order *before* laboratories agree to run a test, there has been no explosion of commercial enterprise catering to consumer demand.

To address the complex interplay of local and transnational issues concerning culture and technology, I am convinced that the most fruitful line of inquiry comes from a particular line of analysis known as co-production theory, in the field of science and technology studies (Thompson 2005; Jasanoff 2004). Rejecting the idea of an autonomous sphere of science, this approach examines how individuals in particular settings use culture and politics for the production and validation of knowledge. It also questions the "given" of social institutions, such as the state or competing interest groups that would necessarily promote self-serving versions of scientific truth. These institutions and interests also have a history, interwoven with local and global influences that include the discovery and dissemination of scientific and technological artifacts. In this arena, as Thompson has aptly pointed out, "Questions about the links between science and democracy, about choice and privacy, about the state versus the individual, and about the international division of labor are growing more, not less pressing" (2005, 50).

Certainly, in Brazil, legislators and public attorneys would not have promoted the broad-scale use of DNA technology without the faith and backing provided by the country's biologists, biochemists, and molecular geneticists. In the early days of DNA research, scientific know-how, as well as costly imported equipment, was nearly all concentrated in university laboratories where professionals invested their energies in basic research as much as, if not more than, in applied technologies. The end of the 1990s brought a reconfiguration of this field, when the convergence of different forces suddenly transformed DNA paternity tests into one of the most lucrative forms of biotechnology in Brazil. Having relied for decades on the government to finance their costly research, scientists suddenly found big money in partnership with the state judicial services. Some, seizing the moment, moved to expand and specialize their university departments. Others splintered off from their original research labs to start their own private enterprises, where they could draw in the extrajudicial demand. In a mirror reflection of DNA's first decade in Brazil, several of these private laboratories, directed by reputable professionals, have since branched out into less lucrative areas of genetic research concerning hereditary disease and genetically modified organisms in agriculture and livestock (Silveira 2001). However, smaller establishments, not to mention mail-order firms from overseas, have continued to proliferate, causing no little consternation among the older crew as to the quality of tests. The 2001 flyer of a private lab based in Porto Alegre alerted the public to the existence of paternity tests in rival labs being run by forest engineers, veterinarians, and even "lawyers in white uniforms."

One might wonder if the Brazilian scientific community doesn't have other misgivings about the spread of DNA paternity tests. Certainly, the five consensual principles concerning the Human Genome Project—autonomy, privacy, justice, equity, and quality (Knoppers and Chadwick 1994)—would be highly relevant to DNA tests. There appears, for example, to be a certain understanding that children at high risk for untreatable genetic disease should not be submitted to presymptomatic tests. The argument here is that such testing would preempt the person's right to, later on, make an adult decision about knowing or not knowing the diagnosis (Zatz 2000). It is obvious that this, as well as many other similar issues, would have strong implications for policies on the DNA paternity test, a situation already rife with the danger of intruding on "basic human dignity and autonomy" and "breaching information privacy" (ALRC 2003).

In fact, in the various national councils concerning bioethics, I encountered scientists who engage in discussions on a wide range of issues including the Genome Project, cloning, gene therapy, and even the forensic uses of DNA for criminal identification. Furthermore, Brazilian scientists and medical doctors are active in various international committees of bioethics, and many are able to cite relevant principles from the Helsinki Conference, the World Medical Association, the World Health Organization, FDA documents in the United States, and parliamentary inquests in the United Kingdom. Yet the tests have nowhere merited particular attention in bioethical debates. One might conjecture that, in this case, the clearly marked boundaries between pure research and its practical applications, more than preserving the disinterestedness of research, have protected its applications from serious ethical examination. Accepted as an inevitable result of technological advancement, commercial uses of the DNA test go unquestioned as they cater to consumer demands.

In conclusion, we may concede that the Brazilian story of DNA has put a certain distinctive twist on the global form of DNA fingerprinting: chronic poverty, inequality, and a historically inefficient state have been responsible for the millions of late birth certificates and the inventive, although irreverent, use of official birth registries by much of the working class. On the other hand, the spread of the use of DNA paternity tests in Brazil, paralleled only by that of North America, prods us to pay special attention to various state-related phenomena these regions might have in common: legislative dynamics, judicial philosophies, and regulatory control over the commercial uses of scientific research. Seen in this light, Brazil's experience would be neither an inevitable, globalized reaction to new technology nor an entirely local phenomenon. The explosion of DNA paternity tests in Brazil, with all its implications for gender relations and family identity, would have less to do with culturally defined machismo or technological determinism than with a particular combination of electoral politics, philosophies of free enterprise, great faith in science and progress, and social policies heavily weighted toward the family. Finally, as the results of our ethnographic research suggest, one must also credit the inimitable way that men and women in particular historical circumstances exert agency to adjust official policy so that it more closely aligns with their own socially defined needs.

Notes

1. In 1997, an estimated 24.8 percent of the children were not registered within the legal time limit. By 2004, these proportions had been reduced to 16 percent.
2. From the desk of Célia Fischer, August 20, 2002, Defensoria Pública do Rio Grande do Sul, Governo do Estado de Rio Grande do Sul, Assessoria de Imprensa, artigo: "RS aumenta o número de exames de DNA."
3. An examination of jurisprudence leaves little doubt about the connection between DNA paternity tests and the latest changes in Brazilian legislation granting married men the practically unrestricted right to challenge their paternal status. See, for example, the decision (194866/RS, 1998/0084082–6) of the Suprema Tribuna de Justiça, emitted by minister Eduardo Ribeiro on April 20, 1999, available on its website, http://www.stj.jus.br.
4. To respect informants' anonymity, I have replaced their names with others, attempting to maintain ethnic or linguistic approximations.
5. Still in 2004, more than 24 percent of the country's adults are considered functionally illiterate.
6. Official statistics show that weddings increase every December, exactly in a month when salaried workers receive their thirteenth month of wages and the economy generally picks up (IBGE 2005).
7. See also Richards 2006 for an analysis of the paternity test's increasing popularity in England.

8. Even in other fields of application, DNA technology seems to exhibit the same "expansionist" tendencies. Johnson and Williams (2003), for example, reporting on the British National DNA Database used in the forensics of criminal justice, point out how DNA fingerprinting, originally conceived for use in extreme cases (rape, murder), gradually became a routine element of many criminal investigations. Improved technology, state investments, and legal readjustments (redefining the mouth as a nonintimate part of the body permitted buccal scrapes without the subject's prior consent) led to the expansion of registers in the data bank from convicted felons to all those suspected of having committed a crime.

PART III

Consequences of Population Movements
for Agency, Structure, and Reproductive Processes

The chapters of part III examine some reproductive consequences of transnational migration. Their overarching themes include the effects of immigration politics and policies on the reproductive practices of migrants and other displaced populations, and the processes that come into play as migrants try to negotiate unfamiliar institutional structures, practices, laws, and regulations.

Mark B. Padilla's contribution, "From Sex Workers to Tourism Workers: A Structural Approach to Male Sexual Labor in Dominican Tourism Areas," offers a framework for understanding the flexible, situationally determined sexual practices of a growing number of working-class Dominican men. His analysis begins with the wide-ranging structural and economic changes that have been transforming this small nation from an agrarian economy to one based on tourism, and shows how these economic and social transformations are being accompanied by new conceptions of masculinity, with health consequences not only for men but for their wives and children as well. In introducing a concept of "regional masculinities," Padilla moves beyond a circumscribed notion of the local to deepen our understanding of the ways in which HIV/STI risks are produced and their consequences for reproduction.

In "Family Reunification Ideals and the Practice of Transnational Reproductive Life among Africans in Europe," Caroline H. Bledsoe and Papa Sow examine some of the contradictory and unanticipated effects of the

European Union's family reunification policies and show that migrants' reproductive lives are often simultaneously determined by legal and other institutional structures and practices both at home and in their host societies. Bledsoe and Sow illuminate some of the reproductive consequences of the countervailing forces at play in the lives of male Gambian migrants living and working in Spain. Their analysis raises provocative questions about how to analytically account for the power of states to affect the reproduction of noncitizen resident groups.

Carolyn Sargent's chapter, "Problematizing Polygamy, Managing Maternity: The Intersections of Global, State, and Family Politics in the Lives of West African Migrant Women in France," similarly examines ways that state immigration policies, in this case in concert with institutionalized biomedical practices, shape the reproductive lives of migrant families in Europe. Like Bledsoe and Sow, Sargent charts the tightening of immigration regulations in relation to marriage and reproduction. Although family reunification has represented a principal route to legal residence in France for African migrants since the 1970s, the recent prohibition of once tacitly accepted polygamous unions has generated conflicts and gendered-based strategic responses as polygamously married women and men seek to retain legal status. She shows how reproduction has become a central component in these marital and family tensions, as well as in national political debates surrounding immigration.

"Lost in Translation: Lessons from California on the Implementation of State-Mandated Fetal Diagnosis in the Context of Globalization," by Carole H. Browner, looks at ways in which a group of Mexican immigrant women interact with, and come to adopt, certain reproductive practices of their host nation, the United States. Like the authors of the previous two chapters, Browner traces the links between broad-scale globalization processes, state policies designed to regulate immigration and reproduction, and male and female migrants' reproductive lives. In discovering and revealing the unexpectedly powerful role that untrained medical interpreters play in the determination of these women's amniocentesis decisions, Browner adds nuance to the meanings of agency, choice, and constraint—and proposes new policy considerations for clinical practice.

In "Reproductive Rights in No-Woman's-Land: Politics and Humanitarian Assistance," Linda M. Whiteford and Aimee R. Eden examine a tragically overlooked consequence of global population movements for women's health and reproduction. They observe that while more than half the world's population lives in disaster-prone areas and that the number of displaced people grows annually, a large proportion of women who are refugees or otherwise displaced are excluded from basic reproductive healthcare by the humanitarian organizations ostensibly overseeing their protection. They conclude their chapter with policy considerations and a call to action.

The third part of this collection expands on the central questions posed throughout: How do global structures and forces shape and reflect state- and local-level dynamics? How does transnational migration generate transformations in marital relations, family ties, and reproductive decision making in diverse locations and situations? In the context of global flows of population, both voluntary and involuntary, how do individuals, families, and other collectivities conceptualize and pursue reproductive goals and strategies, and to what ends?

From Sex Workers to Tourism Workers

*A Structural Approach to Male Sexual Labor
in Dominican Tourism Areas*

I n the following pages, I use the Dominican Republic as a case study
to argue that future reproductive health research, both in the Caribbean and beyond, should seek to develop conceptual frameworks to
understand how structural transformations in men's labor migration
and the resulting reorganization of sexual geographies influence reproductive health outcomes for both men and their partners. The latter half
of the chapter discusses the specific theoretical components of such a
framework as I have applied it to the Dominican Republic.[1] Rather than
relying on the wholesale adoption of static representations of masculinity, the framework is premised on the principle that reproductive health
is best founded on theories that treat gender not as a stable quality to
be described photographically but as an emergent set of cultural practices that should be analyzed in dynamic and processual terms. This
allows us to consider how men's reproductive health is shaped by their
movement through distinct social contexts in which different masculine behaviors and practices are situationally operative. As a research
tool, the framework presupposes a particularly powerful methodological contribution from ethnography, since a truly dynamic analysis of
masculinity in reproductive health requires research that permits the
direct examination of gender as enacted in specific social contexts and
situations—phenomena that are most accessible through the humanistic engagements of participant observation.

While any conceptual framework seeking to summarize complex human phenomena is necessarily somewhat reductive, I use it primarily as
an invitation for colleagues to redress the long-standing failure to turn

the lens of gender theory on to men, a project that is increasingly recognized as essential for the advancement of anthropological approaches to reproductive health (Dudgeon and Inhorn 2004; Gutmann 2003). Indeed, one of the most crucial intellectual priorities of global reproductive health today is engagement in feminist-informed analyses of how masculinity—as a set of culturally inscribed expressions of men's gendered practices—shapes the reproductive health of men and their partners, families, and communities. As argued by a growing theoretical literature on masculinity, the linkages between gender and power are distinct for men, and among men, between different groups, classes, and identities of men (Connell 1995; Gutmann 2003). This may result in disparities in reproductive health that are linked to patterned variations in the practices of masculinity across groups of men, as well as variations in exposure to structural disadvantages across these groups. In an attempt to understand these connections, medical anthropologists need to develop and refine ethnographically grounded frameworks to guide reproductive health research among a broad population of men.

The Caribbean is a rich context for the development of such frameworks, since the region has long attracted anthropological inquiry into cross-cultural variations in the construction of gender and kinship. Much of the early anthropological work in the region sought to explain ethnographically the so-called disorganized and fractured structure of Caribbean families and the apparent attenuation of the marital bond presumably characteristic of these societies (Barrow 1996). A central theme in these discussions was the premise that men were marginal to the household, incorrigible philanderers who shirked their responsibility as fathers and providers, preferring to socialize in all-male peer groups and squandering whatever available cash they had on alcohol and ostentatious displays of (usually temporary) wealth. In contrast, women were depicted within the confines of their roles as mothers and nurturers, largely restricted to the household and limited in their mobility in public space. Such dichotomous gender constructs have tended to produce persistent dualities in the region's literature on gender, exemplified in paradigms such as the *casa-calle* (home-street) distinction (Barrow 1996) and Peter Wilson's (1969) influential framework of "reputation and respectability," which has aptly been described as a "gate-keeping concept" in Caribbean gender theory (Trouillot 1992).

While such frameworks may have been useful in conceptualizing certain dimensions of Caribbean gender relations, more recent anthropological work has problematized the notion of women's confinement to particular moral-spatial domains (Besson 1993; Freeman 2007). Indeed, a growing literature on Caribbean women's work has now thoroughly documented the rapid increases in formal wage work among women resulting from the confluence of neoliberal policies, the expanding service sector, and the growth of export processing zones (Brennan 2004; Browner and Leslie 1996; Freeman 2000; Kempadoo 1999; Safa 1995). Yet while women have increasingly been incorporated into wage work, lower-class men have been gradually but consistently pushed out of traditional sources of formal work, and growing numbers of them are being incorporated into the informal and service sector economies (Murphy 1990; Safa 1995). In my ethnographic research in tourism areas of the Dominican Republic, for example, I have described the diverse forms of informal tourism labor in which young, mostly unemployed or underemployed men engage in resort enclaves, such as the tourist town of Boca Chica on the south coast (Padilla 2007). While Caribbean scholars have rightly criticized recent suggestions in popular discourse that such changes in men's labor are generating a "crisis" in Caribbean masculinity (Lewis 2004), it is beyond debate that men throughout the region are now facing broad structural changes that have inevitable, if unpredictable, consequences for the meanings and practices of masculinity in the region. Tracing the connections between the broad political and economic changes that have occurred in recent decades and men's gendered practices is a key objective of future ethnographic work in the region.

This chapter aims to contribute to this project by illustrating how the contemporary meanings and practices of Dominican masculinity can be linked to regional variations in the social context of masculinity resulting from the expansion of coastal tourism areas, and by suggesting how these regional masculinities may contribute to marital risk for HIV and other STIs. Focusing on a specific group of lower-class Dominican men who work in the country's expanding tourism industry, I challenge the static gender binaries that have dominated discussions of Caribbean men, and focus instead on the dynamic processes whereby different cultural models of masculinity reshape the meanings and practices of gender as migrant male tourism workers move between tourism enclaves and home communities. This approach shifts the analytic goal from one of developing an exhaustive list of defining features of masculinity among apparently static groups or classes of men to one of understanding how the social and contextual characteristics of specific regions or spaces shape the enactment of masculinity. The latter is a remarkably distinct approach to the analysis of gender and reproductive health, which aims to avoid the traditional depiction of men as the mere vessels of gendered meanings rather than as gendered actors engaging and responding to changing contextual or structural circumstances. Further, since this approach seeks to continually contextualize men's practices and to trace their linkages to reproductive health outcomes, it is a more theoretically parsimonious way of representing the complexities of masculinity and reproductive health in the profoundly globalized Caribbean of the contemporary era.

While this chapter centrally addresses the changing contexts of gender as they relate to HIV risk, men's stories demonstrate the applicability of this approach to reproductive health more generally. Indeed, given the ways that masculinity functions across a range of social contexts, the gender imperative for men to provide economically for their families may ironically increase the chances that female partners and children will be affected by the AIDS epidemic as male labor migrants engage in high-risk sexual practices for instrumental purposes while geographically separated from families and communities. These complex linkages between sexual risk practices and reproductive health outcomes further illustrate the need to break down conceptual divisions between reproductive and sexual health to examine instead the linkages between these phenomena within the larger social and material structures in which people are embedded.

Men's Tourism Work in the Caribbean

In the Dominican Republic, where I conducted ethnographic research among men who exchange sex for money in the cities of Santo Domingo and Boca Chica, a growing number of men are turning to informal labor in the tourism sector as a means of coping with diminishing work options (see Padilla 2007 for methodological detail). Orlando explained:[2]

> I've gone for about ten or twelve years without work. . . . Here in the Dominican Republic things are really hard, so since there are some opportunities with some guys who come from abroad, and they offer you money or something to be with them, you grab it, you understand? It's the easiest way to get money. That's what's going on.

Many of the two hundred participants in the survey portion of the study—more than half of whom had already fathered children, despite an average

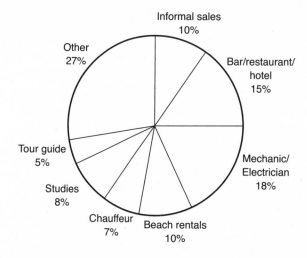

Informal sales
10%

Other
27%

Bar/restaurant/
hotel
15%

Tour guide
5%

Studies
8%

Mechanic/
Electrician
18%

Chauffeur
7%

Beach rentals
10%

FIGURE 1
Income-generating
activities in addition
to sex work (N = 124).
Created by author.

age of only twenty-four—commented that work in the tourism economy
was the most convenient, and often the most profitable, way to provide for
their families amid the shrinking work options available to them. Often
contrasting the work options in tourism enclaves with those in rural parts
of the country, men made comments such as "there is nothing there" or
"there is no way to make money there" when discussing their rural home
communities. Such comments illustrate that men's decisions regarding migration and work are constrained by transformations in the marketplace
for male labor as a consequence of the country's tourism-based development strategy and the concurrent demise of the male-dominated industries.
Among study participants—most of whom had engaged in a wide range
of tourism jobs (see figure 1)—migration to the tourism area led them
to consider the possibility of engaging in sex-for-money exchanges with
tourists, one of the most lucrative economic options within the informal
tourism economy.

Frequently, participants recalled encountering severe economic constraints in their home communities, leading men ultimately to migrate to the
tourism area in search of work. Initial encounters with tourists often occurred through friends already integrated into the world of sex work or by
chance encounters with tourists in the course of conducting other forms
of tourism work. The economic impetus to migrate often led to separations from families and partners while simultaneously facilitating men's integration into a normative social environment in which sexual-economic

exchanges with tourists are highly normalized. Indeed, tourism areas are teeming with businesses that—directly or indirectly—facilitate utilitarian exchanges between locals and tourists. Emphasizing the latter point, Truong aptly observes in his analysis of the tourism industry in Southeast Asia, "For the international tourism conglomerates, the availability of sexual services as an exotic commodity functions as a source of tourist attraction and helps to fill airplane seats and hotel rooms" (Truong 1990, 128). Further, as discussed in detail later, social science research on tourism suggests that the very nature of tourism and the symbolic meaning of the "getaway vacation" may foster a normative climate of sexual escapism, as global consumers of tourism services increasingly oscillate between contexts of labor in the developed world and places of recreation or abandon in the developing world.

Yet tourism areas are not only points of arrival for foreigners, despite their frequent depiction as such in the social science literature on tourism; they are also significant draws for migrant laborers seeking employment in a diverse array of labor markets. In my research, the extent of rural–urban migration among male tourism workers is evident in the results from the surveys. Of the 191 who were residing in either Santo Domingo or Boca Chica at the time of the interview, 98 (51 percent) were originally from other, mostly rural, parts of the country. This pattern of migration and the result-ing familial dispersal that it produces are important themes in the life histo-ries of male tourism workers. Some told stories of moving from the *campo* (countryside) alone, perhaps becoming *niños de la calle* (street kids) or maybe first finding an intermittent informal sector job as a *limpiabotas* (shoe shiner) or *chiripero* (street vendor) in a tourism area. Importantly, these men rarely described migrating with the original intention of exchanging sex for money with tourists, but had subsequently encountered such exchanges as a regular or intermittent source of supplemental income within the tourism environment. In sum, evidence from this sample of Dominican male tour-ism workers strongly suggests that the country's shift from a development model based on agricultural exports (particularly sugar) to one based funda-mentally on a tourism economy has contributed to demographic changes in men's mobility patterns, resulting in migratory pathways linking rural com-munities and tourism areas. Narratives of migration also demonstrate that men's own understandings of rural poverty, migration, and engagement in sexual-economic exchanges are consistent with the conclusion that Dominican tourism dependence has fundamentally changed the social context of labor and the sexual behavior of a growing population of migrant men (Padilla et al. 2008).

Elsewhere I have argued that labels such as "sex worker" are inadequate to capture the kinds of utilitarian exchanges and the fluid context of labor that characterizes these men's experiences (Padilla 2007). This is not only because these men rarely describe themselves as sex workers but also because they engage in a diverse set of income-generating activities that defy such simple, static characterizations. Indeed, it is more parsimonious to conceptualize these men's involvement in sexual-economic exchanges as a reflection of the ways that structural transformations of the Dominican economy have shaped the practices of gender and sexuality among a broad cross section of men, rather than partition certain ones off from their social peers because of their engagement in a particular expression of commerce. Sexual exchanges in the tourism economy are for these men a viable option for income generation in the context of otherwise highly constrained economic options, albeit one with unique social and legal consequences.[3] Viewed in this light, reproductive and sexual health interventions in tourism areas should be cautious with labels such as "sex workers" or "MSM" that divide up and cordon off the communities they serve. Men who engage in sexual commerce, perhaps particularly in its more intermittent or irregular forms, are not significantly different from their non-sex-working peers, many of whom are also informally employed migrant tourism workers. This urges us to move beyond notions of fixed categories and population-based thinking in global reproductive health, particularly in areas of rapid globalization and transformation of local economies, gender relations, demographic patterns, sexual partnering patterns, and labor structures. Under such conditions, we need to develop new ways of thinking about reproductive health outcomes not as properties possessed by easily separable bodies but as manifestations of the various social contexts through which bodies move and the ways differently positioned individuals move through these contexts.

At the same time, since migrant populations such as the men considered here often traverse different social contexts in the course of their migration between tourism areas and home communities, their gendered practices in one environment are not necessarily consistent with those in another. Thus the analytic exercise becomes one of understanding how actors negotiate the multiple meanings and practices of masculinity across social contexts, rather than one of cataloging presumably stable behaviors or masculine norms to which men presumably prescribe. Indeed, the very notion of norms or beliefs that often inform thinking about reproductive and sexual health is problematic not only in its tendency to neglect the multiplicity of gendered meanings across social environments but also in its presumption that a particular gender norm influences behavior in the same way across all contexts. For example, Dominican tourism workers expressed a strong desire to have children and to fulfill the masculine expectations of providing materially for them. While such desires reflect rather traditional notions of Dominican masculinity, when men arrived in tourism areas, these masculine expectations often motivated highly nonnormative, stigmatizing practices, since the masculine pressures of household obligations contributed to decisions to engage in sexual commerce within the tourism area. Eighty-three percent of the two hundred fathers surveyed indicated that they used their sex work income to help support their children and that the cost of raising children was a primary reason for participation in sex work. Martín, thirty-three, expressed this when asked whether his income from sex work covered all his expenses: "No, but it helps me to take care of my children, which is the most important thing."

In sum, the theoretical approach advocated here is one that views reproductive and sexual health outcomes as the product of men's movement through distinct social contexts but does not seek thereby to reduce men's gendered practices to a kind of vulgar "contextual determinism," since masculine expectations are not simply donned and shed, like articles of clothing, as an individual moves from one context to another. Instead it becomes an empirical question in need of investigation to consider to what degree specific gender norms and practices are more or less sensitive to context, and to understand the social, cultural, and economic bases of observed variations. The analytic and methodological challenge for reproductive and sexual health is therefore to understand how diverse sets of gendered meanings and practices intersect with specific health behaviors as individuals negotiate unique social contexts across time and space. More holistic and dynamic frameworks are a necessary first step in meeting this challenge in the contemporary globalized world.

Beyond Structural Violence: Operationalizing Structure through a Focus on Tourism Areas

A key implication of the arguments developed in the previous sections is that reproductive and sexual health interventions among tourism workers must move beyond static notions of risk groups or populations to develop more dynamic frameworks for understanding how structural changes are reshaping the gendered social contexts through which individual bodies move. A corollary is that we should not seek to target static or stereotyped categories of "risky men"—an approach that, if history is our guide, is more prone to demonize them than to improve reproductive health—but turn our analytic attention to the ways that men move in and out of risky social contexts. Drawing on the large social science and public health literature on tourism, along with my own empirical research, I argue that tourism areas are particular kinds of risky social contexts, the basic features of which are only beginning to be understood. In this section, I draw on distinct literatures on tourism, sexuality, and HIV/AIDS to take stock of current scientific knowledge and identify key features of tourism areas that may justify our considering them risky social contexts.[4]

Despite significant evidence dating back to the 1980s suggesting a linkage between the tourism industry and HIV transmission, sustainable HIV interventions are almost unknown in the Caribbean tourism sector. In the Dominican context, for instance, researchers have observed elevated risk for HIV among a wide range of populations with frequent contacts with tourists, including men who have sex with men (MSM) (De Moya and Garcia 1998; Padilla 2007; Ramah, Pareja, and Hasbún 1992; Silvestre, Rijo, and Bogaert 1994; Tabet et al. 1996), female sex workers (Kerrigan et al. 2001, 2003), and hotel and resort employees (CEPROSH 1997). Second, a growing number of qualitative and ethnographic studies have described the cultural and symbolic importance of the tourism industry in shaping contemporary Dominican sexuality, often highlighting the potential for tourism to contribute to HIV transmission (Brennan 2004; Cabezas 1999; De Moya and Garcia 1996, 1998; Padilla 2007). On the whole, the evidence for an epidemiological association between HIV and tourism is fairly robust and strongly suggests not only that tourism was a primary means by which HIV was initially introduced into Caribbean societies but also that tourism continues to function as an important source of new infections. Nevertheless, a weakness of the existing public health literature is that it has focused almost exclusively on particular risk groups—such as MSM or sex workers—and then noted the association between tourism labor and risk behavior rather than examining more upstream questions in the causal chain, such as: How does the rapid growth of the tourism industry reshape the social context of risk among a broad cross section of tourism laborers? What are the defining social and contextual features of tourism areas that shape reproductive and sexual health outcomes?

Answering such questions requires us to move beyond traditional approaches to HIV prevention in global health and to cast a broader theoretical net. In medical anthropology, a growing body of literature has argued for moving away from exclusively individual or cognitive-behavioral models of HIV/AIDS risk and toward an examination of the structural factors that shape HIV risk (Farmer 1992, 2003; Farmer, Connors, and Simmons 1996; Parker, Easton, and Klein 2000; Parker 2001). Such structural approaches to HIV/AIDS examine how large-scale economic factors and social inequalities influence patterns of HIV risk by creating resource disparities and conditions of vulnerability—processes that have been described as "structural violence" (Farmer, Connors, and Simmons 1996). For example, in the Dominican Republic, the reproductive health of male tourism workers is shaped by political-economic processes such as regional development initiatives, state policies and legislation, the structure of taxation and incentives for foreign tourism conglomerates, demographic trends, and institutional supports for organized labor. From a structural perspective, the state's nearly absolute dependence on tourism—now the most important single industry in the country—has contributed to a scenario in which migrant tourism workers provide the cheap labor that is necessary to sustain the flow of foreign dollars from coastal resort enclaves. The inequalities generated by the combination of these structural factors are therefore the primary drivers of disparities in reproductive health indicators, such as HIV/STI prevalence rates.

Nevertheless, while such structural approaches show great promise in highlighting how economic and political factors can shape HIV risk, the actual social processes through which these factors translate into differential disease patterns can be vague and difficult to specify (Poundstone, Strathdee, and Celentano 2004), limiting the policy and programmatic impact of concepts such as structural violence. I suggest that examining social contexts of risk is conceptually useful as a means of operationalizing the otherwise amorphous notion of structure. By looking at specific social contexts of risk, we can move beyond the imprecise assertions of structure that have tended to dominate the HIV/AIDS literature in medical anthropology, allowing us to examine instead how structural processes are actually manifest and experienced within specific social environments. In the case of tourism, we are fortunate to have a significant and growing ethnographic and theoretical literature from which to draw in suggesting some key features of tourism areas that may characterize these "risky social contexts." A review of the scholarly literatures on HIV/AIDS and tourism suggests that tourism areas potentially contribute to risk owing to the confluence of at least five factors: (1) "sexual escapism," that is, the tendency for visitors to engage in sexual activities that are distinct from their typical repertoires (Conway 1993); (2) marked social inequalities between tourists and locals, which produce power differentials that can promote risk taking and diminish protective behaviors (Kinnaird, Kothari, and Hall 1994; Smith 1978); (3) availability and affordability of alcohol, drugs, and sexual-economic exchanges (Forsythe 1999; Forsythe, Hasbún, and Butler de Lister 1998; Kempadoo 1999); (4) isolation of most tourism areas from the home communities and conjugal households of both tourists and workers, which in combination with labor migration may significantly diminish sources of social support (Cohn et al. 1994; Padilla 2007); and (5) use of sexual eroticism as an implicit or explicit marketing tool by tourism businesses, which may result in explicit or implicit pressure on workers to engage in sexual interactions and multiple partnering (Mullings 1999; Truong 1990).

These five key features of tourism areas are integrated into the conceptual model described later in this chapter, and are suggested as possible contextual characteristics of tourism areas that are likely to influence reproductive and sexual health outcomes for individuals who live and work in these environments. Taken together, the empirical support for these factors from a range of disciplinary perspectives strongly suggests that tourism should be examined for its confluence of behavioral, social, and structural features that contribute collectively to reproductive and sexual health vulnerabilities.

Regional Masculinities and Marital HIV Risk

At the outset I showed that contemporary ethnographic studies of Caribbean gender and kinship have tended to foster static representations rather than examining how masculinity and femininity are enacted in specific social contexts and situations. Now I take this argument a step further by suggesting that the notion of regional masculinities not only allows for a more dynamic view of how the meanings and practices of masculinity vary across space, but also reveals potential linkages between gender, work, and HIV risk among male tourism migrants and their wives. Further, I argue that this approach has clear benefits over prior approaches in that it seeks not to identify and target specific groups of "risky men" but to ameliorate the contextual factors that may promote reproductive and sexual health among tourism workers and their partners.

Here I develop the idea of regional masculinities in dialogue with a grow-ing ethnographic literature that examines how gender and sexuality change as individuals move between different communities or social environments (Carrillo 1999; González-López 2005; Hirsch 2003). This literature has drawn attention to the fact that most social research on gender has focused on relatively confined geographic areas and has paid little or no attention to regional variation in the social organization of gender. González-López re-cently argued that concepts such as "regional patriarchies" can call attention to diversity within countries in the ways that social geography and access to resources shape men's experiences of gender (González-López 2005). Here I borrow and extend this approach to suggest that the notion of regional masculinities provides a lens through which to consider intra- or interre-gional differences in constructions of gender that may be linked to reproduc-tive and sexual health vulnerabilities among male tourism workers and their partners. I draw on three bodies of literature in developing this notion: (1) the international literature on migration and AIDS, (2) ethnographic studies of gender and space in the Caribbean, and (3) anthropological theo-ries of gender as situational and contingent.

MIGRATION AND AIDS

Numerous studies in a wide range of international settings have shown that men who migrate for work are often at increased risk for HIV infection, as measured by both frequencies of sexual risk behaviors and HIV infection rates, and that the stable female partners of male labor migrants are often at particularly high risk for HIV and other STIs (Bronfman 1998; Broring and Van Duifhuizen 1993; UNAIDS/IOM 1998). For example, many scholars have discussed the potential risk-taking effects of extended separations from home communities, which may combine with a new normative social climate that encourages sexual risk taking or substance use within the labor area (Bronfman 1998; Wallace et al. 1997). UNAIDS has recently emphasized the need to understand how HIV risk within heterosexual partnerships is shaped by variations in the process and timing of labor migration, such as the periodicity of trips between the home community and the labor area, and the duration of spousal separation during migratory labor (UNAIDS/IOM 1998).

ETHNOGRAPHIC STUDIES OF GENDER AND SPACE IN THE CARIBBEAN

As mentioned at the beginning of the chapter, the Caribbean ethnographic literature has generally focused on describing two contrasting expressions of gender: (1) the domestic and conjugal spaces of the household (considered feminine spaces), and (2) the public and street environments of homosocial male groups (considered male spaces). The regional masculinities framework allows us to move beyond such static and binary ethnographic formulations by putting models of masculinity into motion and allowing the examination of how migrants move through different social contexts of masculinity. For example, participation in "reputational" activities—such as drinking in all-male groups or sexual-economic exchanges—may dominate the normative environment of certain tourism areas, but periodic trips home may promote more "respectable" masculine behaviors and practices. The theoretical benefit of regional masculinities, then, is that the concept allows us to foreground how the meanings and practices of reputation and respectability operate at particular times and places, rather than as presumably fixed characteristics of individuals or groups. The framework advocated here represents reputation and respectability as a continuum of gendered meanings and practices that are differently expressed depending on the social context.

GENDER AS SITUATIONAL AND CONTINGENT

At the same time that distinctions such as "reputation" and "respectability" are useful analytically, it is important to recognize that recent research has criticized static definitions of masculinity, such as the concept of machismo (Gutmann 2003). Instead research should explore how men draw on the meanings and practices of masculinity situationally as they navigate through a variety of social contexts in the course of their daily lives. This fluidity of masculinity is even more likely in areas such as the Caribbean, where intense

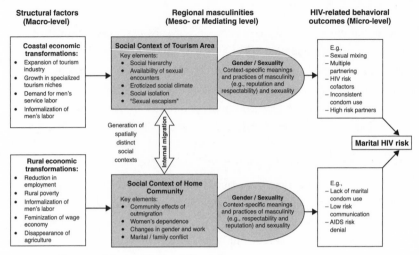

Structural factors
(Macro-level)

Regional masculinities
(Meso- or Mediating level)

HIV-related behavioral
outcomes (Micro-level)

Coastal economic transformations:
- Expansion of tourism industry
- Growth in specialized tourism niches
- Demand for men's service labor
- Informalization of men's labor

Social Context of Tourism Area
Key elements:
- Social hierarchy
- Availability of sexual encounters
- Eroticized social climate
- Social isolation
- "Sexual escapism"

Gender / Sexuality
Context-specific meanings and practices of masculinity (e.g., reputation and respectability) and sexuality

E.g.,
- Sexual mixing
- Multiple partnering
- HIV risk cofactors
- Inconsistent condom use
- High risk partners

Generation of spatially distinct social contexts

Internal migration

Marital HIV risk

Rural economic transformations:
- Reduction in employment
- Rural poverty
- Informalization of men's labor
- Feminization of wage economy
- Disappearance of agriculture

Social Context of Home Community
Key elements:
- Community effects of outmigration
- Women's dependence
- Changes in gender and work
- Marital / family conflict

Gender / Sexuality
Context-specific meanings and practices of masculinity (e.g., respectability and reputation) and sexuality

E.g.,
- Lack of marital condom use
- Low risk communication
- AIDS risk denial

FIGURE 2   Conceptual framework. Created by author.

processes of mobility, migration, and economic transformation contribute to the regular movement of people between rural, urban, and transnational social spaces (Basch, Schiller, and Blanc 1994).

Earlier in the AIDS epidemic, anthropologists made important contributions to public health approaches by highlighting the importance of questioning the assumed congruency between sexual identity and sexual behavior —a theoretically informed perspective that has broadened how public health practitioners conceptualize and address HIV risk practices (Parker 1986, 1987, 1992). Nevertheless, public health has scarcely begun to grapple with the anthropological view that the meanings and practices of gender are flexible and can and do change from place to place, situation to situation.

A PROVISIONAL FRAMEWORK FOR THE STUDY OF
REGIONAL MASCULINITIES AND HIV/AIDS

Integrating each of these literatures, the conceptual model in figure 2 represents the interaction of three levels that are theorized to influence marital HIV risk among migrant tourism workers and their partners: (1) structural factors (macro-level), including the economic changes that have occurred in the Dominican Republic; (2) regional masculinities (meso-level), which we define as regional variations in the social contexts of masculinity; and (3) HIV-related behavioral outcomes (micro-level). A visual schematic of the conceptual framework is shown in figure 2.

Through its theorization of regional masculinities, this approach seeks to move beyond the static view of gender that has tended to dominate considerations of the relationship between gender and HIV, and instead incorporates a key theoretical insight borrowed from gender studies: gender, as a contingent social process, must be examined as a context-dependent phenomenon. Only then can the complex linkages between structural transformations, the contingent practices of gender and sexuality, and reproductive health outcomes be thoroughly understood.

Conclusion

As the global AIDS pandemic has expanded and become entrenched in the poorest and most disadvantaged populations in the developing world, both social scientists and public health practitioners have become increasingly critical of the constraints of traditional theoretical approaches to sexual health. Collectively, structural and political-economic analysts of AIDS have argued strongly for abandoning exclusively micro-level models of sexual risk that, at their worst, mask the operation of more fundamental causes responsible for disparities in health indicators across the lines of gender, class, race, and nationality (Link and Phelan 1995). At the same time, and somewhat ironically, such approaches may have contributed to a marginalization of ethnographic analysis in applied public health, since master tropes such as structural violence have implied that sociocultural factors, such as the meanings of masculinity, are less important in the analysis of health disparities than poverty and material conditions. Yet such approaches commit a more serious error in their theoretical representation of human behavior, since they do not permit a multilevel explanation of HIV risk that combines large-scale structural forces with the intimate meanings and practices that inform everyday behavior. A wealth of ethnographic data attests to the fact that cross-culturally variable constructions of gender and sexuality can have consequences for HIV risk behavior. Rather than seeking to replace a cultural level of analysis with a vulgar economic determinism, contemporary reproductive and sexual health initiatives need to be informed by conceptual frameworks that elucidate the intersections of structural processes and the local meanings and practices of gender and sexuality.

The development of the concept of regional masculinities represents a preliminary attempt to develop such a multilevel framework to understand the linkages between structural changes in Caribbean economies and the regionalization of masculinity across rural areas and tourism zones. It draws on ethnographic, epidemiological, and economic sources, within a structurally informed theoretical framework, to posit that the spatial separation of distinct social contexts of gender may contribute to marital HIV risk among male tourism workers and their wives. As migrant men move between these spaces in the course of making a living, the ways that they relate to others—both socially and sexually—are informed by the specific characteristics of each social context. Mobile populations and labor migration have always been central in the AIDS epidemic, and the accelerated growth of the travel and tourism industries certainly does not bode a decline in this regard. Future work in global health therefore needs to be oriented toward the development of dynamic conceptual frameworks to guide research aimed at understanding how the large-scale transformations brought about by structural processes are shaping the sexual and reproductive vulnerabilities of developing-world populations who are, in most cases, the underclass of globalization.

Notes

I wish to thank Fulbright IIE, the National Science Foundation, the Wenner-Gren Foundation for Anthropological Research, the Fogarty AIDS International Training and Research program, and USAID/AccionSIDA (Dominican Republic) for generous financial support and the many men who confided their stories to me in the course of the research.
1. I am indebted to Jennifer Hirsch for her insightful comments on many of the ideas developed in this chapter, and for our engaging conversations during my tenure in the Department of Sociomedical Sciences at Columbia University.

2. Pseudonyms are used to protect confidentiality.

3. While prostitution is not formally prohibited by the Dominican penal code, abuses by the authorities are common, resulting in significant financial losses by sex workers who are regularly forced to pay bribes to police.

4. Social scientists have correctly questioned the problematic social and moral construction of risk in public health, which has been particularly pronounced in the area of HIV/AIDS. Here I do not engage directly in such critical interventions in favor of developing a rhetorical and theoretical argument that considers risk contextually; nevertheless, it is worth noting that uncritical notions of "risky social contexts" could themselves be in danger of conceptual and discursive misuse.

Family Reunification Ideals and the Practice of Transnational Reproductive Life among Africans in Europe

In the European Union, as in much of the industrialized world, family life is quietly becoming the battleground of immigration struggles. It is doing so through the logics generated by family reunification, now a key mode of legal entry into Europe. Looking through the lenses of recent anthropological interests in transnationalism and reproduction, this chapter examines the spread of global humanitarian conventions that have shaped family reunification, and their consequences for African marital and reproductive life in Europe. We suggest that family reunification doctrine, like any ideological system, can work against people as much as for them. Indeed, despite humanitarian claims to protect the family as the moral core of human relations, the same measures that were designed to bring families together can divide them along precisely the same fault lines they were intended to safeguard.

To address the dynamics surrounding transnational marriage and parent-child relations, we join theoretical strands of social agency to the idea of population to argue that the contours of future exclusionary practices can often be found at the core of categories of inclusion. To the extent that the state seeks to include outsiders, we believe, it is likely to take a tolerant approach to immigrant efforts to bring family members to live with them. Under pressures to exclude, however, state efforts to tighten regulatory scrutiny may center on attempting to enforce the various pieces of logic—age, relationship, quantity—that underlie each reunification position. Because each position in fact rests on different assumptions about identity and the relationships that should connect people, the result is very likely to be separate pathways for family members. For citizens of poor countries, social relationships and even age itself can become commoditized entities that people try to use by selecting individuals for migration whose attributes will most likely pass family reunification muster. In this way, families may seek to accommodate a narrowing set of entry demands structured by state policies. The outcomes, representing varying mixes of opportunity and hardship, produce versions of family life that range from minor variations on business as usual to harsh distortions of social practice.

To illustrate these points, we draw on an ethnographic/demographic project titled "Transnational Vital Events," conducted from 2004 to 2007, which centered on three African groups in Europe: Moroccan youth in Spain, Cameroonian men and women in Germany, and Gambian families in Spain. The project, conceived around an explicitly anthropological theme, centered on in-depth interviews and small surveys with immigrants and their families. Beyond these features, however, the project had few of the conventional contours of anthropology. Not only was it multisited; it was conducted by a multipersoned team of multiple nationalities, some of whom performed technical statistical analyses of national censuses and municipal registers in ways that sociocultural anthropologists, especially since they usually work alone, seldom do. Within this team individuals developed their specific subprojects, but each drew on the skills and expertise of others. When the opportunity permitted, the more demographically oriented re-searchers (Andreu Domingo from Spain, René Houle from Canada, and Gunnar Andersson from Sweden) joined forces with the more ethnographi-cally ones. The anthropologist Caroline Bledsoe and the geographer Papa Sow (himself a Senegalese-born Spanish resident with a highly transnational life), conducted periodic fieldwork in Spain and The Gambia, and two anthropology Ph.D. students conducted several months of ethnographic fieldwork in Europe and Africa (Annett Fleischer in Germany and Cam-eroon; Núria Empez in Spain and Morocco).

Variation infused not only researchers' skills and backgrounds but also the countries studied. In Germany, the postwar *Gastarbeiter* (guest worker) period from the 1950s to the 1970s, when the nation actively sought outside labor, has long since ended. The same is true for Germany's liberal treatment of appeals for asylum in the post-reunification 1990s, through which many people came, especially from the former Soviet Union. The country has now tightened its entry requirements to such an extent that the few Africans who are able to come legally are almost entirely those with offers of admission to technical training institutes or jobs in highly technical fields or those who come as family members of established residents.

Spain's immigration context is entirely different. Spain is now the leading European host country, proportionate to its national population, for immigrant arrivals. However, geography and economy give rise to sharp dilemmas (Domingo and Houle 2005). Situated at the edge of the EU, with vast tracts of borderland exposed to the external world and an economy that has been heavily reliant on agriculture, construction, and tourism, this "interface" country is caught between pressure from its European neighbors to tighten its borders and the risk of excluding immigrant labor that, until recent recession struck, has been much needed.

Confronting the challenges faced by these highly disparate groups in countries with such different immigration profiles brings into sharp relief some otherwise obscure discordance in the logics underlying family reunification. After describing the background of reunification policies, we examine social practices surrounding marriage and reproduction that shape African immigrant life in Europe.

Background

As a topic in the age of transnationalism,[1] the conduct of life across more than one national context, reproduction has drawn surprisingly little explicit attention in anthropology or sociology.[2] In demography, the topic has sparked debates over whether immigrants' youthful age pyramids might solve the economic and care crises posed by a rapidly aging Europe (United Nations 2000; Coleman and Rowthorn 2004; Kulu 2005). As for anthropology, the fact that family reunification policy has been shaped by the language of international law and humanitarian doctrine has appeared to deflect ethnographic attention to its growing import. Not only does family reunification produce or reconnect an immigrant family through transnational mobility, at least in theory; the fact that family reunification has become a significant source of youth in a rapidly aging continent means that its dynamics can no longer be ignored in the study of migration in Europe.

For immigrants themselves, however, especially those from poor countries, concerns about reproductive life differ from those that preoccupy most

European government officials. Birth remains an event of potentially mortal consequence not only in poor countries where women may have begun their reproductive years; women and children in states that do not recognize them as legal residents can drop below the horizon of national healthcare (e.g., Reed et al. 2005). More generally, a transnational existence means that a state to which individuals do not belong can set the terms by which their reproductive lives must transpire. While American tourists can enter Europe with a passport and the 1985 Schengen Agreement allows EU citizens, legal residents, and tourists to travel internally without visas or passport control, shifts in law and policy can undermine the predictability for conducting a work or reproductive life that established residents take for granted (Bledsoe 2004b). Citizens of "high migration potential" countries are required to obtain expensive visas and undergo intensive scrutiny (e.g., Král, 2006). Knowing how difficult reentry will likely be, those without documentation are reluctant to travel internationally, a fact that swells the population of undocumented immigrants in Europe.

The Legal Architecture of Family Reunification

The twentieth century has seen an explosion of international law on human rights,[3] including that governing family reunification: the joining of previously separated or newly acquired ties to people whom society defines as a family. The most basic tenet of the human rights legal corpus is that all people, irrespective of citizenship, ethnicity, religion, or gender, have certain rights simply because they are human beings. After World War I, calls for such measures were among the principal inspirations for the League of Nations. In the late 1940s, after World War II, the United Nations Charter advocated "respect for human rights and for fundamental freedoms for all without distinction as to race, sex, language or religion" (Art. 1, para. 3). The UN's Economic and Social Council ordered its new Commission on Human Rights to draft an "International Bill of Human Rights,"[4] urging signatory governments "to provide for all human beings a life consonant with freedom and dignity and conducive to physical, mental, social and spiritual welfare." Prominent among the bill's expressed ideals was the right, irrespective of national boundaries, to a shared family life.[5]

Family reunification doctrine, based on the humanitarian right to marry and "found" a family (in the wording of international conventions), declares that certain relatives of a legal migrant, whether they became kin before or after the migrants' move, should be allowed to join him or her in the new country of residence. Insisting on the family as the core unit of society, this doctrine gives the family precedence even over the nation-state, which is charged to maintain the family's integrity. If any element in humanitarian doctrine trumps the individual's right to family life, however, it is the "best interests of the child," spelled out most explicitly in the 1989 UN Convention on the Rights of the Child (CRC).[6] The CRC, now adopted by all countries except Somalia and the United States, bestows on children, regardless of their nationality or whereabouts, the right to the care and company of a family: particularly of both parents, if possible, whether defined biologically or by formal adoption. Children thus have not just special rights but special rights to live with their parents, and a CRC signatory state in which an unaccompanied child appears is obligated to facilitate this reunification. If the family cannot be found or is deemed unsuitable, the state is itself bound, through assuming the role of guardian, to constitute the parent to which the CRC declares the child is entitled.

Family Reunification in Practice

Despite the best of intentions, human rights measures spark debate. Disputes center on tensions between individual versus collective rights and universal standards (including what some see as a Western patriarchal ideology) versus local cultural values,[7] and the financial hardship that upholding the conventions may impose on countries. Further, because each signatory state is expected to implement and enforce the principles through its own governance structures and civil codes, interpretation and enforcement standards among states vary greatly (Bhabha 1998). Spain, for example, enacts international human rights and family reunification measures through its seventeen Autonomous Communities, whose internal administrations themselves differ in their interpretation and implementation of the rules. Further, for various reasons, there is considerable slippage between signature and practice. As with most legal measures, the various human rights bills and instruments are themselves complex and ambiguous. Covenants, statutes, protocols, and conventions are considered binding for their signatory states; declarations, principles, and guidelines, though they were intended to provide implementation and moral guidance, are not.[8] And states may adhere selectively or attach impossible conditions to the principles they have pledged to uphold, or they may simply ignore them.

For citizens of poor countries, bringing anyone at all to a distant nation is a daunting proposition. The costs alone are enormous, not just for transportation but for middlemen, translators, and lawyers, and there is every risk of encountering belligerent immigration officials and of being deported. One of their key challenges in bringing family members to Europe, however, is the state's power to define precisely what a family is, within its jurisdiction, and who can belong to it—especially as EU pressures to exclude shrink qualifications for family reunification to a core of highly circumscribed ties with tight age windows and few allowable variations in sexual preference and marital status. Most countries follow the UN Convention on the Rights of the Child, defining childhood in temporal and dependency terms: an unmarried dependent younger than eighteen usually stipulating a minimum age of eighteen for a spouse and less than eighteen for a child.[9] Other restrictions govern number of partners.[10] European countries are monogamous by law, and their family reunification policies follow suit: only one spouse at a time can have a social security card, a health card, and a legal residence permit. Additionally, conjugal unions are increasingly policed to rule out what host countries see as immigration convenience (De Hart 2006).

Further struggles center on the parent-child relationship. Some European countries, while they set strict chronological boundaries between those who would qualify for reunification and those who would not, have tried to shrink the temporal boundaries of childhood, alleging difficulties in incorporating older children: the EU Court of Justice as recently as 2006 reaffirmed states' rights to conduct mandatory "integration tests" for children twelve and older.[11] States also reduce childhood to a biological condition, deploying sophisticated medical technologies to exclude those who do not qualify. According to Núria Empez (personal communication, 2005), the first order of business for Spanish authorities who encounter newly arrived unaccompanied Moroccan youths is often to take them to a hospital, less to ensure their welfare than to identify, through bone density scans, those who can be sent back immediately because they do not biologically qualify as "children." The state may also challenge claims to parenthood. It may demand DNA tests for parents and children.[12] It may also deny reunification for foster children who are not legally adopted, children suspected to be victims of trafficking, and children whose parents are deemed unable to meet state standards of stable employment or adequate income and accommodation.

Conceptualizing Family Reunification Practice:
Selecting Commoditized Attributes

These descriptions paint a bleak picture of normative and state oppression for Africans seeking to enter European states. As in any lived experiential context, however, one finds multiple arenas of negotiation and tacit agreement to look the other way. To grasp a more rounded view of humanitarian doctrine and the family reunification dynamics it generates, we draw on Strathern's (1988) notion of the "partible self," which sees personal identity as a collection of single attributes. Gender, height, residence locale, family name, skin color; anything of possible social significance can be distinguished and treated as relational and meaningful only with respect to other people. The notion of the partible self has particular utility when joined to a second notion: commodification, in which an entity is dissociated from its original context, designated as a universally exchangeable good that can be marketed for sale to the highest bidder (Appadurai 1986). Possessing a personal attribute with external value may be advantageous for, say, special loans or training, but it may also produce risk. A woman's sexual attributes, for example, can make her vulnerable to exploitation in the commercial sex trade, a domain of exchange over which she has little control (Gates 1996; Sharp 2000).

The notion of the self as a set of discrete, commodified facets finds ready application in immigration and family reunification practice. Immigration policies implicitly partition the self—whether according to gender, job skills, or a nationality that is subject to political persecution elsewhere—into personal characteristics that can be converted to transactable immigration value. For the case of family reunification, several points about the characteristics that qualify an individual for inclusion deserve mention. First individuals' characteristics have conversion value only relative to another person. Second, family reunification policies demand "otherness": personal characteristics must be converted across a national boundary, in a country to which these individuals do not belong. Third, characteristics of potential family reunification value are conceived in quantitative terms. While the role of child can be plural, having multiple simultaneous holders, EU rules limit the spouse position to one. Though multiple individuals can circulate through this position over time, it is effectively a slot that just one person at a time can occupy.

Finally, the legal bases underlying each family reunification position differ: each family reunification position, because it relates differently to that of an established migrant, implicitly orients to a distinct pathway of mobility. When pressures to exclude intensify, it should not be surprising that the categories laid out so carefully by human rights idealists themselves become the fault lines along which family splits may occur.

The idea of a self-composed family of state-defined, commoditized attributes is a useful way to frame family reunification for social science analysis. The problem is that few states achieve anything close to pure domination or even governmentality (Foucault 1979), which exacts compliance less by force than by enrolling individuals into disciplines of the self. Missing from such visions is a sense of the interplay between structure and individual action. Combining the idea of selection from statistics (Heckman and Smith 1995) and agency perspectives from the social sciences, the notion of "acts of selection" (Bledsoe 2004a) acknowledges that individuals inevitably act with reference to structure. However, they try to shape the future less by responding post hoc to the structural constraints of the groups in which they find themselves than by prospectively emphasizing those of their partible or commoditized attributes that qualify them for membership in groups offering the most desired pathways of opportunity.[13] This they may do through language or physical movement and with respect to groups that are either fleeting or long-standing. Applied to family reunification, this means that individuals may try to select themselves—or, of course, others—into family relationships that offer immigration advantage. One notable example is the case of U.S. citizens who seek lower taxes abroad; such individuals may select themselves into foreign populations by drawing on attributes that would qualify them for citizenship elsewhere.[14] At the same time, with U.S. citizenship at such a global premium and other means of entering closing rapidly, being the mother of a U.S. citizen has become a heavily commoditized attribute for women from geographically proximate Mexico. Not only do they seek benefits of education and work for their children; they know that such children, once they reach age eighteen, may apply to reunify their family in the U.S. Each year, therefore, many pregnant Mexican women try to select their children into the population of U.S. citizens by giving birth on U.S. soil, a guarantee of citizenship for their child under the Fourteenth Amendment to the Constitution, whether by undertaking dangerous desert or river crossings or by scheduling a caesarean section during a three-day visa stay.[15] Whereas individuals may see such pressures as problematic, they may also conclude that the advantages outweigh the risks.

Generating Forms of Transnational African Family Life in Europe

The mixes of selection, labeling, and maneuvering sketched in the previous sections hint at the convoluted world of immigration struggles that increasingly turn on the international language of family reunification. Here we turn to two broad patterns that have emerged among African groups seeking security in Europe. We will suggest that as state immigration restrictions press up to or even spill over the edges delineated by human rights rules, social formations assemble around the inner perimeters of the allowable family reunification categories, producing both distortion and opportunity.

"The Best Interests of the Child": Unaccompanied Moroccan Minors

Núria Empez's work on Moroccan boys who manage to cross the Strait of Gibraltar from Tangier in speedboats or under trucks that board ferryboats reveals a complex story (Empez, personal communication, 2005; Empez and Galea Montero 2005).[16] According to Empez, all actors, from the Spanish state to Moroccan boys and their parents, have come to draw on the international human rights language of childhood vulnerability and family reunification in their struggles over whether boys who manage to arrive in Spain must return to Morocco. Under Spanish law, the state can send back individuals under age sixteen on the grounds that it is acting in the "best interests" of children too young to have made a key life decision like migration. Individuals over eighteen, on the other hand, are labeled adults, and those who arrive without papers can be deported. In the case of undocumented children who fall into the residual age category, from sixteen to seventeen, the Spanish Childhood Protection System is supposed to take in those who are "unaccompanied" as its wards, giving legal residence at eighteen to those who have been in its care for nine months, during which they are to have undergone proper socialization that would prepare them to enter Spanish society. As legitimate means for adults to enter Europe disappear, however, bizarre arenas of boundary construal emerge. Many impoverished Moroccan youths, feeling the weight of family responsibility, try explicitly to go to Spain as unaccompanied minors, and they do so at exactly age sixteen to try to fit into the narrow temporal window of legal opportunity. Further, as Empez shows, Spanish officials use "best interests of the child" language to reunite the boys with their families; but back in Morocco, the boys may be spurned as failures by their families or met at the port by police who beat them, load them onto buses, and deposit them in the desert far to the south. Moroccan parents and their representatives, ironically enough, may use the same language, but with the opposite intent. When Spanish authorities first contact the parents to report their sons have turned up, parents, through the advice of NGOs and lawyers, may cite the best interests of the child as the reason the family should *not* be reunited. Describing themselves as incompetent, abusive, and too poor to care for children properly, such parents hope to oblige Spain to take on the role of legal guardian to their sons.[17]

The Law of Monogamy: Cameroonians in Germany and Gambians in Spain

Just as the case of Moroccan boys in Spain highlights ironies surrounding definitions of who is a child and who is an appropriate parent in family reunification policy, the logic of spousal singularity produces dilemma as well as opportunity for many Africans in Europe. The cases of Cameroonians in Germany and of Gambians in Spain will illustrate.

Germany's determination to minimize its modes of entry has led Cameroonian immigrants now to orient their marital and reproductive lives in Germany more toward Germans than toward their compatriots. Faced with sharp exclusionary pressures in the German labor market, Cameroonians who try to come to Germany find that almost the only way they can stay and earn money to send home is to create a family life in the host country: specifically to marry or reproduce a German citizen.[18] The divergent pathways that German immigration policies take shape for immigrants from places like Africa are striking illustrations of the trade-offs. Cameroonian women find the best way to gain residence in Germany is by bearing a child by a German man who will acknowledge biological parentage; Germany requires no long-term paternal obligations of men who father single women's children. Using German Federal Statistical Office figures, Fleischer (2010) found that although Cameroonian men in Germany outnumbered Cameroonian women by about two to one in 2004, far more of the 332 live births that occurred that year involving a Cameroonian parent were to Cameroonian women than to men (240 versus 92). Among the children born to married couples, just 49 (23 percent) were born to parents who were both

Cameroonian, while 165 were born to a Cameroonian and German conjugal pair: mostly to Cameroonian women and German husbands.

For most Cameroonian men, the pathway to legal residence is entirely different. Most German women who are willing to strike up relationships with them are substantially older than they are, and are unable or unwilling to have a child. Still, a Cameroonian man improves his chances of being allowed to stay in Germany by contracting a marriage to a German woman and sustaining it for three years, after which he may qualify for residence.[19] So strong are the pressures on Cameroonian men to marry a German woman, according to Fleischer, that there were 163 binational marriages in 2004 between a Cameroonian and a German in Germany (mostly Cameroonian men and German women), but just six marriages between Cameroonian men and women. Further complicating things, many Cameroonian men in these unions desire children. Facing limited chances to bear a child and the logic of singularity on which European marriage rests, some Cameroonian men quietly maintain a marriage with a woman back in Africa by whom they have borne children, or ask their families to find a wife they can visit periodically and eventually join permanently.[20]

Despite the advantages that beckon to many Cameroonians in moving to Germany, German fathers of Cameroonian women's children are often a fleeting presence, and many marriages between Cameroonian men and German women are troubled.[21] Even if a binational couple marries out of genuine affection, the surveillance and harassment they experience from authorities suspecting marriages of convenience can quickly erode a relationship. In a reversal of the usual unidirectional assumptions about development and the West, a Cameroonian man who seeks a marriage with a German woman as a temporary necessity may thus come to see his African marriage as his "real" union and his German marriage as the temporary distortion.

Taking the logic of spousal singularity in a different direction, the case of Gambians in Spain lays bare the paradoxical potential of family reunification to break up families by separating spouses from one another and children from their parents.[22] The number of registered Gambians in Spain is small: just 17,393, according to the 2007 Spanish Municipal Register.[23] Unlike most immigrant groups in Spain, many Gambians, first arriving in the late 1960s on a labor contract in the growing Spanish economy, continue to maintain close ties to rural areas of a high fertility polygynous homeland. In 2005 they appeared to have the highest total fertility rate for any group in Spain: 3.57 children per woman, compared to 1.4 children for all of Spain (Bledsoe, Houle, and Sow 2007).

For a group like this, the conflicting logics of quantity that generate family reunification positions appear in stark relief, and in two ways. First, state exclusion pressures have the effect of increasing the value of those reunification positions that people do manage to create, leading families to try to keep these positions filled independently of the identity of the original occupant. Second, and more specifically, is the tension between multiplicity and singularity that underlies the two core relationships of marriage and filiation in EU family reunification policy: a married pair can bring all children it shares as a couple, but an adult can have only one legal spouse at a time.

Though monogamy is the law of the land in Spain, the pragmatic need to maintain mobility for family members means that men may try to rotate multiple holders through the singular position of legal spouse. This means that a man who wants to bring another wife should do so only if his first wife dies or if the couple divorces. At the very least the first wife should return to Africa. In fact, however, his first wife may take up residence separately, or she may stay in the house and effectively disappear from the official record. In other cases, a man may send a wife with a new baby back home to nurse it, and rotate her back to Spain when his second wife, herself having just given birth, is ready to head back to The Gambia, a pattern with clear parallels to birth interval practices in polygynous areas of Africa. Some Gambian unions thus have a serial character, with co-wives alternating two or three year periods in Spain. To be sure, the husband may not support a woman he sent back to Africa as promised, or he may not bring her back at all, especially if the co-wife relationship has been rivalrous. Where a dynamic of substitution emerges for wives, though, the pathways of children with educational and health institutional roots in Spain follow a cumulative dynamic. Irrespective of where their mothers end up, children born in or brought to Spain usually either remain there or come back eventually. Whether a wife is sent away at her wishes or despite her resistance and whether she remains in the house-hold below the official horizon or leaves the country, Spain's insistence that immigrants comply with the inherently discrepant premises underlying family reunification positions increases the likelihood of separating Gambian children from their mothers. If older women risk exclusion and isolation, however, and children are set onto independent trajectories from their parents, such things do not happen because of traditional norms such as those surrounding polygyny. Rather, the implicit "quantity" elements that separate the legal positions of spouses and children in Europe transform routine patterns of circulation in the homeland into more sharply bifurcated pathways in Spain.[24]

Discussion

We have argued that the press toward exclusion in Europe reduces family reunification to one of the few remaining windows of transnational mobility for people from poor regions. In doing so, it creates incentives to offer up for speculation those relationships or pieces of a partible self that have the greatest transactable human rights value in a foreign country. Because of an increasing migration premium on characteristics with family reunification value, attempts to enforce the rigid letter of the law underlying the separate legal pathways of these positions can drive family members apart or select for migration members whose attributes will best qualify for entry.

Africa itself, to be sure, has long-standing, commonplace practices of polygyny and fosterage that rotate children and wives through households over time. And none of our findings suggest that immigrants are helpless in the face of these measures. Ellie Vasta (2008) recounts in vivid detail how migrants in London countered escalating surveillance and regulation by buying, renting, and fabricating identity cards, driving licenses, passports, visas, work permits, and National Insurance numbers, and obtaining help from members of their local communities. Indeed, we learned of an American woman who agreed to marry an African man—not despite his wife and two children back home but because of her concern for their plight. This man, rendered "undocumented" when his student visa expired, needed to stay in the United States and work to support his family, but he could not risk visiting them, lest he be unable to reenter. By marrying the man, the American woman became a kind of family member to them all. Just as his African wife had pressed for the marriage that would legalize her husband in monogamous America (first a green card and then, after three years of marriage, citizenship), his American wife would eventually press for the divorce that would finally allow him to bring his African family.

Though the new geographies of immigration that appear to divide Africa from the West increase the potentials for both risk and advantage, our interest has focused on the paradoxical outcomes that human rights doctrine on family reunification can generate. As one of the great humanitarian legacies of the twentieth century, human rights initiatives were hardly intended to become weapons. Nor did EU countries set out to produce—through their increasing efforts to control family-based immigration by conceding only the most narrowly defined family reunification requests—patterns among immigrants that seem more traditional than those found back in the homelands today. In the case of people from rural Gambia, this would mean early marriage, high fertility, rotating marital partners, and significant numbers of older women with no marriage partners. But no principles stand on their own as self-contained, autonomous forces; even measures created with the most benevolent of intents can become weapons of restriction. In this case, however, it is the very forms of family integrity that human rights doctrine aimed to safeguard that become the lines on which individuals may be excluded or exploited. When family reunification and the special rights conferred on children become the means of last resort to reach a destination, a migration premium will inevitably be placed on people whose attributes can be construed as allowable, and certain people will be delegated to make the move on the basis of their age and relationships.

Few would argue that some would-be immigrants are using human rights and family reunification provisions in ways that smack of manipulation of the social categories and relationships that Western cultures hold as most sacred. The argument we have presented here would suggest that people seeking to ensure the well-being of their families must try to fit into whatever categories are available, and that state attempts to enforce compliance with the letter of the law merely intensify efforts to maneuver around them. At the same time, we can hardly avoid noting that EU citizens can move to Spain with no pretense at all to a family relationship. Non-EU citizens applying to join a spouse in many European countries are now held to standards of attachment that few EU citizens themselves could meet (see also Fleischer 2010), especially those entailed in the highly conservative models of marriage and childhood that family reunification policies increasingly stipulate.[25] The more Europe, in effect, tries to seal out, the more outsiders who seek legitimacy within it must appear to conform to the most rarified, archaic—if not mythical—models of the European family past.[26]

With so much at stake now on the definitions of family drawn up under international humanitarian doctrine, the categorical boundaries of family reunification have become an immigration battleground. Indeed, in our view, to the extent that exclusionary efforts tighten, they will continue to generate more maneuvering, not less, around children and reproduction by myriad national, international, and family players.

Notes

This project has been supported by the Max Planck Institute for Demographic Research in Rostock, Germany, the Woodrow Wilson Center for Scholars in Washington, and by a grant by the Generalitat de Catalunya to the Centro d'Estudis Demogràfics in Barcelona. We are indebted as well to many individuals for their insights. Among them are Gunnar Andersson, Yussuf Badji, Jalika Bojang, Anna Cabré, Adama Bojang, Jennifer Cole, Bully Diawara, Andreu Domingo, Núria Empez, Annett Fleischer, Jennifer Johnson-Hanks, René Houle, Adriana Kaplan Marcusán, Boury Marianne Rosalie Mendy, Vicens Galea Montero, Dan Rodríguez García, Adela Ros Hijar, Mohamad Saybo Silla, Alassane Silla, and Montse Solsona. Special thanks to Rafaél Bellon-Gómez and Alaina Dyne for research help.

1. Glick Schiller, Basch, and Blanc-Szanton 1995; Ong 2002; Vertovec 2001; Levitt and Glick Schiller 2004.

2. See, however, Ginsburg and Rapp 1995; Hondagneu-Sotelo 2002; Hochschild 2000; Cole and Durham 2006.

3. See, for example, the 1990 International Convention on the Protection of Rights of Migrant Workers (Office of the High Commissioner for Human Rights 1990), though this measure has been accepted largely by "sending" nations and not countries of destination that most migrants favor.

4. For a historical summary, see Office of the High Commissioner for Human Rights 1990.

5. See "The Right to Family" on the Human Rights Education Associates website (http://www.hrea.org/learn/guides/family.html) and Jastram 2003. The EU "Proposal for a Council Directive on the Right to Family Reunification" declares family reunification necessary to the successful integration of lawfully residing third-country nationals and, by enabling them to lead a "normal family life," a way to stabilize and deepen the roots of immigrants (see "Proposal for a Council Directive on the Right to Family Reunification," COM/99/0638 final–CNS 99/0258, on the EUR-Lex website, http://eur-lex.europa.eu/).

6. "Convention on the Rights of the Child," Unicef (http://www.unicef.org/crc).

7. For example, see Wallerstein 1995; J. W. Scott 1996; and Mutua 2002. See Merry 2005 and Ticktin 2006 for critical anthropological perspectives on human rights and humanitarianism.

8. For an overview, see the charter of the United Nations (available at http://www2.ohchr.org/english/law/). See also Watson 1999.

9. Efforts to protect girls from early marriage are part of the intent in banning the reunification of wives younger than eighteen, a concern that Denmark used in 2002 to raise the age of family unification for spouses to twenty-four. See the UN's "Report of the Committee on the Elimination of Discrimination against Women" on the website of the Universal Human Rights Index website (http://www.universalhumanrightsindex.org/).

10. Though France used to allow multiple spouses to immigrants, Pasqua laws banned this possibility (Sargent and Cordell 2003).

11. See the directive, "Council Directive 2003/86/EC of 22 September 2003 on the right to family reunification," on the EU's website, http://europa.eu.

12. Molly Moore, "French Plan to Screen DNA of Visa-Seekers Draws Anger," *Washington Post*, September 21, 2007.

13. See Johnson-Hanks 2006 for an exceptional analysis of intentionality in demographic action.

14. Doreen Carvajal, "Americans Abroad Are Giving Up Citizenship for Lower Taxes," *New York Times*, December 17, 2006.

15. "A Different Kind of Border Cross," *Chicago Tribune*, April 30, 2003.

16. Moroccan numbers in the 2007 Municipal Register were still the largest of any immigrant group in Spain: 563,012. This section describes the situation largely before 2006, when Spain toughened entry requirements for children.

17. Empez's work shows also that northern Moroccan families impoverished by EU policies of exclusion increasingly try to produce children for export to Europe.

18. For a general description of Germany's immigration policies, see the "Zuwanderung in Deutschland" website (http://www.zuwanderung.de).

19. After two years, a foreign spouse of a German citizen can apply for independent residence; after three years he or she can receive temporary residence and apply for permanent residency. However, authorities continue to exert surveillance on these marriages and may even investigate cases of divorce after three years.

20. Striking parallels are found in serial monogamy in Africa, in which an influential man may marry several women over time or a young man may try out several unions before defining one as a marriage (see Comaroff and Roberts 1977). In this case, many German wives, often coming from a previous union, are technically practicing serial monogamy. And a Cameroonian man who seeks to resume a reproductive life back home is effectively circulating in space as well as time through legally monogamous marriages.

21. Luraschi (2007) reports that in Italy, the structure of immigration policies provides much wider grounds for Cameroonians to marry and partner with each other.

22. See also Kaplan Marcusán 1998; Rodríguez 2001; Sow 2004; Bledsoe, Houle, and Sow 2007; and Bledsoe 2006.

23. Padrón Continuo, Instituto Nacional de Estadística (http://www.ine.es). For some calculations, we use 2005 rather than 2007 because the register began to drop people without permanent legal residence from the records if they had not reregistered within the last two years, a move that would strongly affect Africans in Spain.

24. See Azoulay and Quiminal 2002 and Sargent and Cordell 2003 on Malian women who come to Paris for marriage.

25. Like the rest of Europe, Spain has seen the advent of informal unions and a rising age at first marriage for women in recent decades. Spanish women now have one of the highest ages at first marriage in the world: 30.06 in 2008 (Instituto Nacional de Estadística, http://www.ine.es).

26. For parallel observations, see Raissiguier 2003. For a biological model that parallels such reductionisms, see "DNA Tests Offer Immigrants Hope or Despair," *New York Times*, April 10, 2007.

Problematizing Polygamy, Managing Maternity

*The Intersections of Global, State, and Family Politics in
the Lives of West African Migrant Women in France*

In the context of transnational migration, issues such as the tensions
between reproductive agency and structural constraints challenge anthropologists to identify the complex intersections among the personal,
the state, and the global. In my research with West African migrants in
Paris, I have been particularly concerned with how reproductive decisions, especially the use of contraception, may be contested between
spouses, among co-wives in polygamous marriages, and between the
migrant and biomedical communities. Interpretations of Islam figure
prominently in the debates on contraception among Muslim migrant
men and women in Paris and in their communities of origin.

Drawing on research with migrants from Mali, Senegal, and Mauritania in Paris conducted between 1998 and 2007, I will examine the
critiques of marriage and fertility that have dominated French political
and popular discourse concerning North and West African immigration. In addition, I will demonstrate how the contradiction between the
foundational republican political philosophy and the politics of discrimination plays out for women seeking care in the public health
arena. The maternity care system, in particular, has served as a central forum for the negotiation of identities and reproductive strategies
among immigrant women. Following the work of the French scholar
Didier Fassin (2001), I suggest that women's bodies have become one
site of inscription for the politics of discrimination in France directed at
Muslim immigrants.

Historical Context

Media coverage of immigrant uprisings in France in 2005 and 2007, replete with images of burning cars, police confronting suburban immigrant youth, and impassioned polemics across the political spectrum, has obscured the historical complexities of West African transnational migration. Certainly the increasingly anti-immigrant public and political discourse in France and the call for zero immigration have obscured the significant French initiative in recruiting labor migrants during the so-called *trente glorieuses*, the years of economic prosperity between 1947 and 1974 (La Documentation Française 2006).

In the postwar period of reconstruction, the French government recruited French colonial subjects (legally French citizens after 1946), for whom there were no legal obstacles to employment. Among these, Soninke from the Senegal River Valley region (Senegal, Mali, Mauritania) dominated the migrant flow from West Africa to France until the mid-1980s and continue to represent a significant proportion of labor migrants and their families.

The historian François Manchuelle argues persuasively that in contrast to widely accepted assumptions that this migration resulted from economic and social disruptions produced by colonialism, Soninke migration to France was an extension of urban migration within Africa since at least the nineteenth century (Manchuelle 1997, 215). Thus, in his interpretation, the Soninke formed the vanguard of a larger movement of transnational migration from urban sub-Saharan Africa whose causes and channels were both economic and social. The particular histories of Soninke labor migration relevant to the contemporary dynamics of migrant integration in French society include the shift from migration by those in upper social echelons, already French speaking and urbanized, to a migration stream comprising primarily subordinate groups (former slaves, and young rural residents).

Scholars such as Manchuelle have suggested that because of the time depth of these migrations, the migrant populations in France have been (and continue to be) characterized by strong communal solidarity, occupational specialization, and a general disinterest in integrating with the host society (1997, 225). Although his call for the analysis of African labor migration in global perspective is beyond the scope of this chapter, attention to the complex features of West African labor migration to France between the nineteenth century and the present without question enhances our understanding of the politics of immigration in France today.

Methodologically, a compelling question involves the extent to which historical analysis is requisite to comprehend how state institutions have structured transnational migration and the local reception of migrant populations since the formal suspension of labor migration in 1974. In addition, a historical perspective illuminates the subjective experiences of migrants in the current hostile social climate so much in contrast to the open-door immigration period. Central to the history and evolution of Senegal River Valley migration to France is the legislation regulating family reunification dating to April 29, 1976 (Barou 2002; La Documentation Française 2006). This decree established the conditions under which migrants residing in France—almost always male labor migrants—could legally bring spouses, children, and other relatives to France. Family reunification policies were a response to the suspension of labor migration, which in turn limited the possibility of circulatory migration between France and West Africa and its corollary, the separation of work and family.

Between 1946 and 1974, male migrants who lived as "bachelors" in French worker hostels customarily returned to their communities of origin, where their spouses and children remained, sometimes for months at a time. With the advent of more restrictive immigration regulations after 1976, advocates argued that migrants had the "right to a normal family life" and supported more humane policies of family reunification (Barou 2002; La Documentation Française 2006). Retrospectively, one can date much of the shift in public opinion concerning immigration and in the state management of immigrant populations to family reunification and its economic and social implications.

Contemporary Tensions and Debates

France has long taken pride in promoting a republican model of integration based on principles of equality and universal human rights and ignoring ethnic differences (Sargent 2006). At the same time—and increasingly since 1974—the state has paradoxically discriminated against immigrant populations, leading, for example, to riots in numerous French cities that erupted in the fall of 2005 and 2007.

Discriminatory practices affecting migrants from the Senegal River Valley also continue to be implicated across a broad spectrum of everyday life.

Migrants confront frequent restrictions in regulations concerning work permits and long-term residence authorization, as well as high unemployment, housing shortages, insalubrious lodgings, and growing public hostility, especially from those favoring zero immigration. Marriage itself, rather than constituting a stable structure in a shifting environment, is often problematized by numerous regulations concerning legal marital unions and immigration status (Ministère de l'Emploi et de la Solidarité 2002).

The public dissension surrounding polygyny, for example, has generated considerable conflict for numerous migrant families. Polygyny was tacitly permitted under French immigration law until 1993, when new legislation (the Loi Pasqua) stipulated that a residence card could not be delivered to a foreigner in a polygynous union—whether the husband or his "conjoints" (wives). A card delivered "unknowingly" must be withdrawn (Law no. 93-1027, Article 15, August 24, 1993). Given that many (precise numbers unknown, but an estimated twenty to thirty thousand unions) polygynous families had been admitted before the Pasqua Law, enforcement was problematic and resulted in a Ministry of the Interior circular (no. 477, April 25, 2000) amending the 1993 law to allow for polygynous families with a history of "long residence" in France to receive a temporary residence card, identifying the holder as a visitor. Renewal of the card was based on demonstrating the intention of "leaving polygamy." In reality, the options for "leaving polygamy" include divorce, wives returning to the society of origin (willingly or not), or abandonment of wives other than the wife formally designated as "first," to allow the possibility of residence permits for the husband and one wife. Moreover, reproductive rivalries among co-wives play out in the context of these pressures to retain legal immigration status as women strategize to protect their marital, financial, and legal situations.

Managing Maternity: Transnational Migration and Contested Reproduction

Between 1998 and 2005, I interviewed 176 women of reproductive age at diverse research sites including two public hospitals, a public family planning center, and six maternal and child health clinics. I administered structured interviews to women attending prenatal or gynecology consultations, women hospitalized on the high-risk pregnancy unit or on the postpartum ward, and mothers consulting at the maternal and child health centers. The interviews elicited demographic data, reproductive histories, narratives of contraceptive use, immigration and employment information, and perspectives on religious doctrine regarding contraception, childbearing, and women's autonomy.

To obtain male perspectives, I interviewed forty-five men in focus groups consisting of four to six migrants residing in nine worker hostels. The hostels are extremely overcrowded (for example, one officially has two hundred beds but is housing six hundred men). Recommendations from hostel leadership led me to rely on focus groups, rather than individual interviews. Because many residents were undocumented, anonymity was a highly important consideration for them in agreeing to an interview. I raised two issues with each focus group: (1) the pros and cons of bringing one's wife to live in France in relation to French concepts of autonomy for women; and (2) interpretations of Islam with regard to contraception, childbearing, and child rearing.

Based on my experiences shadowing midwives in prenatal clinics and postpartum wards, I heard many spontaneous comments by the staff on the excessive fertility of African and Muslim women and how beneficial contraception would be for them. An older, more senior group of midwives who were reaching retirement age and were highly critical of current hospital policies described a widespread anti-immigrant philosophy among nurses, doctors, and many midwives, which plays out in strong recommendations for use of contraception or handing out of prescriptions for the pill, without explanation, in a stack of prescriptions at discharge. These midwives argue that the intent implicit in these practices is to limit the reproduction of the African immigrant population.

The actual presentation of information on contraception was erratic, often indifferent to the presence of men in the room, and presented in French, regardless of the language competence of the client. Few midwives call for an interpreter, and the majority stated that they are able to use gestures and pantomime effectively to convey the desired message.

My observations of incidents where midwives used interpreters suggest that the interpreters had their own agendas for translation (cf. Browner, this volume). One interpreter described how she had developed a routine for discussing contraception based on her sense of how migrants should adapt to life in Europe. She says that Paris is not "the village"; there is no help with children from the extended family. Women need to rest, space their children, avoid anemia, and also consider the problem of crowded housing. She said she usually concludes by saying, "So take the pill." She added that if she is not available for translation, the prescription for the pill may be added to the stack of prescriptions a woman receives at discharge, without explanation. Although this practice disturbed her, she had not protested because she felt it was unlikely that her opinion would be influential.

Another interpreter said, "I can give all the advice myself [that the midwives do]; all I need is the degree." She also emphasized the differences between African village life and parenting in Paris that should encourage child spacing. These interpreters may see themselves as representing the requirements of "modernity" to a less-educated and more-traditional population of women who need to become more independent and assertive and have fewer children.

For a minority of midwives, encouragement of contraception appears to be linked to a concern for women's levels of fatigue, the need for child spacing to ensure the well-being of the children, and an appreciation of the difficulties of raising numerous children on small incomes in inadequate lodging. In contrast are those practitioners whose rhetoric is much more critical of high fertility among African women, echoing the National Front's anti-immigrant platform, with remarks about irresponsibility, traditionalism, and willful failure of integration.

Essentializing the diverse ethnic populations targeted by the public hospital system was the norm in conversations with hospital personnel (for instance, a midwife might describe North African women as submissive or overly modest, and West African women were characterized as "traditional" or "laying hens"). In this regard, biomedical practitioners' assessments resonate with political discourse and the realities of everyday life for many West Africans who contend with racism across multiple institutions in France—housing, employment, education, and the immigration authority. The public hospital and social welfare systems are by no means immune to these same political currents.

In analyzing biomedical perspectives on contraceptive use by African women and the strategies of migrant women themselves, it became clear that the role of Islam as an influence on women's reproductive decisions is central. However, some hospital practitioners are not aware that their Malian or Senegalese patients are probably Muslim, associating Islam with North African immigrant populations. For those who are, the turbulent national debate concerning the politicizing of Islam and the perceived correlation between Islam and terrorism may shape interactions with Muslim women. The strong secular, humanist, and anticlerical tradition in France also influences responses to religious issues that may affect reproductive decisions (Sargent 2006). Because it is widely considered inappropriate, if not illegal, for official personnel such as midwives to pose questions about religious observances, they are unlikely to explore how interpretations of Islam may shape migrant women's decisions concerning cesarean delivery or contraception.

Accordingly, few midwives had any awareness of religious controversy surrounding contraception, and they were unaware of the widespread marital conflicts over the issue and debate in the broader Muslim communities on this topic. Malians and other women from the Senegal River Valley, on the other hand, expressed firm views on religion and its consequences for family planning. When I asked them what Islam had to say about contraception, the dominant view was that Islam opposes its use, despite the reality that Islamic jurisprudence has generated diverse judgments on the issue.

Recent legal opinions by Islamic theologians allow contraception, whether unequivocally or under limited conditions. In contrast, I found that some authorities, such as the imam of the Mosque of Paris, strongly opposed family planning as a policy, while allowing for the possibility of unique cases where contraception would be permissible. Leaders of neighborhood mosques in Paris expressed varied opinions, including vigorous support from some based on the argument that "the Prophet himself used it."

I also found a significant difference of opinion between men and women on the issue. Although approximately 70 percent of women surveyed had used a contraceptive method, almost half of the sample said that their husband did not approve, that it was none of his business, or that he didn't know about it. Specifically, almost half of those whose husbands disapproved of using contraceptives were currently using contraception anyway, often in secret.

Men interviewed in worker hostels often responded to queries concerning marriage, fertility, and religion by addressing the dilemma of long-term celibacy. Although living as "bachelors," the term used to describe them in government and scholarly documents, as well as by social service officials, many of the hostel residents are *célibataires mariés*. That is, they are living in France with wives "at home" in West Africa.

In all the focus group discussions, men mentioned the challenge to a devout Muslim of lengthy periods of sexual abstinence, and the perils of adultery. One recounted how both his and his wife's family objected to her following him to France, fearing that family ties would be permanently ruptured. However, he reminded them of the temptation of adultery if he remained without his wife. The families relented, and she joined him. Informally, some men commented on the hostel residents' ready access to sex with women from the on-site cooking teams; in fact, the cooks are reputed to belong to prostitution rings. At the same time, many men stated that they practice abstinence using "magical" products obtained from a *marabout* (ritual specialist in Paris or in West Africa) to "break sexual desire," as well as religious practices suggested by Islamic leaders to avoid adultery.

Men were almost unanimous in their conviction that Islam does not allow contraception. For most of these men, using contraception is merely one of the problematic ideas that women are exposed to in Europe. As one elder migrant on the verge of retirement said, "Bring a woman to Europe and she catches ideas." Thus these men attributed marital tensions and extended family conflicts to women's decreasing respect for the husband as head of household and final arbiter of important decisions such as contraceptive use.

In general, both men and women concurred that Islam prohibits the use of contraception except under exceptional circumstances (illness of the woman or illness of another child). Men were more likely to argue against contraception on religious grounds, but women, while accepting this argument, used contraception nonetheless. To justify this stance, many women complained of fatigue from numerous pregnancies or short birth intervals, and the difficulties of child rearing in France. Thus the embodied experience of reproduction and the pragmatics of everyday life in France contribute to women's autonomous decisions to delay or space births, men's opposition notwithstanding.

Regardless of religious devotion, Islam may serve both as doctrine and as a philosophical framework for negotiating the social transformations experienced by migrants in diasporic Muslim communities. The flow of information and critique from midwives and social workers regarding contraception has produced a gendered debate, framed in Islamic terms, but expressing tensions and uncertainties surrounding women's enhanced autonomy in France.

The Case of Yassa

The following narrative evokes some of the central issues raised by my research. This account begins with Mr. Fofanna, forty-eight, who emigrated from Mali in 1980. Initially he lived in a worker hostel but soon found a job as a motorcycle delivery person for a small business, a job he has held ever since. He rented a one-room apartment in a coveted location in central Paris and eventually married. His wife became a cook at one of the worker hostels and, he says, turned to prostitution. Having found her in his own bed with a hostel worker, he divorced her. After years of "celibacy," he phoned his brother in Bamako, asking for assistance in finding "a serious girl" to marry, which he received.

The young woman in question, Yassa, was at the time twenty-two, divorced from a brutal alcoholic husband, and had formal custody (very rare) of her four-year-old daughter. She accepted Mr. Fofanna's proposal, married in Bamako, left her daughter with the elderly woman who had raised her, and came to Paris in 2003. She arrived pregnant (she had had two miscarriages before the birth of her daughter) but had a pre-term delivery at six months of pregnancy. It was then that I met her, after the psychologist for the maternity service at the public hospital where I was working asked me to participate in Yassa's therapy consultations. Advised by the psychologist, Mr. Fofanna decided to bring Yassa's daughter to France.

Why had he not done so previously? Possibly he did not want a stepchild to deal with. But his primary expressed concern was to act in accordance with reunification regulations. As he noted, since his arrival in France, he had always "done everything correctly." He had come to France as a recruited worker and brought Yassa properly, "with papers," under the family reunification policy. To bring his stepdaughter to live with them, he had to demonstrate that he was in compliance with financial and space requirements. Unfortunately, when the mayor's official came to his apartment to measure it to determine whether the size was adequate to add a relative, it was found to be twenty-three square meters. This was deemed sufficient for two individuals, but not three, and his petition to bring the child was denied. However, when relatives phoned from Bamako to say that the little girl was old enough for genital cutting, Yassa (with the help of social workers and other advocates) succeeded in persuading the French embassy in Mali to give the child a visa, and she joined her mother and stepfather. Soon thereafter, Yassa became pregnant again and delivered a premature baby weighing 600 grams. The baby was hospitalized for a year; she visited him daily from 9 a.m. to 6 p.m., and he is now home—an energetic and vocal toddler with no apparent deficits.

Did this story end happily? Actually, no. Yassa got a job as a home health worker for the elderly, her French improved, she opened two savings accounts for the children and a burial account. She began to take birth control pills. Her husband wanted her to get pregnant again, but she refused, citing financial problems, fatigue, and a sickly baby to care for. He told her she had gotten a swelled head in Europe. Her analysis of the situation is that her husband is jealous of her financial success and confidence and how well she has learned French. She is no longer the shy young woman who feared to take the subway and cried constantly. Fearful of jealousy-generated sorcery (by her husband, his family in Mali, or her maternal aunts), she has become a close friend of the wife of the neighborhood imam, who provides her with protective ritual objects and medicines.

This excerpt from the lives of one Malian couple in Paris evokes a number of the central themes in my chapter:

1. The historical shifts from worker recruitment to family reunification and the increasing constraints on legal reunification.
2. The important role of state policies and institutions such as the prefecture and public hospitals, designated to implement statutes and circulars, in shaping family and gender relations.
3. Contested reproductive relations between spouses but strong support from midwives, psychologists, and others at one of the major public hospitals in Paris.
4. Religious observances (Islam, sorcery protection) implicated in reproductive relations.
5. The issue of women's agency and autonomy (e.g., "getting a swelled head") as sources of conjugal and extended family tensions.

Problematizing Reproduction

For West African migrants in Paris, widely shared understandings of marriage, family, and gender relations have been disrupted in the context of French immigration policies, biomedical protocols, and religious tensions. Indeed, these broader state and institutional structures have explicitly problematized reproduction in the course of debates surrounding the perceived costs of immigrant fertility to the social welfare system. Such issues, contested at the level of national political discourse and discriminatory practices, play out in the everyday lives of West African migrants. Gendered controversies on topics such as the use of contraception have the potential to profoundly disrupt conjugal and family relations, spurred by biomedical and philosophical agendas of midwives, social workers, and interpreters. As women's and men's narratives have shown, the gendered debate on contraceptive use is often framed in Islamic terms but fundamentally references significant uncertainty regarding women's autonomy in France. Women's bodies have come to represent the site at which multiple political agendas concerning immigration converge. Migrant women's fertility, in turn, has become a defining issue in the politics of immigration. During the immigrant uprisings in the fall of 2005, media and political discourse increasingly redefined the violence as a cultural product, rather than as a response to fluid and restrictive immigration policies, a failed political ideology, and rampant unemployment among immigrant suburban youth. Among the cultural analyses of the riots are commentaries by prominent politicians such as the following (Ligues des Droits de l'Homme 2006; translations mine):

> Certainly, the youths responsible for this urban violence are completely French legally, but let's tell things as they really are: polygamy and the acculturation of some families leads to greater difficulties integrating a young French person of African origin than one of another origin.
> —Nicolas Sarkozy, minister of the interior

> Family reunification explains the crisis of the suburbs.
> —Jacques Chirac, as mayor of Paris, 2005

> Insofar as one segment of society demonstrates this antisocial behavior [polygamy], it is not surprising that some of them have trouble finding work. . . . If people are not employable, they won't be employed.
> —Gerard Larcher, minister for professional "insertion" of youth

This emphasis on the cultural underpinnings of urban violence diverts attention from the politics of discrimination at the core of immigrant alienation. National political dynamics, influenced by postcolonial relations between France and its former West African colonies, have shaped the policies and politics of state institutions, such as the public health system, that play important roles in managing immigrant populations. Women from the Senegal River Valley region routinely negotiate these structures of inequality.

The problematizing of polygamy and its symbolic representation of the immigrant crisis has influenced the experience of maternity for many migrant women. Internal politics (cf. Ortner 1995) within families affected by anti-polygamy laws generate reproductive rivalries between co-wives and tensions between spouses. At the level of the hospital maternity service, implicit and explicit policies to reduce the supposed excessive fertility among African immigrants further produce conflicts within families and between migrants, midwives, and other hospital staff. Crosscutting these contested negotiations, diverse and gendered interpretations of Islam shape migrants' reproductive decisions. Thus resistance and negotiation figure prominently in the management of maternity, in spite of significant structural constraints.

I have not addressed reciprocal relations between migrants and their communities of origin in this chapter. However, with the proliferation of satellite and cell phones, faxes, audiotapes, and Internet access, frequent communications allow intense mutual involvement in everyday decisions at both sites (Sargent, Larchanche, and Yatera 2007). Migrants report the intervention of sisters, mothers, mothers-in-law, and myriad friends and relations who offer solicited and unsolicited counsel, mediate disputes, and advise on the contested reproductive and marital issues discussed here. Anthropologists working to identify the links among global processes, state structures, and individual subjectivities face daunting methodological challenges as they explore the internal politics of resistance as well as the broader power structures that shape reproduction in this immigrant population.

Lost in Translation

Lessons from California on the Implementation of
State-Mandated Fetal Diagnosis in the Context of Globalization

Globalization processes invariably involve large-scale population movements that transform every level of sending and receiving societies (Acker 2004). Yet while ethnography's greatest contribution is to reveal how such large-scale social processes shape quotidian activities, ethnographers all too often assume the links between such macro- and micro-phenomena rather than demonstrating what they actually entail. My theoretical objective is to consider how the reproductive behavior of recent immigrants comes to mirror those of women in a host society (Wingate and Alexander 2006). The analytical framework is inspired by co-production theory (Jasanoff 2004) and its premise that the nature of the scientific knowledge produced and validated in a given social setting is a manifestation of the histories, cultures, and politically derived positionalities that key stakeholders bring to that interactional domain (see also Jordan 1997). I focus on immigrants from historically high fertility Mexico to much lower fertility southern California (NVSS 2005). I analyze California's state program, which, since 1986, has mandated that fetal diagnosis be offered to all pregnant women so that they may have the option of terminating an affected pregnancy.

The research objective was to understand how a group of women from Mexico who did not speak English and had only limited formal education made sense of the offer of fetal diagnosis and decided whether to accept an amniocentesis after they had been told they were at elevated risk for a birth anomaly based on the results of a blood screening test (see Browner, Preloran, and Cox 1999 for methods and main findings). Any amniocentesis decision can be momentous because of the difficult issues it may evoke about the prospect of ending the pregnancy should the amniocentesis reveal an anomaly. But amniocentesis decisions by working-class women reared in Mexico can be even more fraught, given that their society has historically not placed much emphasis on formal prenatal care, and the notion of preventing birth defects by selective abortion of defective fetuses remains quite alien. I will show that many of the women in our study who were offered amniocentesis through an interpreter, whether a relative, friend, or a clinic staff member, received information about the test's benefits and risks that was shaded to reflect the interpreter's own views about the woman's best course of action.

While many contextual factors contributed to the patterns I describe, my emphasis will be on the micro-interactions between English-speaking clinicians and Spanish-speaking women, as well as any friends and family members also present during clinical encounters where the amniocentesis offer was made. I focus especially on the extraordinary influences of husbands serving as interpreters and non-medical-professional clerical workers pressed into service as interpreters. Within the large social science literatures on healthcare decision making and barriers to successful cross-cultural clinical communication, virtually no systematic attention has been paid to the influence of interpreters, despite their potential centrality in such situations (Angelelli 2004). And while Rapp's pathbreaking work on the cultural construction and social impact of amniocentesis in the United States brilliantly explicates many sources of miscommunication between prenatal genetic counselors and clients of diverse ethnic and social class backgrounds, such as counselors' use of specialized language and jargon, preexisting prejudices or biases on the part of both groups, and divergent expectations of the purpose and preferred content of prenatal care, she does not consider the additional complexities involved in situations where amniocentesis is offered through an interpreter (Rapp 1988, 2000).

In some sectors of the U.S. population, fetal diagnosis has become a well-established, if not routine, part of prenatal care (Sharpe and Carter 2006). In contrast, many of the women in our study had never heard of fetal diagnosis, let alone been seeking it. I will show that not knowing the best course of action—or even how to go about choosing one—left them particularly vulnerable to the wills of others with stronger opinions.

Most U.S. medical settings provide interpretation services through on-site interpreters (often with no formal interpreter training and other primary job responsibilities such as clerical or nursing). Patients with limited English may also be accompanied by a family member or friend who ostensibly speaks English better than the patient. Either alternative can present its own difficulties, as reflected hereafter in examples illustrating how an interpreter can actually impede comprehension and compromise informed decision making. I then offer quantitative data that show how on-site interpreters' interpretative approaches can indeed influence women's amniocentesis decision making.

The Contours of Fetal Diagnosis in California

Most babies born in the United States today are routinely screened for the most common birth anomalies, but the infrastructure for doing so varies from state to state (Cunningham and Tompkinson 1999). In California, the 8 percent of pregnant women who screen positive (i.e., at increased risk for a birth anomaly) are referred to a state-certified center where they are offered a consultation with a certified genetic counselor and additional testing, ordinarily a high-resolution ultrasound and, if indicated, an amniocentesis. The typical genetic consultation follows a standard protocol that includes a woman's reproductive and family medical histories; the mathematical probability of a fetal anomaly based on the screening test result and other known risk factors; options for additional testing; risks of amniocentesis; and the woman's right to accept or decline the test. The role of the genetic counselor is to get and give information and answer questions—not to offer recommendations or personal opinions.

My research team and I conducted semistructured face-to-face interviews with 120 Mexican-origin women (and, when meaningful and possible, their male partners) who were offered amniocentesis after having screened positive, 27 Mexican-origin women who had separated from partners while participating in the study, and 9 Latinas of non-Mexican backgrounds, also including the male partners when appropriate. Study participants were recruited from eleven state-approved prenatal diagnosis centers in Southern California. We also interviewed a heterogeneous, opportunistically recruited sample of sixty staff members who worked at these centers, twenty-three of whom served as ad hoc interpreters.

As the state of California mandates that amniocentesis be offered in the context of a prenatal genetic consultation with a certified genetic counselor, my research collaborator, Dr. Mabel Preloran, and I conducted systematic observations of the genetic consultations of 102 Mexican-origin women referred for prenatal genetic counseling because they had screened positive (most were the same women described earlier). Amniocentesis was offered through an interpreter in seventy-three of these consultations. We designed two paper-and-pencil instruments to record data including information conveyed, questions asked, content, and affect of interaction among participants (appendixes A and B).

We used an inductive analytical approach to analyze the observational data (Patton 2001). The narratives of seven pilot observations were analyzed toward identifying commonly occurring behavioral and interactive characteristics that could be used as a checklist in subsequent observations of similar interactions. We scored the seventy-three genetic consultations according to the presence or absence of the nineteen most commonly noted characteristics (the remaining observations did not involve an interpreter). We recorded these ratings live during the observations (appendix C) and subsequently reviewed the field notes and observational data for each interaction and categorized them based on the global dynamic between client and interpreter.

When, Why, and How Interpreters Can Influence Amniocentesis Decisions

While 60 percent ($n = 93$) of interviewees agreed to amniocentesis, 40 percent ($n = 63$) declined, a refusal rate significantly higher than most other U.S. groups (Cunningham and Tompkinson 1999).[1] There were few quantitative correlates of amniocentesis acceptance or refusal (table 1). The two groups had similar reproductive, personal, and family histories of birth anomalies, and there was no association between amniocentesis decision and whether the woman screened triple marker[2] positive high or low.

There were just three quantitative correlates of amniocentesis acceptance: being born in the United States rather than in Mexico, believing there were justifiable circumstances for abortion, and attending the genetic consultation accompanied by a male partner (Browner and Preloran 1999). While the first two might be unsurprising, the last was completely unexpected and cued us to the potential importance of interactional dynamics during prenatal genetic consultations.

In fact, a surprising 86 percent of women said they arrived at the genetic consultation undecided about whether to have the test. English speakers were as likely as Spanish speakers to say they were undecided beforehand.

TABLE 1 Background characteristics

	Accepted amniocentesis $n = 93$	Declined amniocentesis $n = 63$
Mean age	28	27
Education		
≥ 6 years	24%	24%
7–9 years	55%	48%
≤10 years	21%	28%
Household income		
< $20,000 per annum	69%	77%
> $20,000 per annum	31%	23%
Mean years in United States (for immigrants)	12	10
Religion		
Catholic	88%	81%
Other (Evangelist, Jehovah's Witness, etc.)	7%	16%
None	5%	3%

But when male partners also acted as interpreters, they could clearly be influential in shaping the women's decisions, as the following examples demonstrate. Although both couples described their amniocentesis decisions as jointly made, in each case, the information the men got from the clinicians was reshaped in translation to achieve their own desired outcome.

Husbands as Interpreters

Elisa, twenty-nine, a housewife married to Hector, an insurance salesman, wanted Hector with her at the genetic consultation and requested he serve as her interpreter.[3] In our subsequent interview, she explained that he had been extremely involved in the pregnancy, including accompanying her to all her prenatal visits. Regarding the amniocentesis offer, she said, "At the [genetics] clinic, he explained all the pros and cons of the test and later when we were relaxed at home, I could see things more clearly." There, she said, they had talked "about all the advantages of the test," the most important being "the opportunity to be reassured," something Elisa said her husband told her the counselor had mentioned several times during the consultation. Elisa said that talking with her husband enabled her to see that the "small risk" of amniocentesis was worth taking.

Lia, twenty-eight, was employed part-time and married to Pedro, a full-time college student. Both raised Catholic, they had left the church but had recently returned to become active adherents of their faith. They were thrilled by the prospect they would soon become parents, having tried unsuccessfully for several years. While both feared miscarriage, Pedro seemed the more anxious about the miscarriage risk associated with amniocentesis. He said he would abide by his wife's amniocentesis decision but also explained that he was committed "to helping her to decide by considering all the facts, especially that she might lose this baby." He said he advised her to take time and think because "now that we belong to the church, we can't just do whatever we want, and in the church, they say one could kill his own child with that test. I made her realize that that is the truth."

On-site Interpreters

Family and friends serving as interpreters constituted about 8 percent of the cases; most amniocentesis offers were made through twenty-three on-site interpreters, none of whom had formal training in medical interpretation, nor was it a formal part of any of their jobs. Rather, they were among the growing corps of receptionists, nurses, clerks, and other bilingual personnel in U.S. medical facilities enlisted to help out with interpretation as needed. The following example illustrates how interactional dynamics introduced by an interpreter can play a determining role in a woman's amniocentesis decision.

Rosalia, in her mid-twenties, with no family history of disabilities, had lived in the United States for three years before the interview, had completed high school in Mexico, and was married to a man twenty years her senior, but attended the consultation alone. Feeling her command of English was insufficient, she requested an interpreter. A secretary was called away from her usual duties to translate (but was not unaccustomed to providing this service in that setting).

The Genetic Consultation

Assisted by the interpreter, the genetic counselor asked Rosalia about her family's medical history. The interpreter translated the conversation literally.

Rosalia reported no problems on her father's side but indicated that her younger half sister's (with her mother's second husband) legs were "semi-paralyzed" as a child. Hearing this, the counselor probed to learn more about the half sister, but her questions, when translated literally (e.g., "Estaba retardada?" [Was she retarded?]), sounded harsh and crude, and Rosalia appeared discomfited. Eventually the counselor turned to the interpreter to discuss how the questions could be asked without further upsetting Rosalia. This exchange was not translated, and throughout the continuing consultation, the interpreter looked mainly at the counselor, only once making eye contact with Rosalia. At one point, Rosalia repeated that her sister had improved, as though she wanted to convince the genetic counselor that her sister's medical condition should not be of concern: "She is walking well now," Rosalia asserted, "she only has to use special shoes." But the interpreter said only: "She said her sister is okay now." Rosalia seemed to notice that her words were not being faithfully conveyed, enlarging her sense that she was being disregarded.

The counselor then explained that the ultrasound showed the pregnancy was dated correctly and she would therefore like Rosalia to consider amniocentesis. Rosalia appeared doubtful. She replied that she would "perhaps prefer to consider" the test later because at the moment she was not feeling all that well, adding that she had recently had the flu and had been eating poorly when she had the blood screening. The counselor explained that the flu would not cause a positive blood test and urged Rosalia to decide as soon as possible because her pregnancy was very advanced. Rosalia responded: "If you want to do it because of my sister, she is well now. My mother says she was a little behind [*quedada*] when she went to school, but she is walking well now. She only has to use special shoes." The interpreter again translated this by saying: "She said her sister is okay now." Instead of responding, the counselor sighed and changed the subject, suggesting that Rosalia use the office phone to discuss the situation with her husband. Rosalia replied that she would talk with him when she got home. She did not return to the clinic for an amniocentesis.

Post-consultation Interview

When the ethnographer asked Rosalia whether she had had difficulty understanding the information, she said no, but that she disliked the way the counselor and the interpreter interacted with her: "They were talking to each

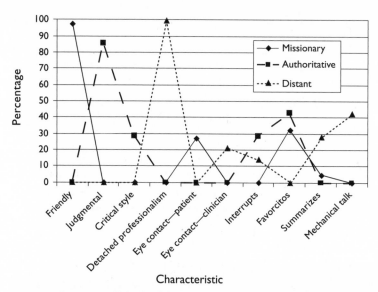

FIGURE 1   Percentage of behavioral characteristics observed across interpreter-patient interactions by interpreter approach (*n* of observed interactions = 61). Drawn by Eli Lieber. (See appendix C for coding.)

other, not to me. . . . I told her about my sister, she only needs special shoes. [The interpreter] didn't say 'shoes'; I think she didn't say anything [about that]." She added that she knew the English word for shoes and complained that they were "very impolite" in excluding her from the interaction, adding that she strongly preferred her neighborhood clinic where everyone spoke Spanish and was friendlier and less intimidating. Each time Rosalia was asked how well she felt, the information about fetal diagnosis had been conveyed; instead of answering she shifted the conversation back to the interpreter's shortcomings and the strong negative reactions they produced.

Impact of the Interpreter's Approach

Variations in the interpretative approaches used by different on-site interpreters became apparent as the research progressed, and I came to suspect that an interpreter's approach itself might influence a woman's amniocentesis decision. Subsequent analyses revealed that each interpreter adopted a generally consistent approach and that three distinct styles could be identified. These were labeled "missionary," "authoritative," and "distant" (figure 1). Data analysis supported the hunch, revealing a statistically significant

TABLE 2 Decisions about amniocentesis by interpreter approach
($n < 73$ due to missing data)

Number of observations	Interpreter approach	Amniocentesis acceptance
40	missionary	75%
7	authoritative	57%
14	distant	21%

Chi-square (2) = 12.5, p = .002 between interpreter type and amniocentesis decision.

For pair-wise comparisons between groups, patients with missionary interpreters accepted amniocentesis testing significantly more often than those with neutral-distant interpreters (z = 2.57, p = .0104).

link between interpreter approach and amniocentesis decision (table 2): interpreters using approaches that sought to build rapport and engender trust were associated with a higher likelihood of amniocentesis uptake.

Missionary Approach

Missionary was the label borrowed from an interpreter who defined her job as a "mission" to ensure adequate healthcare for U.S. Latinos. The missionary approach was the most common in the sample. All but one of the ten missionaries were in their mid-twenties to early thirties and were U.S. born to immigrant parents. All were satisfied with their jobs and the opportunities to serve Latinos, especially recent immigrants.

Figure 1 shows that the statistically significant features of this approach include high levels of friendly engagement with patients throughout the consultation; making relatively frequent eye contact with patients; listening without interrupting; providing relatively frequent offers of assistance (*favorcitos*, e.g., with paperwork); using a relaxed, warm tone; asking personal, rapport-building, nonjudgmental questions (e.g., "Did you know about this test when you were pregnant the last time?"); employing gestures conveying emotional support (e.g., touching a patient's hands if she showed distress); and using a directive approach built on *personalismo* (e.g., "I wouldn't offer you something I wouldn't consider for myself").

While missionaries were invariably friendly and empathetic, the hallmark of their approach went beyond simply facilitating communication. A typical example was the interpreter who walked a patient to the parking lot after her amniocentesis and stayed with her until she felt ready to drive. More extreme was the missionary interpreter who collected donations from coworkers for a pregnant patient to finance her trip to Mexico to bury her two-year-old daughter.

EXAMPLE

Ana, twenty-eight, a full-time typist-clerk, was helping forty-five-year-old Rocio, who had a family history of hereditary illness. Although Rocio arrived at the clinic intending to have amniocentesis, during the more than five hours she spent there, she changed her mind twice before finally consenting to the procedure.

While waiting for her amniocentesis, Rocio told the ethnographer that she felt no rapport with Kelly, the monolingual English-speaking genetic counselor, whom she found too skeptical of Rocio's accounts of her family's medical history, adding that the counselor's words of comfort sounded false: "If everything is going to be okay, why would they send me to do that [amniocentesis]?" Instead she preferred the directness of the interpreter, with whom she "could talk." Asked whether this was because she and Ana shared a common language, Rocio said it went beyond that. Unlike Kelly, Ana did not challenge Rocio's explanation of the cause of the hereditary illnesses in her family and, when talking privately, told her openly that while things could go wrong (e.g., a miscarriage), she should have amniocentesis if she wanted to be reassured. Rocio said that Ana's "frankness" inspired her trust ("Esa franqueza [de ella] me dio confianza"). She added that being so uncertain about what to do, she felt relieved and supported when Ana "pushed her a little" to agree to amniocentesis.

Throughout Rocio's long stay at the clinic, Ana was observed not only helping her with interpretation but also patiently listening to her, comforting her, and bringing orange juice from time to time: all actions characteristic of the missionary approach.

Authoritative Approach

The authoritative label came from a fieldworker's observation that some interpreters presented genetic information as "gospel." "It's like they believe they *own* the truth," she noted. The six authoritative interpreters were significantly older than the missionaries, ranging from their mid-forties to mid-sixties; all were born outside the United States. All expressed dissatisfaction with their jobs, feeling overloaded and unappreciated; five said they had held higher-status jobs in their native countries.

Figure 1 shows that the authoritative approach involved engaging with patients in a superior, openly judgmental manner (e.g., often using the word "must"); infrequent eye contact with both patient and clinician; intermittently interrupting the consultation; frequently offering patients help with a task; asking personal questions in a critical manner (e.g., "Your husband won't be the one to take care of the baby [if something goes wrong], right?"); making directive, seemingly defiant remarks (e.g., "If you want [the test], do it; after all, it's your body"); and making directive comments (e.g., "Don't pay attention to what [your sister] says [about amniocentesis]. People don't know. Doctors know, the genetic counselor knows").

EXAMPLE

Susana, a sixty-five-year-old receptionist, translated for twenty-two-year-old Lucia; this was Lucia's first pregnancy. The genetic consultation lasted forty minutes, and Lucia subsequently interacted for fifteen minutes more with only the interpreter while searching for information about her medical insurance coverage.

Her sister drove Lucia to the clinic and stayed with her during the genetic consultation. The sister looked much older than Lucia and seemed extremely protective; she held Lucia's hand and, on a couple of occasions, answered questions for her. Both agreed that Lucia should have an ultrasound, but when the sister left for work before they could perform it, she made it clear that she did not like the idea of amniocentesis, at least "before having a second opinion." When Lucia's ultrasound proved inconclusive and she was offered amniocentesis, she told the genetic counselor she wanted "to think about it." However, after briefly talking alone with Susana, the receptionist-interpreter, Lucia agreed to have the test.

Asked by the ethnographer why she decided not to wait, Lucia explained, "I'm convinced that having it today is best. I can't imagine having this [decision] on my mind all weekend." She added that although she was worried about her sister's reaction, she was comfortable with her decision. "When I arrived, I was not sure what to do [about amniocentesis]. Later, I thought I should follow my sister's advice of not doing it until getting a second opinion. But the lady [the interpreter] told me so strongly that it was for my own good, that I felt like it was my mother talking [to me]. Now I believe the sooner, the better."

The interaction during the genetic consultation between Susana and Lucia was observed, as well as their subsequent informal interaction. Susana acted somewhat impatient and interrupted Lucia twice when she tried to convey her fears about the test, and again when she brought up concerns about the extent of her insurance coverage and the possibility of losing more than a day's work due to the procedure. Susana often used a tone of voice that sounded judgmental, such as when she suggested that Lucia, "as a mother [to be], should take responsibility" and not take the amniocentesis offer "lightly." She also went out of her way to help Lucia understand her insurance coverage, characteristics all consistent with an authoritative approach.

Distant Approach

The distant label was used for interpreters who communicated information in a detached, mechanical, almost rote manner, devoid of emotional involvement. Seven interpreters used this approach and were the youngest in the sample. All were U.S. born, five, the grandchildren of immigrants. Unlike the others, distant interpreters were often volunteers. All were somewhat satisfied with their work, valuing the chance it offered to be in a medical environment, but all to some degree felt underappreciated by coworkers and clinicians.

Figure 1 shows that those who adopted a distant approach were quite disengaged from patients during most of or the entire encounter; made infrequent eye contact with patients, although somewhat more with clinicians; made infrequent interruptions but provided relatively frequent summaries; and talked in a relatively mechanical manner, not asking personal questions or offering words or gestures of support but using a neutral approach, perhaps built on some sense of "professionalism" (e.g., "It's your decision; the counselor said you may call her if you have questions").

EXAMPLE

Irma, a twenty-one-year-old nursing student—volunteering as a medical assistant—interpreted for Marta, a thirty-year-old in her twenty-third week of pregnancy. Marta's situation on the day she received genetic counseling was greatly complicated by family problems. As the observation began, Irma was mechanically translating a description of the amniocentesis procedure. She intermittently made eye contact with the genetic counselor, but never with Marta.

Marta explained that she thought she wanted the amniocentesis but could not decide because she was preoccupied with a long list of problems, which she proceeded to detail.[4] The most pressing was the need to move from her home the very next day. Irma translated only by summarizing, "She's concerned because she needs to move tomorrow." Seeing Marta's indecision, the counselor left her alone to think things over.

While waiting, Marta told the ethnographer that she wanted the amniocentesis but was not sure she could do it today as the counselor urged. Asked her opinion of the genetic consultation so far, Marta expressed dissatisfaction. She said she was finding it difficult to communicate with the counselor "because she is in a hurry and doesn't speak Spanish" and that the interpreter was "not very helpful" when Marta told her about her living situation. Being preoccupied with immediate problems, she said, made it difficult to decide about amniocentesis. She added, "But the doctor [as she referred to the genetic counselor] didn't say anything. . . . And when she left I asked [the interpreter], 'What do you think?' and she said nothing. . . . I asked, 'And what happens if I have to pack for the move? You said I can't lift heavy things [right after the amniocentesis], what can I do?' And all she said was, 'I don't know, I don't know, you can talk with the counselor later.' Well, I know I can talk with the counselor later, but I was trying to talk to [the interpreter] now!"

Just then, Irma (the interpreter) looked into the room. Marta jumped to her feet, saying, "It's taking too long, and my boys are [home] alone. . . . I can't wait any longer." Irma responded flatly that there were two patients ahead of her. Frustrated, Marta answered, "But they told me she will see me before them," to which Irma mechanically responded, "I don't know," and walked away. At Marta's request, the ethnographer left to see what she could learn about the situation, and when she returned, Marta was gone.

During the interaction between Irma, Marta, and the genetic counselor, Irma seemed impatient and avoided eye contact with Marta. When Marta asked Irma to speed up her wait, Irma left the room rapidly without offering additional help. Irma's approach was to be virtually uninvolved when she repeatedly met Marta's questions and requests with "I don't know," all characteristics of a distant interpretative approach.

Discussion

The overarching question animating the foregoing analysis is a demographic one: how do global processes and micro-level interactions become implicated when immigrants adopt the reproductive practices of their new society? To answer this, I chose to highlight the unacknowledged but extremely important role of informal medical interpreters. A corollary question I considered concerns the place of universal fetal diagnosis in routine prenatal care. Might it create as many, if not more, problems than it solves—and is there even a meaningful calculus to determine this?

In drawing on co-production theory, I focused on the micro-interactions that occurred during clinical encounters in which a group of recent Mexican immigrants were informed that their pregnancy might be defective and offered an amniocentesis to determine whether indeed this was the case. In doing so, I sought to show that a type of actor regarded as all but invisible, in fact, held enormous power. We saw that prenatal genetic counselors generally adhered to their professional mandate of nondirectiveness and neutrality: they successfully resisted patients' efforts to elicit more emotional involvement or greater guidance. But into this void stepped family and on-site interpreters, many of whom brought with them their own agendas as to whether an amniocentesis was in the pregnant women's best interests.

That husbands could have their own agendas when interpreting for their wives might not seem all that surprising, nor that this was also the case when other relatives or friends were enlisted (or volunteered) to serve in the same capacity. More startling was the finding that two of the three on-site interpreter groups also had agendas that extended beyond simple medical interpretation. We saw that the missionaries and authoritatives were staunchly pro-amniocentesis—and pro-biomedical authority in a larger sense—in that they regarded their clinics as benign guardians of patients' interests: if amniocentesis was the standard of care for pregnant women in the United States, they didn't want "their" patients left behind. That in so doing they were helping implement California's state mandate to reduce birth defects through selective abortion was not foremost in their thinking. Instead they considered reassurance—in and of itself—the main purpose of the test.

These findings add depth and nuance to the meanings of choice, agency, and constraint in the context of medical decision making (Ortner 2006, 131–34). That women who were offered amniocentesis through a distant interpreter were significantly less likely to agree to the procedure adds yet another layer to our understanding. And, perhaps ironically, although women assigned distant interpreters reported much lower satisfaction with their interactions than those assigned to the other two groups, those distant and detached interpreters were in fact adhering more closely to the professional standard of medical interpreters, who are trained to be neutral. Moreover, in the end, it was the distant interpreters who inadvertently created the space for women to decide on their own about amniocentesis.

Conclusions

The analytical strength of co-production theory lies in its ability to problematize the most fundamental categories of social science, including macro and micro, and structure and agency (Jasanoff 2004). As such, it provides a potent framework for disentangling the interwoven dynamic processes through which particular social uses of scientific knowledge come to prevail. In this regard, co-production theory opens a window on to how the dialectical nature of globalization processes, in interaction with state policies, is played out in a given social domain, in this case, reproduction.

Global flows of people, technologies, and information are dramatically reshaping everyday experience, including immigrant women's experiences of pregnancy and prenatal care. Although the agonizing burden of decisions about genetic testing and abortion will continue to fall on pregnant women—as, of course, they should—textured ethnographic accounts such as this will help advance our understanding of some of the emergent issues at the nexus of globalization processes, population movements, state demographic agendas, and women's reproductive health.

Appendix A: Observation Instrument

Informant ID # _____   Date of Consultation: ____ - ____ - ____

Site:

Tick One: 1 woman   2 man   3 couple

A. REPRODUCTIVE HISTORY

A.20 PREVIOUS AMNIOCENTESIS

_____   0   no

_____   1   yes

A.21 CHILDREN BORN WITH ANOMALIES?

_____ 0 no

_____ 1 yes; which? _____

A.22 CHILDREN DIED?

_____ 0 no

_____ 1 yes; of what? _____

A.23 FAMILY WITH DISABILITIES?

_____ 0 no

_____ 1 yes: who, which? _____

W. INTERACTION WITH MEDICAL PERSONNEL

W.21 VERBAL INDICATIONS THAT COUNSELOR SEEKS TO ENCOURAGE AMNIOCENTESIS:

_____ 0 "It's logical."

_____ 1 "It reassures you."

_____ 2 "It's your decision, but . . ."

_____ 3 other _____ ; _____

_____ 4 neutral

W.22 PHYSICAL INDICATIONS THAT COUNSELOR SEEKS TO ENCOURAGE AMNIOCENTESIS:

_____ 0 smile

_____ 1 tone of voice; if so, describe _____

_____ 2 other _____ ; _____

_____ 3 neutral

W.23 VERBAL INDICATIONS THAT COUNSELOR SEEKS TO DISCOURAGE AMNIOCENTESIS:

_____ 0 _____

_____ 1 neutral

W.24 PHYSICAL INDICATIONS THAT COUNSELOR SEEKS TO DISCOURAGE AMNIOCENTESIS:

_____ 0 _____

_____ 1 neutral

W.25 COUNSELOR ALLOWED TIME FOR INTEGRATION OF INFORMATION?

_____ 0 no

_____ 1 yes

X. PARTICIPATION IN DECISION MAKING

X.1 WOMAN ASKS COUNSELOR QUESTIONS

_____ 0   no

_____ 1   a little

_____ 2   somewhat

_____ 3   a lot

Specify: _____

X.2 WOMAN APPEARS TO BE ACTIVELY PARTICIPATING IN CONSULTATION

_____ 0   no

_____ 1   a little

_____ 2   somewhat

_____ 3   a lot

Describe: _____

X.3 MAN ASKS COUNSELOR QUESTIONS

_____ 0   no

_____ 1   a little

_____ 2   somewhat

_____ 3   a lot

What? _____

X.4 MAN APPEARS TO BE ACTIVELY PARTICIPATING IN CONSULTATION

_____ 0   no

_____ 1   a little

_____ 2   somewhat

_____ 3   a lot

Describe: _____

X.5 DECISION MADE ON THE SPOT

_____ 0   no

_____ 1   yes

Notes: _____

X.7 DECISION

_____ 0   refuse

_____ 1   accept

_____ 2   undecided

Y.1 DO YOU KNOW WHY YOU CAME?

_____ 0 no

_____ 1 yes

Patient's explanation: _____

Counselor's explanation: _____

Z. SIGNS OF INTENT TO ACCEPT OR DECLINE

Man: _____

Woman: _____

ZZ. INFLUENCE ON EACH OTHER'S DECISION

ZZ.1 MAN TRIES TO INFLUENCE WOMAN

_____ 0 no

_____ 1 tried, didn't succeed

_____ 2 succeeded

ZZ.2 WOMAN TRIES TO INFLUENCE MAN

_____ 0 no

_____ 1 tried, didn't succeed

_____ 2 succeeded

Appendix B: Additional Observation Guidelines for Prenatal Genetic Consultations Involving Interpreters

A. UNDERSTANDING

A1. DID PATIENT ASK QUESTIONS OR MAKE COMMENTS ABOUT THE INFORMATION SHE WAS RECEIVING?

_____Yes _____No _____Somewhat

Explain: _____

A2. DID CLINICIANS ACCURATELY ANSWER QUESTIONS WITHOUT MISINTERPRETATION INTRODUCED BY INTERPRETER?

_____No questions

_____Yes _____No _____Somewhat

Explain: _____

B1. DESCRIBE BROAD DYNAMICS OF GENETIC CONSULTATION:

_____

B2. BASES FOR ASSESSMENT:

_____

Appendix C: Most Frequently Observed Interpreter Behaviors

Observation ID: _____ Mark each behavior observed

1. Engages with patient in friendly manner.*
2. Engages with patient in judgmental manner.*
3. Makes frequent eye contact with patient.
4. Makes infrequent eye contact with patient, more frequent with clinician.*
5. Listens without interrupting.
6. Interrupts patient often.*
7. Does not interrupt patient but summarizes interpretation.*
8. Offers help (*favorcitos*) (e.g., making a phone call).*
9. Uses relaxed and warm tone.
10. Talks fast and looks irritated or annoyed.
11. Talks mechanically.*
12. Asks casually informal questions (e.g., "Do you live nearby?").
13. Asks personal questions in a challenging or critical manner.*
14. Gives emotional support.
15. Gives support in a defiant manner.
16. Makes directive, "personalistic" comments (e.g., "I wouldn't offer you something I wouldn't consider for myself").
17. Makes directive comments (e.g., "Don't pay attention to what [your sister] says [about amniocentesis]; people don't know. Doctors know; the genetic counselor knows").
18. Makes distant or detached comments ("It's your decision; the counselor said you may call her if you have questions").*
19. Goes in and out of interpreter role (when alone with patient acts like the genetic counselor).
* = varied significantly among groups.

Notes

The research was funded by NIH-NCHGR, the Russell Sage Foundation, UC-MEXUS, and the UCLA Centers for the Study of Women and for Culture and Health. Throughout our long collaboration, Dr. H. Mabel Preloran has been a constant source of guidance, patience, and wisdom; no words can sufficiently convey my gratitude. Maria Christina Casado, Irma Herrera, Carolina Izquierdo, Nancy Monterrosa, Jesus Montoya, Jeffrey McNairy, and Ricardo Rivera helped with data collection, and Casado, Monterrosa, and Rivera assisted with data analyses. Richard M. Rosenthal helped clarify and strengthen the arguments. Some data were published in a different form in Preloran, Browner, and Lieber 2005 and in Browner et al. 2003.

1. All but two amnioceteses were negative; both women with positive amnioceteses aborted their pregnancies. Level 2 ultrasounds of two women who refused amniocentesis indicated the likelihood of problems. One miscarried, and the other bore a baby with multiple anomalies.

2. The triple screen test, also known as the triple test, multiple marker screening, and AFP, plus looks for specific substances (AFP, hCG, and Estriol) in the maternal blood. The results are analyzed in conjunction with a number of other factors (e.g., age, ethnicity) to estimate the likelihood of a fetal abnormality. These tests are not diagnostic but rather signal the need for further testing.

3. Pseudonyms are used throughout.

4. Rapp (2000) shows that an amniocentesis offer can have extremely low salience for many women chronically facing many more immediate sources of life stress.

Reproductive Rights in No-Woman's-Land

Politics and Humanitarian Assistance

In 1999, the volcano that looms over Baños, the jewel of a tourist town nestled between the Andean peaks and the river that leads to the Amazon, began to explode. Soon the eruptions of steam and gas were replaced by expulsions of burning rocks and boulders. The authorities predicted an explosion of lava, lahars, and the potential destruction of the town and its inhabitants. The Ecuadorian government ordered a complete evacuation of the town and the surrounding communities. Two months later, while the community was still evacuated, a colleague and I (Whiteford) began a six-year project of analyzing the consequences of the volcanic eruption and the ensuing political activities on the lives and health of those evacuated, displaced, and dispossessed. This chapter takes the reproductive experiences of women like those displaced in Ecuador as the starting place to analyze how ideology, history, and tradition conspire to create arenas of constraint in which women's agency is redefined in liminal statelessness. Here we (Whiteford and Eden) investigate the role of global forces as they are played out on a stage where the authority of the state is nebulous at best and, at its worst, absent. The analysis of this failure to provide the most elementary and critical protection and care for women who are stateless and whose survival depends at least partly on global assistance led us to a chain of influence, ideology, and politics.

We see anthropology as providing the methods and theories to deconstruct and demystify the complex forces that render women invisible or, worse, visible but unimportant. We ask why women refugees have been allowed to be raped and discarded while in the care of humanitarian agencies, and why the knowledge of this fails to produce outrage. To answer these questions, we have drawn on our own research and the research of others. We have conducted interviews with policymakers and providers, shelter givers, and those being sheltered. Using a critical medical anthropological perspective, we have privileged political and economic data as pivotal to our understandings, but our analysis is also shaped by the words of women as they describe their experiences and actions. In this chapter we examine the local reality of being displaced, the multinational reality of provisioning, and the national and global challenge to provide reproductive healthcare to women who need humanitarian aid. Sadly enough, our chosen topic—the reproductive health and rights of women in shelters and camps— tragically demonstrates how displaced women are caught in the global vortex of ideological blackmail.

The Local Reality

The Ecuador study that stimulated our research was conducted by a geographer (Graham Tobin) and one of the authors of this chapter (Whiteford), a medical anthropologist. In the course of that research, we studied people living in shelters: those who were relocated and those who, in time, returned to live in the shadow of Mount Tungurahua. Over six years we conducted 697 interviews, sixteen focus groups, countless interviews with political and civic leaders, and months of observations (Whiteford and Tobin 2002, 2004).

We asked women about their responses to their experience of being evacuated, living away from their community, and what effect it had on them. Earlier research in reproductive health (e.g., Whiteford and Manderson 2000; Whiteford and Poland 1989) stimulated questions about women's reproductive experiences and how displacement affected them. Several women said they delayed having children. One woman said that before the explosions and evacuations, she and her husband had planned to have a third child. But when they were evacuated and had to live with her mother, a sister, and her brother and his family, they reassessed having another child. Under stressful conditions, it is not uncommon for women to become amenorrhetic and cease menstruating, worrying them about their ability to conceive in the future.

In 2006 the volcano again erupted, destroying communities as pyroclastic flows rolled down the flanks of the volcano, consuming everything in their path—livestock, homes, gardens, fields, pets, and people. Within hours of the destruction, we interviewed families in shelters. The shelters were quite minimally adequate, located in schools, churches, and abandoned buildings. Few had any privacy; families lived with only curtains separating them from the next family, or with no physical separation at all. Some of the larger shelters had weekly access to a nurse, but there was no reproductive health (RH) care provided. The failure to provide for women's RH in Ecuador stimulated questions about women's experiences in shelters elsewhere and whether they were also were denied reproductive care.

Clearly, women's need for contraceptive or other types of reproductive care does not cease when they become displaced. The Ecuador shelter research presented a microcosmic view of what women around the world experience during and following disasters or complex emergencies when they are removed from their extended families and support networks, removed from their sources of income, and placed in shelters where gender roles—of the administrators as well as of the displaced women themselves— may remove them from access to decision making or resource distribution.

Women as Internally Displaced People and Refugees: The Global Reality

Who are these women, and why do they need our attention? The 1951 United Nations Convention's definition of a refugee as a person who "owing to a well-founded fear of being persecuted for reasons of race, religion, nationality, membership of a particular social group or political opinion is outside the country of his nationality" and cannot return to it is still in use today (UNHCR 2005). Internally displaced persons (IDPS) were defined formally in the *Guiding Principles on Internal Displacement* in 1992 as persons forced or obliged to flee, "in particular as a result of or in order to avoid the effects of armed conflict, situations of generalised violence, violations of human rights or natural or human-made disasters, and who have not crossed an internationally recognized State border" (IDMC 2006). While the term *refugee* enjoys its status as a legal definition offering protection, the definition of IDP does not offer the same legal protection. Despite these differences, in this chapter we use these terms interchangeably.

According to the U.S. Committee for Refugees and Immigrants, there were approximately 32.8 million refugees and IDPS in the world in 2004 (USCRI 2005), with women of reproductive age (15–49 years) making up an estimated 20 percent of refugees and IDPS who, along with children, are the most vulnerable because they are separated from their support systems and their families (Hynes et al. 2002, 595). These women and girls face many RH risks, such as sexual violence, HIV/AIDS and other sexually transmitted infections, unwanted and high-risk pregnancies, and unsafe abortions (Krause 2004).

Displaced women are marginalized from power structures that may have protected them. Forced to move by environmental factors (famine, hurricanes, floods, volcanic eruptions), development displacement (resettlement due to dam construction), civil wars, and other complex emergencies (Bosnia, the Sudan), women too often are moved into a "no-woman's-land" without protection. Moreover, the rights of displaced women to RH shift with changing global politics; however, their physical needs do not change just because they are displaced. Regardless of shifts in global powers, women need protection from sexual violence and from sexually transmitted infections, and they need access to prenatal care and pregnancy termination.

Despite widespread reports of women and girls being raped as they leave refugee camps in search of firewood or other items critical for survival, little psychological or physical attention is provided for violated women. Here we ask why humanitarian agencies responsible for protecting these women are unable to protect them, and why, when these women are violated, they are not treated. The crimes are known and acknowledged, but why are women not at least provided emergency contraception (EC) and offered safe pregnancy terminations? Even in the best of circumstances, life in camps and shelters is traumatic, and every pregnancy puts the woman at increased risk of malnutrition, infections, and exhaustion. We believe that all women, but particularly those displaced through war and disasters, should be provided access to RH care, including EC and abortion. To understand some of the reasons why this inhumane treatment occurs, we need to situate our questions in the context of global politics, flows of power, wealth, and history.

Reproductive Care for Women Refugees: Multinational Reality

It was not until the mid-1980s that women refugees began to receive attention as needing protection while under protective care. While women were not deliberately marginalized, camps are most often administered by men, governing councils often consist exclusively of men, and leadership roles in the camps are mostly occupied by men. In addition, the daily activities of women that put them at risk were unacknowledged, and many UNHCR staff members believed that rape and sexual violence were "regrettable side effects" of complex emergencies, an "inevitable incident" in refugee life

(Berthiaume 1995). We believe that such "side effects" and "regrettable incidents" are not inevitable, but are abuses of human rights.

The history of RH services in emergency situations extends back only to 1992, when Marie Stopes International (MSI) developed the first reproductive health kits during the Bosnian crisis. In 1994 the Women's Commission for Refugee Women and Children published the seminal report *Refugee Women and Reproductive Health Care: Reassessing Priorities* based on first-hand research on RH needs among refugee women in six camps and with internally displaced women in two countries (Schreck 2000). Since then, UNFPA, UNHCR, WHO, the Inter-Agency Working Group on Reproductive Health in Refugee Situations (IAWG), and the Reproductive Health Response in Conflict (RHRC) have worked to establish new RH policies and practices during and following emergencies. Despite this growing attention, little change has occurred in the last decade to protect and provide for refugee women.

Reproductive Health in Refugee Situations: An Inter-agency Field Manual is considered the most comprehensive and in-depth document guiding RH in emergency situations, but it fails to provide explicit guidance on politically contentious issues such as abortion and the use of emergency contraception —two elements critical to RH. And providers are difficult to find, so services are not provided (Schreck 2000). UNFPA also offers a set of prepackaged RH kits for crisis situations, but because they must be purchased with the agency's own funds, doing so may disqualify the agency for aid from the United States (as of 2008).

Despite the general international human rights treaties, humanitarian law, and the more specific refugee law established in the 1951 United Nations Convention relating to the Status of Refugees, the agencies and organizations that are primarily responsible for providing refugees with RH services often simply do not comply with them. The UNHCR encourages its partner NGOs to provide RH services during emergencies, but does not require them to do so, and does not offer recommendations on how to resolve the problem of the religious or ideological barriers to providing RH to the women they serve.

The National Becomes Global: U.S. Resistance
to Women's Reproductive Rights

Regardless of the global recognition of the raping of displaced women, women in conflict-affected settings still do not have access to comprehensive

RH services. What services are available to them depends on a variety of interrelated factors such as "which agency services them, whether they are in a camp or non-camp setting, whether they are refugees or internally displaced. Their care also depends on the donors who fund services in their area, and on the geopolitical importance of the conflict that has uprooted their lives" (McGinn and Purdin 2004, 237; Whiteford 2009). In short, while rape may be "an unavoidable element of camp life," comprehensive reproductive care is not.

In places such as Bosnia, Darfur, the Democratic Republic of Congo (DRC), and increasingly in other parts of the world, rape is not simply a consequence of conflict or "undisciplined troops" but is a tool of that conflict. Often the very protectors are unable or unwilling to intercede when women and girls are raped. The rapist rapes with impunity, and the camps insufficiently provide either protection or prevention for women and girls in their care. A Masalit woman from Darfur told Amnesty International in Chad that "the AU [African Union Mission in Sudan, AMIS] is not interested in the displaced. . . . When girls are raped in the neighbourhood of the camp, the AU's only action is to bring the girl back to the camp. They do not carry out any investigation into the event" (Amnesty International 2006).

How can we understand why this is allowed to happen? Policy is not politically or ideologically neutral. Despite significant strides in terms of the international provision of RH, progress is constantly threatened by politics and globally powerful ideologies (Krause 2004). To understand this process, we turn our attention to the recent history of U.S. foreign policy and the influence of private interests such as the Christian Right.

The U.S. government's role in global RH programs is not recent; the overtly negative impacts of U.S. policies extend back at least thirty-five years, when Jesse Helms authored the 1973 Helms Amendment prohibiting the spending of federal money on abortions outside the United States. In 1984, President Reagan presented the Mexico City policy, known as the "global gag rule" by its opponents. The effect of the rule, which pulled USAID funding from nongovernmental organizations that used funds, even from other sources, to address abortion (including counseling, referrals, and lobbying), was to effectively undermine international reproductive health policies. Opposing the policy, President Clinton reversed it on his first day in office in 1993, and George W. Bush reinstated the policy almost immediately after taking office in 2001. Later in his administration, Bush extended the policy to prohibit the Department of State from funding NGOS overseas that even discussed abortion as an RH issue. Bush's actions expanding this global family planning policy represented "a disturbing example of a conservative moral export that has become ever more problematic, contributing to both HIV infections and deteriorating women's health" (Wildman 2004).

Indeed, it appears that "whatever funding streams it is attached to, the gag rule forces indigenous NGOS providing RH care to the world's poorest women to make a terrible choice: sacrifice their ability to provide legal abortion-related services in their own country and their ability to advocate to stem the public health crisis of unsafe, clandestine abortion throughout the developing world, or sacrifice their eligibility for U.S. funding to provide desperately needed family planning services" (S. Cohen 2003, 3). But not only indigenous NGOS were affected; the impact on U.S. organizations and the consequent impact on refugee RH have been far-reaching. Because the policy required U.S. agencies to investigate their partner organizations in the field, critical healthcare programs proven to reduce rates of maternal and child mortality were delayed or terminated (Sandbaek 2004). President Obama rescinded the ban in his first month in office in 2009, but the funding lost by the International Planned Parenthood Federation alone over the eight years of the Bush administration could have prevented an estimated 36 million unplanned pregnancies and 15 million abortions globally (IPPF 2009).

Specifically targeting refugee populations, the Bush administration withdrew an offer of $650,000 to RHRC, funds that were earmarked for an initiative addressing HIV/AIDS and the RH of youth in conflict-affected areas of the world. Based on unsubstantiated accusations of involvement in forced abortions and involuntary sterilizations in China, the Bush administration also denied funding to MSI, a Consortium member organization. The Consortium decided not to accept any further U.S. funding, noting that "allowing the Administration's decision 'to remain undisputed,' would be more harmful in the long term to refugee populations than actually losing the funding" (Brocato 2003, 3).

At the same time as the Bush administration cut funding from comprehensive RH initiatives, it increased funding for foreign abstinence-only-until-marriage programs, including the Global AIDS Bill (Brocato 2003). The failure of such U.S. foreign policies to consider the realities of refugee women's lives (which might involve not only rape but sex for resources, coerced sex, etc.) makes the implementation of abstinence-only programs dangerous and unethical. President Bush, for instance, appointed the inexperienced and politically conservative politician Ellen Sauerbrey as assistant secretary of state for the Bureau of Population, Refugees, and Migration while Congress was in recess in January 2006. Many stakeholders, including advocates and relief workers in the refugee community, opposed Sauerbrey's nomination to a department responsible for formulating the U.S. response to global refugee crises, concerned that her opposition to sex education and sexual health services would negatively affect millions of refugees (SIECUS 2006).

The influence of the Christian Right on global public health policies increased with Bush's "faith-based initiative," which allowed religious groups to receive federal grants while exempting them from civil rights statutes. The controversial initiative's impact on foreign public health assistance has not yet fully been documented, but implications for global RH are clear: the *Boston Globe* reported that the percentage of USAID dollars allocated to faith-based groups had doubled by 2005. In addition, of the over $2 billion of federal money provided to religious groups, the Bush administration gave 98 percent of the faith-based foreign-aid money to exclusively Christian groups (Stockman, Kranish, and Canellos 2006). The Global AIDS Bill allows faith-based groups who receive funds to exclude information about contraceptive methods, including condoms, if such information is not consistent with their religious teachings. While the Bush administration gave faith-based organizations the power to determine their approach to RH services through the bill, with the global gag rule it simultaneously stripped the NGOs that provide a variety of family planning options of the ability to freely provide such information and services if they wished to continue receiving U.S. funding.

Because the Christian Right and other pro-life organizations shape conservative policies for RH access and options for women around the world, it is important to understand how these groups frame the issue and the ways in which they affect policy. They have been diligent in making public their argument that the right to life is a basic human right, so that RH (since it includes access to abortion and other forms of contraception) *cannot* be considered a basic human right. To position themselves to promote a "culture of life" globally, pro-life groups are highly vocal critics of the UN and UNICEF in particular for incorporating RH into its missions. The American Life League stated in an online article titled "The Truth about UNICEF" that while monetary contributions to UNICEF "may help to provide food, clothing, medicine or the like, chances are they may also go toward various forms of birth control, abortion and sterilization. . . . 'UNICEF is pro-abortion. They don't want poor children coming into the world.' UNICEF, as originally established, no longer exists. Indeed, UNICEF is no friend of children" (Tignor 2005). These are powerful and misleading statements.

Not only U.S.-based Christian groups attempt to impact global RH policies. The Vatican has also used its political influence to discourage abortion and, by extension, to affect refugee RH. In 1996 the Vatican suspended its annual symbolic support to UNICEF largely because of the organization's backing of the *Inter-agency Field Manual* (UNFPA 1999), which supports the RH rights of women and specifically addresses the needs of women who are victims of rape as an instrument of war (Crossette 1996; S. Cohen 1998). In 2000 the Vatican opposed the use of so-called morning-after pill emergency contraception for rape victims in Kosovo refugee camps (Eckstrom 2000).

Too often, the globalization of health policies results in a poor fit with culturally determined local needs. Certainly, global policies should make available variations in local practice in recognition of local needs and local contexts. To do that, a range of services needs to be derived from overarching global policies. The local context of women and girls being routinely raped while in the "protection" of humanitarian agencies would suggest that something is terribly wrong. Likewise, failure to provide the option of emergency contraception or abortion places women's and girls' lives at grave risk during pregnancy and birth.

Hiding the Problem: Multinational and Women's Responses

As we try to unravel the reasons for the failure to provide RH to refugee women, and seek to expose the underlying fabric of deceit and denial, confounding issues—methodological, conceptual, and theoretical—become evident. Simply locating accurate global estimates of the number of refugees presents one such challenge. According to the U.S. Committee for Refugees and Immigrants, there were approximately 32.8 million refugees and internally displaced persons in the world in 2005 (USCRI 2005). However, the UNHCR reported 19.2 million refugees, asylum seekers, and IDPs at the end of 2004. Discrepancies in the number of refugees often stem from the difficulties in measuring such a population but also are a result of politics. "Politics impinge upon the collection of comprehensive, reliable and up-to-date statistical data on refugees and other groups of displaced people . . . in many different ways and at many different levels of the international refugee regime" (Crisp 1999, 8). In addition to global and national politics, people refuse to report their movements to the very authorities they wish to escape. This is a fluid population with many reasons for hiding: individuals and families may move out of fear of the authorities or out of the perception that conditions might be better elsewhere, or that other refugees in a camp have opposition ties. Not only are absolute numbers difficult to locate, but they sometimes change according to whose interest is being protected. In addition to host country and UNHCR interests, other stakeholders have varying (and sometimes competing) interests, including the different humanitarian agencies (with varying objectives) and the countries from which refugees are fleeing.

Locating accurate numbers is but one of the many problems researchers encounter. Women are active players, and their agency must also be taken into account. They do not choose to be displaced, forced into camps, or excluded from externally administered decision making. Within the contexts available to them, however, they do make decisions about their lives and the options available to them. Hammond describes conflicting viewpoints of refugee displacement: the first considers displacement as deculturing and the displaced as "helpless or dependent on the assistance external actors"; the second "insists that migrants never lose their agency entirely, but must learn to adapt it to their rapidly changing circumstances" (Hammond 2004, 211). Doug Henry, an anthropologist who found himself living in one of the Sierra Leone camps, presents data that movingly describe how women in camps choose to maximize their access to whatever resources may be available (personal communication, 2006).

Earlier we described women as the most vulnerable of refugees. However, social science thinking on "women as passive and vulnerable" has evolved. In the 1990s, much of the social science literature on displaced women presented them as victims. For example, Lipson and Omidian (1996, 6) observed that women are particularly vulnerable to human rights abuses, "especially in cultures in which women must rely on male family members for protection. In the process of flight, families may be separated, and unaccompanied women are at special risk for rape, kidnapping and murder."

This is not untrue, but it frames women as not being active decision makers in their own lives. While this framing of "women as vulnerable" has appealed to humanitarians, and so "was likely a convincing factor in pushing forward a policy on refugee women . . . it also reinforced the passivity and voiceless-ness of refugee women, in addition to silencing the contestations over the root causes of displacement. . . . Focus on the cultural sources of gender persecution masks global and national political, economic and intersecting socio-cultural (such as disability, religion, ethnicity, and sexuality) factors that lead to displacement" (Baines 2004, 38). In her analysis of domestic violence in refugee camps, Carlson (2005) points out that in an African context, humanitarian organizations often view the individual to be acting largely under the influence of tradition and cultural norms, placing less emphasis on the individual's agency. Ethnographic research in Sri Lanka conducted by Rajasingham-Senanayake (2004) uncovers the new roles that women, displaced and affected by the war, perform in their everyday activities, particularly within the changing family and community structures generated by conflict and displacement.

Unraveling the Fabric: Local, National, and Global Threads

How can anthropological research, theory, and methods contribute to furthering the provision of RH services, particularly emergency contraception and abortions, to refugee and internally displaced women in need? How do we connect the global with the local to replace the "fantasy" plans with real provision of services (Whiteford and Manderson 2000)? As Sargent and Browner (2005, 5) have noted, "Anthropological studies of reproduction are particularly rich for exploring articulations between global processes and state policies, and how these are experienced at the individual, household and community levels." In the context of complex humanitarian and other emergencies, where global forces in the form of assistance are nearly always involved, anthropological studies of RH are glaringly absent. While they acknowledge the methodological challenges involved in such research, Sargent and Browner contend that "grounded ethnographic research . . . offers a powerful means to analyze the intersection between the local and global, and to see how the personal, state and transnational interact to shape reproductive behaviors" (5).

Because RH services and technology provided by Western humanitarian aid are often foreign and unfamiliar to the recipients, and because the concept of RH itself is culturally constructed, anthropology can help monitor the progress of global RH programs from a cultural context and clarify the link between the global and the local (Obermeyer 1999). In our review of the anthropological literature, we found a void in research on refugee RH and were struck by the erasure of women even while focusing on them and advocating for them. One way anthropological research can help is by allowing women to speak for themselves, but hearing women's voices and understanding the cultural context is not always easy: "Women will not tell you easily if such a thing happens to them. In our culture, it is a shame, and women will hide this in their hearts so that the men do not hear about it," one female refugee in Chad told Amnesty International in 2003 (Amnesty International 2006).

Also absent were the voices of policy and decision makers. Research like Judith Justice's work on USAID's Child Survival programs demonstrate how anthropological research can bring both those most directly affected and those making the decisions that affect them into the discussion. In our (Whiteford) own work among IDPs, we found that decision makers did not know how to listen to (or perhaps hear) issues that were thought of as women's issues. Reproductive health is certainly thought of as a women's issue, thus perhaps making it easier to dismiss. We argue, however, that the provision of RH is a social issue that underlies the health of the society, since it reflects the health of families. To help policymakers "hear" the most marginalized populations— stateless women—and to address needs that are perceived as theirs alone, we must reframe the issue. Careful ethnographic documentation of both the policymakers and the refugee/IDP women is necessary for that reframing.

Besides the logistical and financial difficulties in providing RH services to refugees, "sociocultural issues can be especially problematic [due to the] status of women, cultural or religious reticence to address reproductive issues, and the intimate nature of reproductive beliefs and practices" (Bartlett, Purdin, and McGinn 2004, 77). Refugee camps and IDP relocation centers are not composed of homogeneous groups of people who share the same cultural beliefs and behaviors. Anthropological analysis of humanitarian aid and its policies, practices, and means of distribution may help broker new communication and provision plans based on perceived similarities rather than the perceived difference.

Anthropologists also need to address the confusing and contested convergence of "cultural relativity" and "universal human rights." Reproductive health, including access to emergency contraception and safe abortion, cannot be both a universal human right and one dependent on local customs and norms. Anthropologists can help policymakers and practitioners understand how to respect cultural variation and diversity while simultaneously respecting the rights of individuals and groups within that culture.

Our last suggestion is for more anthropological research on policy development and application to make clear how ideologies, motives, and political reciprocities underlie the provision of RH—or the failure thereof—penalize vulnerable and marginalized displaced women.

Humanitarian Camps: No-Woman's-Land

Women seeking shelter in IPD and refugee camps are not the only ones violated by the failure to protect them. Women and girls are damaged, but so are men and families who are destroyed because women are forced into a place where no woman should be. Anthropological research can do more than connect the dots in what appears to be a global conspiracy to deny women their voice in reproductive rights. It can provide the larger context in which these decisions to deny are made. It can document the consequences to women and their families of these policies, and it can provide data that humanitarian agencies may use to combat the ideological blackmail that the U.S. government has used on the most vulnerable women during their most vulnerable times.

In this chapter, we have tried to unravel some of the forces that create a no-woman's-land: a place where no woman should be, and yet where women constitute more than 50 percent of the population; a place where a woman's physiological sexual identity marks her as a target for sexual abuse, and yet a place where gender renders her invisible in accessing formal help and resources; and finally a place where political and cultural ideologies erase her rights. We have tried to explain how the organizations originally designed to assist refugees are overwhelmed and understaffed, how they must depend on the vagaries of public opinion for much of their funding, and how the debate in the United States over a woman's right to control her own reproduction is played out on the global stage to the cruel detriment of those most in need.

Anthropological theories and methods allowed us to conceptualize how women in Bosnia and in the DRC share more than they do not, and how their status as women becomes the primary identifying variable as they come into the care of humanitarian organizations. They, as women, give our analysis a starting place from which we scale up from the individual to the family and gender dyads that are critical to the analysis of rape as a weapon, to community lost in conflict, to the shelter of international humanitarian care, and finally to the global political arena where women who have no other choice are denied the right to control their own reproduction. In this complex array of forces, we have tried to show not only the effect of scale but also the mutuality of reinforcing policies and practices shaped by gender roles, cultural expectations and status, statelessness, and international policies as they limit, but never destroy, a woman's agency.

The Mystery Child and the Politics of Reproduction

Between National Imaginaries and Transnational Confrontations

In the midst of an eventless and sunless summer, desperately lacking global tragedies or presidential love affairs, the French were nonetheless captivated by a highly mediatized newspaper saga that journalists quickly titled "The Mystery Child from Marseille."[1] At first the story seemed trivial: a two-and-a-half-year-old boy from a northern suburb of Marseille—a predominantly working-class, immigrant (mostly North African) neighborhood—was found left alone on a playground. After he was brought to the local police station, people started wondering why no one would come to claim him, let alone why nobody in the neighborhood seemed even to know who he was. For a few days, the investigation made no headway. The child was placed in foster care. Both the newspaper and TV media called for witnesses, broadcasting a picture of the child, terrorized and screaming, surrounded by police officers. Finally, after a two-week wait, the mystery was solved. An Algerian woman named Fatma came to the police station to claim the child. Aged thirty-four, Fatma had come to France twelve years earlier to join her husband, from whom she had since separated. Residing in France legally, she had been raising her five children on her own. She explained that she had left for Algeria hurriedly to visit her seriously ill mother. She could take only her four older children with her because the youngest one did not yet have a passport. She thus entrusted the infant to a young woman she knew and paid, and whom she regularly called from Algeria to check on her son. Alerted by a phone call from one of her cousins, who had seen the pictures of the child in the media, Fatma immediately contacted the police and flew back to France. Upon her arrival, child protective services took her four other children away, and she was extensively interrogated by the police. The investigators had discovered something that Fatma, according to her testimony, was unaware of: the baby sitter, although married to a French citizen, had no documents; this is why she had not presented herself to the police station after the child momentarily disappeared from view at the playground. Accused both of encouraging illegal residence by hiring the young woman and of acting irresponsibly toward her child, Fatma was held in police custody. When she was eventually allowed to return home, only her four older children were given back to her: Mohamed, her youngest son, whom she could only embrace for a few seconds in court, was again placed in foster care by child protective services, until it could be determined that Fatma was, in the words of the state prosecutor, "able to properly care for her child." As the case appeared close to resolution, media interest slowly died.

Ten days later, however, drama suddenly resurfaced. DNA tests collected from Mohamed and Fatma showed that they were not biologically related (conversely, Fatma's four other children, who had also been tested, were genetically "authenticated"). The local court immediately ordered further investigation of the mother for "child substitution," an offense carrying a three-year jail sentence and a fine of seven thousand euros. The media unleashed accusatory comments against the defendant, depicting her as a "fake mother," judging her as "predisposed to dissimulation," even going as far as evoking "child trafficking."[2] Accusations poured among bloggers on the newspaper website: it was claimed, for example, that this story perfectly illustrated how immigrants came to France to exploit the benefits of welfare; the deportation of Fatma and her children back to their country of origin was called for to make an example against other potential cheats; the imposition of DNA tests verifying blood relations for all immigrants and their children was also requested. It is important to note here that fathers' responsibilities were never alluded to. Their absence from Fatma's life and her children's was paralleled by their absence in public space.

In contrast to the frenzy displayed by the media, justice, and public opinion, the facts, as they progressively took shape, were quite simple. During one of her trips back home, Fatma had heard of a young woman among her acquaintances who had just had a child and had decided to abandon him. Algerian law, like other legal systems in North Africa, does not recognize adoption but authorizes a type of extended guardianship called *kefala*. According to this legal procedure, although the adopting parent is expected to raise the child, the child cannot be given the parent's family name, nor can he or she receive family inheritance. In an effort to comply with the legal system of children's country of origin, French law does not allow kefala to be transformed into adoption. With this knowledge, let us return to Fatma's story.

As she explained, adopting the child was an opportunity for her to fulfill her desire to give her only son a little brother. This is why she took the child with her to France. But considering the status of kefala under French law, she did not register the child as her own—which, incidentally, prevented her from receiving any social benefits on his behalf, despite the suspicions publicly voiced on that subject. The judge, however, remained oblivious to the situation: setting aside the emotional ties between Fatma and the child, he presented the Algerian state with letters rogatory in an attempt to find Mohamed's biological parents. From then on, Fatma was threatened with a severe jail sentence, and Mohamed was likely to remain in foster care.

Fatma's story is significant from several perspectives. I will, however, circumscribe its relevance to the national imaginary on biological reproduction on the one hand, and to the transnational confrontation between different, at times incompatible, paradigms of reproduction on the other. The national-transnational opposition I am referring to differs from the local-global opposition recurrent throughout this volume. The national-transnational dualism specifically highlights the deeply rooted historical and political dimension of representations and practices surrounding reproduction. In that respect, far from leading to some sort of fluidity, as it is often argued, globalization also tends to consolidate territories, borders, and differences, at both the geographic and ideological levels.[3] Consequently, the national must be apprehended as what is left of a world past and simultaneously transformed, and the transnational must be understood in terms of circulations, but also in terms of confrontations.

The French narrative on reproduction was construed at once on the basis of an outspoken pronatalism (especially since the end of the nineteenth century, as the aging of the population became a permanent, at times obsessive, concern) and on an implicit racial ideal (beyond the racist theories of the nineteenth century, it meant a specific image of the nation at the cultural and biological levels).[4] Hence the ambivalence displayed toward immigrant families as they quantitatively fulfill France's pronatalist desire while qualitatively departing from its racial ideal of the nation. The urban riots in the fall of 2005 shed light on this tension, notably through the discourse of conservative politicians and intellectuals, who interpreted this revolt of the youth—French citizens of African origin in majority—as precisely the consequence of their parents' marriage and reproductive practices, mixing moral judgments with biological explanations and cultural discourses, especially on polygamy.[5] For several decades already, this ambivalence toward the reproductive potential of immigration had translated into increasingly severe immigration control policies. Having initially interrupted labor migration (primarily involving men) in 1974 while sustaining settlement migration (mostly concerning women and children), such policies had made family reunification increasingly difficult after 1984 (thereby reducing the demographic contribution of immigrants to the nation). The fear of otherness had thus finally superseded the fear of depopulation.

We must situate Fatma's story in this context. Raising five children on her own, with only meager resources (from social welfare and part-time jobs), this young woman could have inspired, if not the nation's gratitude,[6] at least admiration for her courage or compassion for her hardships. Instead, every comment about her related back to the often-portrayed image of "undeserving mothers" from the working classes, stigmatized by society and eventually losing their children's custody to social services. Such phenomena have even inspired a series of socially inspired films, from D. W. Griffith's *Intolerance* to Ken Loach's *Ladybird*. Thus the media highlighted the fact that her four children were born from "different fathers" (there were two fathers, to be precise, but the phrasing suggests there could be as many as there are children), evoked the "possibility that welfare support was illegally claimed" (though the adopted little boy was not even registered and therefore known to social services), assessed the mother's intention to "cheat the administration" (when the prefecture's services themselves prevented Mohamed from being legally registered), and asserted evidence that "everything in this case is related to the issue of illegal residence" (although Fatma held a residence permit along with her four children and claimed to be unaware that the baby sitter did not). In the end, Fatma was acknowledged only as a "fake mother" (even references to her as an "adoptive mother" were put in quotation marks). Comments posted on blogs oscillated between xenophobic indignation ("one more who had her little nephew sent from his village to be naturalized in France") and racist irony ("over there, people pass children around, and here's the result"). Never was it suggested that this mother only intended, as she said she did, to adopt a child who was going to be abandoned, that she conformed to Algerian law in taking him in, and that she ran into difficulties with the French administration as she tried to regularize the situation.

Each year, thousands of French citizens have a similar experience as they travel abroad to try to adopt a child, at times by means of extralegal procedures. In their case, adoption is considered an act of love. In Fatma's case, however, bad faith, self-interest, and duplicity were suspected.[7] These contrasted assessments may be considered a sort of moral discrimination. They imply means of disqualifying the mother not only based on her past but also in anticipation of her children's future: by being stigmatized, immigrant mothers thus become dangerous.[8] Besides, by provoking a form of legal (Mohamed) and social (Fatma) exclusion, the political interpretation of such a situation can become performative by actually shaping children's future marginalization, thus producing what is denounced. But the comparison with French adoptive parents unveils a broader perspective on the underlying logics at work here.

The transnational confrontation of the politics of reproduction brings together distinct and even contradictory paradigms. National traditions, far from solving their differences through strategies of reciprocal influence or through subtle negotiations enabling them to harmonize practices between countries, can sometimes result in strengthening oppositions. Yet it is in the differential treatment of the people submitted to these transnational movements that contradictions emerge most violently. On the French side exists a plenary adoption procedure, inherited from Roman law, which secures the adopted child with the same prerogatives as a biological child's, including inheritance. This means, in the legal sense, that family is defined not by blood ties but by social and affective ties. On the Algerian side there is no adoption procedure, in accordance with Islamic law, but there are established ways to care for abandoned children, most of them born out of wedlock, notably in the context of kefala. This means, in the legal sense, that the definition of family rests strictly on biological filiation. The two legal systems thus seem incompatible. For French parents living in North Africa who take in a child following the kefala and go back to live in France, there is no possible means of transforming this guardianship status into legal adoption. A law was thus recently prepared with the aim of authorizing adoption in such cases, to protect the child's rights. It was presented to the Senate on February 21, 2007, but was never put to the vote of its members. In accordance with current French legislation and with the Hague Convention signed by France on May 29, 1993, it is the country of origin that imposes its system of filiation and, in this case, the preeminence of biological ties over social ties. In Fatma's case, the paradox lies in the fact that, in spite of its more generous tradition when it comes to its citizens, France requires biological authentication and refuses official guardianship. While, for French parents, the administration recognizes kefala, and legislators even consider transforming it into simple adoption, the young Algerian woman must be subjected to DNA testing. For the French, the state searches for a liberal interpretation of Muslim law; for Fatma, the Republic acts more Muslim than Islam itself.

Rather than a mere confrontation of national paradigms on reproduction (the biological model in Muslim law versus the elective model in Roman law), this analysis thus reveals an inequality of application in the transnational politics of reproduction (biological model for foreigners versus elective model for the French). The latter evidence (inequality of application) somehow supersedes the former (confrontation of paradigms). Indeed, while attempts are made to find arrangements for the incompatibility of paradigms, through legislation, the discrimination of treatments is only consolidated, even legitimized, by the same legal system. It would be wrong, however, to limit this observation to Fatma's story only and make it an anecdotal or exceptional case. Her story is part of a broader context. "Long live DNA testing," read an enthusiastic comment on a blog in reference to Mohamed. It was followed immediately by another comment: "In the end, one can only regret the bill on DNA testing, which was so criticized by a number of politicians."[9] Indeed, it is in the context of the little boy's genetic identification that one can approach the law of November 20, 2007, concerning immigration restrictions, and more specifically the amendment of the conservative deputy Thierry Mariani. This amendment required that foreigners residing in France and seeking visas for their children in the context of family reunification prove their biological ties through genetic testing. Insofar as this obligation concerns only residents from countries with allegedly no reliable documentation of civil status, the African continent is the almost exclusive target. Beyond the issues of feasibility and cost that have been raised by opponents, the genetic testing proposition means that only biological filiation is recognized for foreigners living in France, particularly for Africans, whereas, at the same time, French citizens take the opposite road in hope of adopting children from the Third World, notably from Africa, with the help of the state's services.[10] Such politics of reproduction, apprehended here in their transnational dimension, appear firmly rooted in what must be called this time a legal discrimination. Under the pretext of controlling immigration flows, only blood ties are accepted as family ties for citizens of poor nations, though the system of foster care is one of the pillars of family organization in many Third World countries, especially on the African continent. But what is required from foreigners does not apply to nationals. For French couples, the state not only covers expenses for medically assisted reproduction technologies, such as artificial insemination, but also facilitates access procedures for adoption, including a recent plan encouraging international adoption.[11] This biologization of immigration, which claims to authenticate the veracity of family ties, most certainly constitutes a regression. In response to those who would read this situation as the never-ending extension of the empire of biopolitics, we should retort, using the same reference to Foucault, that it rather displays a differential and unequal application of these biopolitics, which can be likened to a mitigated form of "state racism."[12] When discriminations target poor Third World populations, more specifically Africans, and when the definition of social relations rests ultimately on biology, one must wonder if racial politics of reproduction are not being reinvented.

I hope not to have left the reader, after this lengthy French detour, with the impression that I was straying from the core problematic of this book. In any case, such an impression would not be justified, since I wrote this piece inspired by the texts that compose the book. It might be, however, a telling impression. For in the end, is an epilogue not an ultimate digression, rather than a concluding synthesis? We can nonetheless draw a few lessons from it. This is what I would like to achieve by offering, in conclusion, three general observations I can draw from Fatma's and Mohamed's story, which intersect, in my opinion, with some of the concerns articulated by the contributors in this book.

First, if it seems self-evident to say that the politics of reproduction have a biological dimension, they cannot be reduced to it: they involve, from a loose interpretation of Marxist theory, all social events through which a society or a group perpetuates itself with some level of stability, especially by maintaining its power structures and relations. They are articulated not only in the spheres of medicine and technologies, of contraception and assisted reproduction, of abortion and pregnancy control, but also more broadly within the social landscape at large, which ideologies they mirror, and which disparities they reproduce. In addition, it should be noted that biotechnologies, biobanks, genetic testing, gynecological consultations, reproduction control programs, and adoption legislations are not neutral instruments. Their application is uneven, at times unequal or even discriminatory, and thus contributes to social reproduction, or, in other words, to how a society or a group treats its members and those who will succeed them.

Second, the politics of reproduction must be understood and construed both as a global phenomenon carried out by international institutions and trivialized ideologies and as a local reality, which, in each particular place, expresses itself and crystallizes dilemmas in a unique fashion. But these politics are also shaped by national narratives; that is, they are set in territories limited by borders and subjected to authorities. In other words, the global is not more powerful at erasing these limits than the local is at unveiling them. The national level thus reveals the role of the state in how these politics are produced, appropriated, and avoided. In this case, the influence of the state is less visible in the management of programs or in the application of techniques—these are largely determined by a globally spread model—than in their manipulation to meet its objectives, such as a protection-of-life ideology, a modernization project, or the control of immigration. Such an instrumental use does not exclude oppositions, contradictions, or failures. In fact, the transnational confrontation of reproduction paradigms can sometimes reveal these through the clash of incompatible models, and perhaps even more efficiently by the inability to make those models coherent to those to whom they are meant to apply: small injustices sometimes effectively enlighten the contempt toward living beings beyond the protection of life, the survival of archaisms behind the modernization project, and the resurgence of racism under the control of immigration.

Finally, the politics of reproduction may also be interpreted in terms of technologies of population regulation, even as the conduct of conducts (to borrow Foucault's wording): population surveys and family planning are thus shaped by a normalizing biopower and enact forms of governance, be they liberal or authoritarian. Yet these politics are not simply ways of acting and behaving; they are politics of life in the sense that they act on life itself and put life at stake. They involve life not merely in the restrictive biological sense—as antiabortion movements or debates on cloning illustrate—but also in the broader and undetermined anthropological sense, relating to life-forms or, more specifically perhaps, to the management of lives, whether they concern AIDS patients, poor peasants, or immigrant women. In that respect, the politics of reproduction relate to democracy, to citizenship—in sum, they relate a way of thinking the reproduction of which is political.

Notes

The translation by Stéphanie Larchanché has been revised by the author.

1. Laura Adda, "Enfant mystère à Marseille," *Le Journal du Dimanche*, August 14, 2008. For a complete analysis of the news item and its significance, see Eric Fassin, "Mohamed et Fatma, immigration subie, mères suspectes," in *Regards*, October 8, 2008 (available at http://www.regards.fr/).

2. Romain Luongo, "Marseille: L'enfant perdu n'avait pas retrouvé sa vraie mère," *La Provence*, September 4, 2008; Claire Angot, "Enfant trouvé, une 'fausse mère,'" *Le Journal du Dimanche*, September 3, 2008.

3. This is how the evolution of Arjun Appadurai's intellectual project could be interpreted, from *Modernity at Large* (1996) to *Fear of Small Numbers* (2006)—from "ethnoscapes" in the first to "ideocides" in the second.

4. Benedict Anderson's "imagined communities" (1983) necessarily involve narratives on reproduction, though he explores this aspect of communities' narratives less than he does others.

5. Thus, as Eric Fassin and I (2006) pointed out, Bernard Accoyer, president of the right-wing group majority at the Parliament, used African families' practice of polygamy to interpret the events; while Claude Imbert, chief editor of *Le Point*, a leading French weekly magazine, accused an "immigration out-of-control, so strange to our beliefs, our customs and our laws, and compromising the long labor of biology required for harmonious integration."

6. The Medal of the French Family was created by decree in 1920 "to honor French mothers who raised several children with dignity." Since 1983, it may also potentially be awarded to mothers who, whatever their nationality, are raising or have raised French children on their own. If the gold medal is reserved for mothers of at least eight children, the bronze medal can be earned with just four or five children. See "Medaille D'honneur De La Famille Française" on the Medailles and Decorations website (http://medaille.decoration.free.fr).

7. We may, like Faye Ginsburg and Rayna Rapp (1995, 3), inspired by Shellee Colen's concept, refer to "stratified reproduction" to analyze these "arrangements by which some

reproductive futures are valued while others are despised." It is well known that in the United States, such a phenomenon applies in particular to "black welfare mothers."

8. As someone commented on an article from LaProvence.com: "These kids, they no longer know who their parents are and what their country is, they will end up as dropouts, thieves, or dealers" ("Marseille: l'enfant perdu n'avait pas retrouvé sa vraie mère," September 4, 2008).

9. Which triggered yet another cry of outrage: "The law on DNA tests will not be voted because people who consider themselves intellectuals will say it is a racist, fascist law, when it is merely protecting the French territory from the massive disembarking of children with no blood ties to their parents" (LaProvence.com, "Marseille: l'enfant perdu n'avait pas retrouvé sa vraie mère," September 4, 2008).

10. This quest for children actually caused several scandals when corruption and deceit cases were discovered of children abducted from their parents. The most mediatized case concerned the Arche de Zoé association, whose members were arrested in Chad in October 2007, just as they were about to take 103 children away, pretending they were orphans from Darfur, when in fact they were Chadian kids abducted from their families. Although he had been informed of this initiative, Bernard Kouchner, the French minister of foreign affairs, did not act to intervene. See "Imbroglio politico-humanitaire," RFI.fr, October 26, 2007.

11. See the interview given by Rama Yade, French secretary of state for human rights, on July 28, 2008 on leParisien.fr: "Des Peace Corps à la française pour aider les familles."

12. For Michel Foucault (1997, 227), racism is "a rupture of a biological nature inside a domain which defines itself as being precisely biological," in other words, as a splitting of biopolitics according to a principle of biophysical difference.

References

Abbasi-Shavazi, Mohammad Jalal, Marcia C. Inhorn, Hajiieh Bibi Razeghi-Nasrabad, and Ghasem Toloo. 2008. "The Iranian ART Revolution: Infertility, Assisted Reproductive Technologies, and Third-Party Donation in the Islamic Republic of Iran." *Journal of Middle East Women's Studies* 4 (2): 1–28.

Abdalla, Raqiya Haji Dualeh. 1982. *Sisters in Affliction: Circumcision and Infibulation of Women in Africa.* London: Zed.

Abdullah, Fareed. 2005. "The Complexities of Implementing Antiretroviral Treatment in the Western Cape Province of South Africa. Development Update: From Disaster to Development; HIV and AIDS in Southern Africa." *Interfund* 5 (3): 245–64.

Abusharaf, Rogaia Mustafa. 1998. "Unmasking Tradition." *Sciences*, March–April, 22–27.

———. 2000. "Revisiting Feminist Discourses on Infibulation: Responses from Sudanese Feminists." In *Female Circumcision in Africa*, ed. Bettina Shell-Duncan and Ylva Hernlund, 151–66. Boulder, Colo.: Lynne Rienner.

———. 2001. "Virtuous Cuts: Female Genital Circumcision in an African Ontology." *Differences: A Journal of Feminist Cultural Studies* 12 (1): 112–40.

———. 2006. *Female Circumcision: Multicultural Perspectives.* Philadelphia: University of Pennsylvania Press.

Acker, Joan. 2004. "Gender, Capitalism, and Globalization." *Critical Sociology* 30 (1): 17–41.

Ahearn, Laura. 2001. *Invitations to Love: Literacy, Love Letters, and Social Change in Nepal.* Ann Arbor: University of Michigan Press.

Ahmadu, Fuambai. 2000. "Rites and Wrongs: An Insider/Outsider Reflects on Power and Excision." In *Female Circumcision in Africa*, ed. Bettina Shell-Duncan and Ylva Hernlund, 283–312. Boulder, Colo.: Lynne Rienner.

Alba, Francisco, and Joseph E. Potter. 1986. "Population and Development in Mexico since 1940: An Interpretation." *Population and Development Review* 12 (1): 47–75.

ALRC (Australian Law Reform Commission). 2003. ALRC 96 *Essentially Yours: The Protection of Human Genetic Information in Australia.* Sidney: Southwood Press.

Amnesty International. 2006. "'No One to Help Them': Rape Extends from Darfur into Eastern Chad." Human Rights Watch, December 2006 (http://www.amnestyusa.org/).

Amuchástegui, Ana. 2001. *Virginidad e iniciación sexual en México: Experiencias y significados*. Mexico City: EDAMEXun/Population Council.

Anagnost, Ann. 1988. "Family Violence and Magical Violence: The Woman as Victim in China's One-Child Policy." *Women and Language* 11 (2): 16–21.

———. 1995. "A Surfeit of Bodies: Population and the Rationality of the State in Post-Mao China." In *Conceiving the New World Order: The Global Politics of Reproduction*, ed. Faye Ginsburg and Rayna Rapp, 22–41. Berkeley: University of California Press.

———. 1997. *National Past-Times: Narrative, Representation, and Power in Modern China*. Durham: Duke University Press.

Anderson, Benedict. 1983. *Imagined Communities*. London: Verso.

Anderson, Kermyt G. 2006. "How Well Does Paternity Confidence Match Actual Paternity?" *Current Anthropology* 47:513–20.

Angelelli, Claudia V. 2004. *Medical Interpreting and Cross-Cultural Communication*. New York: Cambridge University Press.

Appadurai, Arjun. 1986. *The Social Life of Things: Commodities in Cultural Perspective*. New York: Cambridge University Press.

———. 1990. "Disjuncture and Difference in the Global Cultural Economy." *Public Culture* 2 (2): 1–24.

———. 1996. *Modernity at Large*. Minneapolis: University of Minnesota Press.

———. 2006. *Fear of Small Numbers*. Durham: Duke University Press.

Assaad, Marie Bassili. 1980. "Female Circumcision in Egypt." *Studies in Family Planning* 11 (1): 3–16.

Azoulay, Muriel, and Catherine Quiminal. 2002. "Reconstruction des Rapports de Genre en Situation Migratoire. Femmes 'Réveillées,' Hommes Menacés en Milieu Soninké." *VEI Enjeux* 128:87–102.

Baines, Erin K. 2004. *Vulnerable Bodies: Gender, the UN, and the Global Refugee Crisis*. Burlington, Vt.: Ashgate.

Barlow, Tani. 1991. "Theorizing Woman: Funü, Guojia, Jiating." *Genders* 10:132–60.

Barnard, Alan. 2000. *History and Theory in Anthropology*. Cambridge: Cambridge University Press.

Barou, Jacques. 2002. "Les immigrations Africaines en France au tournant du siècle." *Hommes et Migrations* 1239:6–19.

Barrow, Christine. 1996. *Family in the Caribbean: Themes and Perspectives*. Kingston: Ian Randle.

Bartlett, Linda A., Susan Purdin, and Therese McGinn. 2004. "Forced Migrants—Turning Rights into Reproductive Health." *Lancet* 363:76–77.

Basch, Linda, Nina Glick Schiller, and Cristina Szanton Blanc, eds. 1994. *Nations Unbound: Transnational Projects, Postcolonial Predicaments, and Deterritorialized Nation-States*. Amsterdam: Gordon and Breach.

BBC (British Broadcasting Corporation). 2006. "Drug Trials Outsourced to India," April 27.

Becker, Gary. 1976. *The Economic Approach to Human Behavior*. Chicago: University of Chicago Press.

Becker, Gaylene. 2000. *The Elusive Embryo: How Men and Women Approach New Reproductive Technologies.* Berkeley: University of California Press.

Berthiaume, Christiane. 1995. "Refugee Women: Do We Really Care?" *Refugees Magazine,* no. 100 (http://www.unhcr.org/).

Besson, Jean. 1993. "Reputation and Respectability Reconsidered: A New Perspective on Afro-Caribbean Peasant Women." In *Women and Change in the Caribbean,* ed. Janet Momsen, 15–37. Bloomington: University of Indiana Press.

Best, Kim. 2004. *Family Planning and the Prevention of Mother-to-Child Transmission of HIV: A Review of the Literature.* Family Health International Working Paper Series. Research Triangle Park, N.C.: Family Health International.

Bhabha, Jacqueline. 1998. "Enforcing the Human Rights of Citizens and Non-citizens in the Era of Maastricht: Some Reflections on the Importance of States." *Development and Change* 29:697–724.

Bharadwaj, Aditya. 2000. "How Some Indian Baby Makers Are Made: Media Narratives and Assisted Conception in India." *Anthropology and Medicine* 7 (1): 63–78.

——. 2002. "Conception Politics: Medical Egos, Media Spotlights, and the Contest over Test-Tube Firsts in India." In *Infertility around the Globe: New Thinking on Childlessness, Gender, and Reproductive Technologies,* ed. Marcia C. Inhorn and Frank van Balen, 315–33. Berkeley: University of California Press.

——. 2003. "Why Adoption Is Not an Option in India: The Visibility of Infertility, the Secrecy of Donor Insemination, and Other Cultural Complexities." *Social Science and Medicine* 56 (9): 1867–80.

——. 2005. "Cultures of Embryonic Stem Cells." In *Crossing Borders: Cultural, Religious, and Political Differences concerning Stem Cell Research,* ed. W. Bender, C. Hauskeller, and A. Manzei, 325–41. Munster: Agenda Verlag.

——. 2006. "Clinical Theodicies: The Enchanted World of Uncertain Science and Clinical Conception in India." *Culture, Medicine, and Psychiatry* 30 (4): 451–65.

——. 2008. "Biosociality to Biocrossings: Encounters with Assisted Conception and Embryonic Stem Cells in India." In *Genetics, Biosociality and the Social Sciences: Making Biologies and Identities,* ed. Sahra Gibbon and Carlos Novas, 98–116. Oxon: Routledge.

——. 2009. "Assisted Life: The Neoliberal Moral Economy of Embryonic Stem Cells in India." In *Assisting Reproduction, Testing Genes: Global Encounters with New Biotechnologies,* ed. Daphna Birenbaum-Carmeli and Marcia Inhorn, 239–57. New York: Berghahn Books.

——. 2011. *Conceptions: Infertility and Procreative Modernity in India.* Oxford: Berghahn Books.

Bharadwaj, Aditya, and Peter Glasner. 2008. *Local Cells, Global Science: The Rise of Embryonic Stem Cell Research in India.* London: Routledge.

Bhattacharji, S. 1990. "Motherhood in Ancient India." *Economic and Political Weekly,* October 20–27, WS50–WS57.

Bledsoe, Caroline H. 2002. *Contingent Lives: Fertility, Time, and Aging in West Africa.* Chicago: University of Chicago Press.

———. 2004a. "Acts of Selection: Reproduction and Risk in Contemporary America." Paper presented at Conference on the Political and Symbolic Implications of Quantification. Working Group on Anthropology and Population. Watson Institute for International Studies, Brown University.

———. 2004b. "Reproduction at the Margins: Migration and Legitimacy in the New Europe." *Demographic Research*, Special Collection, 3 (4): 87–116.

———. 2006. "The Demography of Family Reunification: From Circulation to Substitution in Gambian Spain." Max Planck Institute for Demographic Research Working Paper 2006–053 (http://www.demogr.mpg.de).

Bledsoe, Caroline H., René Houle, and Papa Sow. 2007. "High Fertility Gambians in Low Fertility Spain: The Dynamics of Child Accumulation across Transnational Space." *Demographic Research* 16:375–412.

Bledsoe, Caroline H., Susana Lerner, and Jane I. Guyer, eds. 2000. *Fertility and the Male Life Cycle in the Era of Fertility Decline*. Oxford: Oxford University Press.

Block, Alan A., and Patricia Klausner. 1987. "Masters of Paradise Island: Organized Crime, Neo-liberalism, and the Bahamas." *Dialectical Anthropology* 12:85–102.

Blyth, Eric, and Ruth Landau, eds. 2004. *Third Party Assisted Conception across Cultures: Social, Legal, and Ethical Perspectives*. London: Jessica Kingsley.

Boddy, Janice. 1982. "Womb as Oasis: The Symbolic Context of Pharaonic Circumcision in Rural Northern Sudan." *American Ethnologist* 9:682–98.

———. 1989. *Wombs and Alien Spirits: Women, Men, and the Zar Cult in Northern Sudan*. Madison: University of Wisconsin Press.

———. 1998. "Violence Embodied? Female Circumcision, Gender Politics, and Cultural Aesthetics." In *Rethinking Violence against Women*, ed. R. Emerson Dobash and Russell P. Dobash, 77–110. Thousand Oaks, Calif.: Sage.

———. 2007. *Civilizing Women: British Crusades in Colonial Sudan*. Princeton: Princeton University Press.

Bolles, A. Lynn. 1992. "Sand, Sea, and the Forbidden." *Transforming Anthropology* 3 (1): 30–34.

Boston Women's Health Book Collective. 1973. *Our Bodies, Ourselves*. New York: Simon and Schuster.

Brambila, Carlos. 1998. "Mexico's Population Policy and Demographic Dynamics: The Record of Three Decades." In *Do Population Policies Matter? Fertility and Politics in Egypt, India, Kenya, and Mexico*, ed. Anrudh Jain, 157–91. New York: Population Council.

Brennan, Denise. 2004. *What's Love Got to Do with It? Transnational Desires and Sex Tourism in the Dominican Republic*. Durham: Duke University Press.

Briggs, Charles L. 2003. "Why Nation-States and Journalists Can't Teach People to Be Healthy: Power and Pragmatic Miscalculation in Public Discourses on Health." *Medical Anthropology Quarterly* 17 (3): 287–321.

Briggs, Charles L., and Clara Mantini-Briggs. 2003. *Stories in the Time of Cholera: Racial Profiling during a Medical Nightmare*. Berkeley: University of California Press.

Brocato, Vanessa. 2003. "SIECUS Fact Sheet: Exporting Ineffective Policy; The Globalization of American Abstinence-Only-Until-Marriage Programs." October. (http://www.siecus.org)

Bronfman, Mario. 1998. "Mexico and Central America." *International Migration* 36 (4): 609–42.

Broring, G., and R. Van Duifhuizen. 1993. "Mobility and the Spread of HIV/AIDS: A Challenge to Health Promotion." *AIDS Health Promotion Exchange* (1): 1–3.

Brown, Barbara B. 1983. "The Political Economy of Population Policy in South Africa." *Women, Health, and International Development*, ed. Margaret I. Aguwa. East Lansing: Office of Women in International Development and African Studies Center, Michigan State University.

———. 1987. "Facing the 'Black Peril': The Politics of Population Control in South Africa." *Journal of Southern African Studies* 13 (3): 256–73.

Browner, Carole H. 1986. "The Politics of Reproduction in a Mexican Village." *Signs* 11:710–24.

———. 2000. "Situating Women's Reproductive Activities." *American Anthropologist* 120 (4): 773–88.

Browner, Carole H., and Joanne Leslie. 1996. "Women, Work, and Household Health in the Context of Development." In *Gender and Health: An International Perspective*, ed. Carolyn F. Sargent and C. B. Brettell, 260–77. Upper Saddle River, N.J.: Prentice Hall.

Browner, Carole H., Bernard R. Ortiz de Montellano, and Arthur J. Rubel. 1988. "A Methodology for Cross-Cultural Ethnomedical Research." *Current Anthropology* 29 (5): 681–701.

Browner, Carole H., and H. Mabel Preloran. 1999. "Male Partners' Role in Latinas' Amniocentesis Decisions." *Journal of Genetic Counseling* 8 (2): 86–108.

Browner, Carole H., H. Mabel Preloran, M. C. Casado, H. N. Bass, and A. P. Walker. 2003. "Genetic Counseling Gone Awry: Miscommunication between Prenatal Genetic Service Providers and Mexican-Origin Clients." *Social Science and Medicine* 56 (9): 1933–46.

Browner, Carole H., H. Mabel Preloran, and Simon H. Cox. 1999. "Ethnicity, Bioethics, and Prenatal Diagnosis: The Amniocentesis Decisions of Mexican-Origin Women and Their Partners." *American Journal of Public Health* 89:1658–66.

Browner, Carole H., and Carolyn Sargent. 1996. "Anthropology and Human Reproduction." In *Medical Anthropology: Contemporary Theory and Method*, ed. Carolyn Sargent and Thomas Johnson, 219–34. Westport, Conn.: Praeger.

———. 2007. "Engendering Medical Anthropology." In *Medical Anthropology: Regional Perspectives and Shared Concerns*, ed. Francine Saillant and Serge Genest, 233–52. Oxford: Blackwell.

Burawoy, Michael. 2000a. "Grounding Globalization." In *Global Ethnography: Forces, Connections, and Imaginations in a Postmodern World*, ed. Michael Burawoy, Joseph A. Blum, Sheba George, Zsuzsa Gille, Teresa Gowan, Lynn Haney, Maren Klawiter, Steve H. Lopez, Séan Ó. Riain, and Millie Thayer, 337–50. Berkeley: University of California Press.

———. 2000b "Introduction: Reaching for the Global." In *Global Ethnography: Forces,*

Connections, and Imaginations in a Postmodern World, ed. Michael Burawoy, Joseph A. Blum, Sheba George, Zsuzsa Gille, Teresa Gowan, Lynn Haney, Maren Klawiter, Steve H. Lopez, Séan Ó. Riain, and Millie Thayer, 1–40. Berkeley: University of California Press.

Cabezas, Amalia L. 1999. "Women's Work Is Never Done: Sex Tourism in Sosúa, the Dominican Republic." In *Sun, Sex, and Gold: Tourism and Sex Work in the Caribbean*, ed. Kamala Kempadoo, 93–123. Lanham, Md.: Rowman and Littlefield.

Calavita, Kitty. 2005. *Immigrants at the Margins: Law, Race, and Exclusion in Southern Europe*. Cambridge: Cambridge University Press.

Caldeira, Teresa, and James Holston. 2005. "State and Urban Space in Brazil: From Modernist Planning to Democratic Interventions." In *Global Assemblages: Technology, Politics, and Ethics as Anthropological Problems*, ed. Aihwa Ong and Stephen J. Collier, 393–416. Oxford: Blackwell Publishing.

Caldwell, John, and Pat Caldwell. 1986. *Limiting Population Growth and the Ford Foundation Contribution*. London: Frances Pinter.

Camara, Bilali. 2001. *Twenty Years of the HIV/AIDS Epidemic in the Caribbean*. Port of Spain, Trinidad: CAREC-SPSTI.

Cambrosio, Alberto, Allan Young, and Margaret Lock. 2000. Introduction to *Living and Working with New Medical Technologies: Intersections of Inquiry*, ed. Margaret Lock, Alan Young, and Alberto Cambrosio, 1–16. Cambridge: Cambridge University Press.

Campbell, Shirley, Althea Perkins, and Patricia Mohammed. 1999. " 'Come to Jamaica and Feel Alright': Tourism and the Sex Trade." In *Sun, Sex, and Gold: Tourism and Sex Work in the Caribbean*, ed. Kamala Kempadoo, 125–56. Lanham, Md.: Rowman and Littlefield.

Carlson, Sharon. 2005. *Contesting and Reinforcing Patriarchy: An Analysis of Domestic Violence in the Dzaleka Refugee Camp*. RSC Working Paper no. 23. Oxford: Refugee Studies Center.

Carrillo, Hector. 1999. "Cultural Change, Hybridity, and Male Homosexuality in Mexico." *Culture, Health, and Sexuality* 1 (3): 223–38.

——. 2002. *The Night Is Young: Sexuality in Mexico in the Time of AIDS*. Chicago: University of Chicago Press.

Carsten, Janet, ed. 2000. *Cultures of Relatedness: New Approaches to the Study of Kinship*. Cambridge: Cambridge University Press.

——. 2004. *After Kinship*. Cambridge: Cambridge University Press.

Casey, Sean. 2005. "Providing Highly Active Antiretroviral Therapy in Cape Town, South Africa: An Interview-Based Case Study of Social Challenges to Treatment Provision." MA thesis, Faculty of the Humanities, University of Cape Town.

Caulfield, Sueann. 2000. *In Defense of Honor: Sexual Morality, Modernity, and Nation in Early-Twentieth-Century Brazil*. Durham: Duke University Press.

CDC (Centers for Disease Control). 2006. "Revised Recommendations for HIV Testing of Adults, Adolescents, and Pregnant Women in Health-Care Settings." September 22. 55 (RR14): 1–17. http://www.cdc.gov.

CEPROSH. 1997. *Proyecto hotelero*. Puerto Plata: Centro de Promoción y Solidaridad Humana.

Chant, Sylvia, and Matthew C. Gutmann. 2000. *Mainstreaming Men into Gender and Development: Debates, Reflections, and Experiences*. Oxford: Oxfam.

Chen, Junjie. 1995. "The Intergenerational Relationship and the Chinese Peasants' Idea of Childbearing: A Social Anthropological Study in the Village of Yue in Eastern China" [in Chinese]. *Population Research* 19 (1): 36–41.

Chen, Junjie, and Guangzong Mu. 1996. "The Chinese Peasants' Needs of Childbearing" [in Chinese]. *Social Sciences in China* 17 (2): 126–37.

Chimere-Dan, Orieji. 1993. "Population Policy in South Africa." *Studies in Family Planning* 24 (1): 31–39.

Chopra, Mickey, and David Saunders. 2004. "From Apartheid to Globalisation: Health and Social Change in South Africa." *Hygiea Internationalis* (http://www.ep.liu.se).

Chu, Junhong. 1995. "The Development of Population Studies and the Establishment of Demographic Science in China" [in Chinese]. *Peking University Learned Journal* 32 (5): 74–80.

Clarke, Morgan. 2006. "Shiite Perspectives on Kinship and New Reproductive Technologies." *ISIM Newsletter* 17:26–27.

——. 2007. "Children of the Revolution: 'Ali Khamene'i's 'Liberal' Views on in Vitro Fertilization." *British Journal of Middle Eastern Studies* 34 (3): 287–303.

——. 2009. *Islam and New Kinship: Reproductive Technology, Anthropology, and the Shari'ah in Lebanon*. New York: Berghahn Books.

Cohen, Lawrence. 1999. "Where It Hurts: Indian Materials for an Ethics of Organ Transplantation." *Daedalus* 128 (4): 135–65.

——. 2000. "The Other Kidney: Biopolitics beyond Recognition." *Body and Society* 7 (2–3): 9–29.

——. 2005. "Operability, Bioavailability, and Exception." In *Global Assemblages: Technology, Politics, and Ethics as Anthropological Problems*, ed. Aihwa Ong and Stephen J. Collier, 79–90. Oxford: Blackwell.

Cohen, Susan A. 1998. "The Reproductive Health Needs of Refugees: Emerging Consensus Attracts Predictable Controversy." *Guttmacher Report on Public Policy* 1 (5): 10–12.

——. 2003. "Global Gag Rule Revisited: HIV/AIDS Initiative Out, Family Planning Still In." *Guttmacher Report on Public Policy* (http://www.guttmacher.org).

Cohn, S. E., J. D. Klein, J. E. Mohr, C. M. van der Horst, and D. J. Weber. 1994. "The Geography of AIDS: Patterns of Urban and Rural Migration." *Southern Medical Journal* 87 (6): 599–606.

Cole, Jennifer, and Deborah Durham, eds. 2006. *Generations and Globalization: Youth, Age, and Family in the New World Economy*. Bloomington: Indiana University Press.

Coleman, David A. 1994. "Fertility and Immigration among Immigrant Populations as Measures of Integration." *Journal of Biosocial Sciences* 26:107–36.

Coleman, David, and Robert Rowthorn. 2004. "The Economic Effect of Immigration into the United Kingdom." *Population and Development Review* 30 (4): 579–624.

Colen, Shellee. 1995. " 'Like a Mother to Them': Stratified Reproduction and West Indian Childcare Workers and Employers in New York." In *Conceiving the New World Order: The Global Politics of Reproduction*, ed. Faye Ginsburg and Rayna Rapp, 78–102. Berkeley: University of California Press.

Collier, Stephen J., and Aihwa Ong. 2003. "Oikos/Anthropos: Rationality, Technology, Infrastructure." *Current Anthropology* 44 (3): 421–26.

Comaroff, John L., and Simon Roberts. 1977. "Marriage and Extra-marital Sexuality: The Dialectics of Legal Change among the Kgatla." *Journal of African Law* 21:97–123.

Connell, R. W. 1995. *Masculinities.* Berkeley: University of California Press.

———. 2005. "Change among the Gatekeepers: Men, Masculinities, and Gender Equality in the Global Arena." *Signs* 30 (3): 1801–25.

Conway, Dennis. 1993. "The New Tourism in the Caribbean: Reappraising Market Segmentation." In *Tourism Marketing and Management in the Caribbean*, ed. Dennis John Gayle and Jonathan N. Goodrich, 167–73. London: Routledge.

Covey, R. Alan. 2007. "Political Complexity, Rise of." In *Encyclopedia of Archaeology*, ed. Deborah Pearsall, vol. 3, 1842–53. Oxford: Elsevier.

Crisp, Jeff. 1999. *"Who Has Counted the Refugees?": UNHCR and the Politics of Numbers.* New Issues in Refugee Research, Working Paper no. 12. UNHCR: Geneva, Switzerland.

Crossette, Barbara. 1996. "Vatican Rebuffs Unicef, Widening a Family Planning Dispute." *New York Times*, November 10.

Crowley, Jocelyn Elise. 2001. "Who Institutionalizes Institutions? The Case of Paternity Establishment in the United States." *Social Science Quarterly* 82 (2): 312–28.

Cunningham, George, and D. Geoff Tompkinson. 1999. "Cost and Effectiveness of the California Prenatal Screening Program." *Genetics in Medicine* 1 (5): 199–206.

Daly, Mary. 1978. *Gyn/Ecology: The Metaethics of Radical Feminism.* Boston: Beacon Press.

Das, Veena. 1995. "National Honor and Practical Kinship: Unwanted Women and Children." In *Conceiving the New World Order: The Global Politics of Reproduction*, ed. Faye Ginsburg and Rayna Rapp, 212–33. Berkeley: University of California Press.

———. 2000. "The Practice of Organ Transplants: Networks, Documents, Translations." In *Living and Working with the New Medical Technologies*, ed. Margaret Lock, Allan Young, and Alberto Cambrosio, 263–87. Cambridge: Cambridge University Press.

Davis, D. E. 1978. "Development and the Tourism Industry in Third World Countries." *Society and Leisure* 1:301–22.

Davis-Floyd, Robbie, and Carolyn F. Sargent. 1997. Introduction to *Childbirth and Authoritative Knowledge: Cross-Cultural Perspectives*, ed. Robbie F. Davis-Floyd and Carolyn F. Sargent, 1–51. Berkeley: University of California Press.

Debert, Guita G., Maria Filomena Gregori, and Adriana Piscitelli, eds. 2006. *Gênero e Distribuição da Justiça: As delegacias de defesa da mulher e a construção das diferenças.* Campinas: PAGU/Núcleo de Estudos de Gênero da UNICAMP.

De Bruyn, Maria. 2004. "Living with HIV: Challenges in Reproductive Health Care in South Africa." *African Journal of Reproductive Health* 8 (1): 92–98.

——. 2005. *Reproductive Rights for Women Affected by* HIV/AIDS: *A Project to Monitor Millennium Development Goals 5 and 6.* Chapel Hill, N.C.: Ipas.

De Hart, Betty. 2006. "Introduction: The Marriage of Convenience in European Immigration Law." *European Journal of Migration and Law* 8 (3–4): 251–62.

De Moya, Antonio, and Rafael Garcia. 1996. "AIDS and the Enigma of Bisexuality in the Dominican Republic." In *Bisexualities and* AIDS: *International Perspectives*, ed. Peter Aggleton, 121–35. Bristol, Penn.: Taylor and Francis.

——. 1998. "Three Decades of Male Sex Work in Santo Domingo." In *Men Who Sell Sex: International Perspectives on Male Prostitution and* AIDS, ed. Peter Aggleton, 127–40. London: Taylor and Francis.

Department of Health. 2004. *Annual Report.* Provincial Government of the Western Cape Metropole District Health Services. Cape Town: Department of Health.

——. 2005. "National HIV and Syphilis Antenatal Sero-Prevalence Survey in South Africa 2004." Pretoria: South Africa.

Domingo, Andreu, and René Houle. 2005. "The Economic Activity of Immigrants in Spain: Between Complementarity and Exclusion." Paper presented at the International Union for the Scientific Study of Population, 25th International Population Conference, Tours, France, July 18–23.

Dorkenoo, Efua. 1994. *Cutting the Rose: Female Genital Mutilation; The Practice and Its Prevention.* London: Minority Rights Group.

Dudgeon, Matthew R., and Marcia C. Inhorn. 2003. "Gender, Masculinity, and Reproduction: Anthropological Perspectives." *International Journal of Men's Health* 2 (1): 31–56.

——. 2004. "Men's Influences on Women's Reproductive Health: Medical Anthropological Perspectives." *Social Science and Medicine* 59 (7): 1379–95.

Eckstrom, Kevin. 2000. "Pro-Choice Catholic Group Challenges Vatican at UN." *Religion News Service*, June (http://www.seechange.org).

Editorial Department of China Population Press (EDCPP). 2000. *An Essential Pamphlet for Leaders of the Family Planning Program* [in Chinese]. Beijing: China Population Press.

El Dareer, Asma. 1982. *Woman, Why Do You Weep? Circumcision and Its Consequences.* London: Zed Press.

El Saadawi, Nawal. 1980. "Creative Women in Changing Societies: A Personal Reflection." *Race and Class* 22 (2): 159–82.

Empez, Nuria. 2007. *Social Construction of Neglect: The Case of Unaccompanied Minors from Morocco to Spain.* WP-2007–007. Max Planck Institute for Demographic Research.

Empez, Nuria, and Vicens Galea Montero. 2005. "Family Strategies and Unaccompanied Migrant Minors." Paper presented at the European Association of Population Studies, Working Group on the Anthropological Demography of Europe, Max Planck Institute for Demographic Research, Rostock, Germany.

Erikson, Susan. 2003. "Post-diagnostic Abortion in Germany: Reproduction Gone Awry, Again?" *Social Science and Medicine* 56:1987–2001.

——. 2007. "Fetal Views: Histories and Habits of Looking at the Fetus in Germany." *Journal of Medical Humanities* 28 (4): 187–212.

Evans, Peter B., Dietrich Rueschemeyer, and Theda Skocpol. 1985. *Bringing the State Back In*. Cambridge: Cambridge University Press.

Ewick, Patricia, and Susan Silbey. 1998. *The Common Place of Law: Stories from Everyday Life*. Chicago: University of Chicago Press.

Express Healthcare Management. 2000. "ICMR's Proposed Prohibition Creates Furore." (http://www.expresshealthcaremgmt.com).

Farmer, Paul. 1992. *AIDS and Accusation: Haiti and the Geography of Blame*. Berkeley: University of California Press.

——. 2003. *Pathologies of Power: Health, Human Rights, and the New War on the Poor*. Berkeley: University of California Press.

Farmer, Paul, Margaret Connors, and Janie Simmons, eds. 1996. *Women, Poverty, and AIDS: Sex, Drugs, and Structural Violence*. Monroe, Maine: Common Courage Press.

Fassin, Didier. 2001. "Biopolitics of Otherness: Undocumented Immigrants and Racial Discrimination in the French Public Debate." *Anthropology Today: Journal of the Royal Anthropological Institute* 17 (1): 3–7.

——. 2002. "Embodied History. Uniqueness and Exemplarity of South African AIDS." *African Journal of AIDS Research* 1 (1): 63–68.

——. 2007. *When Bodies Remember: Experiences and Politics of AIDS in South Africa*. Berkeley: University of California Press.

Fassin, Didier, and Eric Fassin. 2006. *De la question sociale à la question raciale: Représenter la société française*. Paris: La Découverte.

Ferguson, James. 1990. *The Anti-politics Machine: "Development," Depoliticization, and Bureaucratic Power in Lesotho*. New York: Cambridge University Press.

——. 1999. *Expectations of Modernity: Myths and Meanings of Urban Life on the Zambian Copperbelt*. Berkeley: University of California Press.

Financial Express. 2005. "Firms with Good Track Record to Get Stem Cell R&D Aid." (http://www.financialexpress.com).

Fleischer, Annett. 2010. "Making Families among Cameroonian 'Bush Fallers' in Germany: Marriage, Migration, and the Law." Faculty of Political and Social Sciences, Humboldt University, Berlin. Ph.D. diss., Free University of Berlin.

Fonseca, Claudia. 1997. "Ser mulher, mãe e pobre." In *História das Mulheres no Brasil*, ed. Mary DelPriore, 510–53. São Paulo: Editora Contexto.

——. 2003. "Philanderers, Cuckolds, and Wily Women: A Reexamination of Gender Relations in a Brazilian Working-Class Neighborhood." In *Changing Men and Masculinities in Latin America*, ed. Matthew Gutmann, 61–83. Durham: Duke University Press.

——. 2009. "Doubt Is the Mother of All Invention: DNA and Paternity in a Brazilian Setting." In *Assisting Reproduction, Testing Genes: Global Encounters with New Biotechnologies*, ed. Daphna Birenbaum-Carmeli and Marcia C. Inhorn, 258–84. London: Berghahn Books.

Ford Foundation. 1991. *Reproductive Health: A Strategy for the 1990s: A Program Paper of the Ford Foundation.* New York: Ford Foundation.

Forsythe, Stephen. 1999. "HIV/AIDS and Tourism." *AIDS Analysis Africa* 9 (6): 4–6.

Forsythe, Stephen, Julia Hasbún, and Martha Butler de Lister. 1998. "Protecting Paradise: Tourism and AIDS in the Dominican Republic." *Health Policy Plan* 13 (3): 277–86.

Foucault, Michel. 1977. *Discipline and Punish: The Birth of the Prison.* New York: Vintage.

———. 1978. *The History of Sexuality.* Vol. 1. *An Introduction.* New York: Vintage.

———. 1979. "Governmentality." *Ideology and Consciousness* 6:5–21.

———. 1997. *Il faut défendre la société.* Hautes Etudes. Paris: Gallimard/Seuil.

Franklin, Sarah. 1997. *Embodied Progress: A Cultural Account of Assisted Reproduction.* London: Routledge.

———. 2003. "Ethical Biocapital: New Strategies of Cell Culture." In *Remaking Life and Death: Toward an Anthropology of the Biosciences,* ed. Sarah Franklin and Margaret Lock, 97–127. Santa Fe, N.M.: School of American Research Press.

———. 2005. "Stem Cells R Us: Emergent Life Forms and the Global Biological." In *Global Assemblages: Technology, Politics, and Ethics as Anthropological Problems,* ed. Aihwa Ong and Stephen J. Collier, 59–78. Oxford: Blackwell.

Franklin, Sarah, Celia Lury, and Jackie Stacey. 2000. *Global Nature, Global Culture.* London: Sage.

Franklin, Sarah, and Maureen McNeill. 1988. "Reproductive Futures: Recent Literature and Current Feminist Debates on Reproductive Technologies." *Feminist Studies* 14:545–60.

Franklin, Sarah, and Helena Ragoné, eds. 1998. *Reproducing Reproduction: Kinship, Power, and Technological Innovation.* Philadelphia: University of Pennsylvania Press.

Freeman, Carla. 2000. *High Tech and High Heels in the Global Economy: Women, Work, and Pink-Collar Identities in the Caribbean.* Durham: Duke University Press.

———. 2007. "Neoliberalism and the Marriage of Reputation and Respectability: Entrepreneurship and the Barbadian Middle Class." In *Love and Globalization: Transformations of Intimacy in the Contemporary World,* ed. Mark B. Padilla, Jennifer S. Hirsch, Miguel Muñoz-Laboy, Robert E. Sember, and Richard G. Parker. Nashville, Tenn.: Vanderbilt University Press.

Front National. 2003. "Famille: Accueillir la vie." Programme (http://www.frontnational.com).

Gal, Susan, and Gail Kligman. 2000. *The Politics of Gender after Socialism: A Comparative-Historical Essay.* Princeton: Princeton University Press.

Garmaroudi, Shirin. n.d. "Kinship Intimacy in the Age of Assisted Conception: An Ethnographic Account of the Assisted Reproduction Technologies in Iran." MA thesis, Institute of Social Anthropology, University of Berne, Switzerland.

Gates, Hill. 1996. "Buying Brides in China—Again." *Anthropology Today* 12:8–11.

Geertz, Clifford. 1983. *Local Knowledge: Further Essays in Interpretative Anthropology.* New York: Basic Books.

Giddens, Anthony. 1979. *Central Problems in Social Theory.* Berkeley: University of California Press.

Gilmartin, Christina, Gail Hershatter, Lisa Rofel, and Tyrene White, eds. 1994. *Engendering China: Women, Culture, and the State*. Cambridge: Harvard University Press.

Ginsburg, Faye D., and Rayna Rapp. 1991. "The Politics of Reproduction." *Annual Reviews of Anthropology* 20:311–43.

——, eds. 1995. *Conceiving the New World Order: The Global Politics of Reproduction*. Berkeley: University of California Press.

Glenn, Evelyn Nakano, Grace Chang, and Linda Rennie Forcey, eds. 1994. *Mothering: Ideology, Experience, and Agency*. New York: Routledge.

Glick Schiller, Nina, Linda Basch, and Cristina Blanc-Szanton. 1995. "From Immigrant to Transmigrant: Theorizing Transnational Migration." *Anthropology Quarterly* 68:48–63.

González-López, Gloria. 2005. *Erotic Journeys: Mexican Immigrants and Their Sex Lives*. Berkeley: University of California Press.

González Montes, Soledad. 1999. "Los aportes de las ONG a la salud reproductiva en México." In *Las organizaciones no gubernamentales mexicanas y la salud reproductiva*, ed. Soledad González Montes, 15–51. Mexico City: El Colegio de México.

Greene, Margaret E., and Ann E. Biddlecom. 2000. "Absent and Problematic Men: Demographic Accounts of Male Reproductive Roles." *Population and Development Review* 26 (1): 81–115.

Greenhalgh, Susan. 2003. "Planned Births, Unplanned Persons: 'Population' in the Making of Chinese Modernity." *American Ethnologist* 30 (2): 196–215.

——. 2008. *Just One Child: Science and Policy in Deng's China*. Berkeley: University of California Press.

Greenhalgh, Susan, and Edwin Winckler. 2005. *Governing China's Population: From Leninist to Neoliberal Biopolitics*. Stanford: Stanford University Press.

Gruenbaum, Ellen. 1982. "The Movement against Clitoridectomy and Infibulation in Sudan." *Medical Anthropology Newsletter* 13 (2): 4–12. Reprinted in *Gender in Cross-Cultural Perspective*, ed. Caroline Brettell and Carolyn Sargent, 2nd ed., 441–53. Upper Saddle River, N.J.: Prentice Hall, 1997.

——. 1991. "The Islamic Movement, Development, and Health Education: Recent Changes in the Health of Rural Women in Central Sudan." *Social Science and Medicine* 33 (6): 637–46.

——. 1996. "The Cultural Debate over Female Circumcision: The Sudanese Are Arguing This One Out for Themselves." *Medical Anthropology Quarterly* 10 (4): 455–75.

——. 2001. *The Female Circumcision Controversy: An Anthropological Perspective*. Philadelphia: University of Pennsylvania Press.

——. 2005. "Feminist Activism for the Abolition of Female Genital Cutting in Sudan." *Journal of Middle East Women's Studies* 1 (2): 89–111.

——. 2006. "Sexuality Issues in the Movement to Abolish Female Genital Cutting in Sudan." *Medical Anthropology Quarterly*, n.s., 20 (1): 121–38.

Gu, Baochang. 2002. "On the Reform of China's Family Planning Program" [in Chinese]. *Population Research* 26 (3): 1–8.

Gupta, Akhil, and James Ferguson, eds. 1997. *Anthropological Locations: Boundaries and Grounds of a Field Science.* Berkeley: University of California Press.

Gutmann, Matthew C. 1996. *The Meanings of Macho: Being a Man in Mexico City.* 10th anniversary ed. Berkeley: University of California Press.

———. 2003. *Changing Men and Masculinities in Latin America.* Durham: Duke University Press.

———. 2007. *Fixing Men: Sex, Birth Control, and AIDS in Mexico.* Berkeley: University of California Press.

Hale, Sondra. 1996. *Gender Politics in Sudan: Islamism, Socialism, and the State.* Boulder, Colo.: Westview Press.

———. 2005. "Activating the Gender Local: Transnational Ideologies and 'Women's Culture' in Northern Sudan." *Journal of Middle East Women's Studies* 1 (1): 29–52.

Hammond, Laura C. 2004. *This Place Will Become Home: Refugee Repatriation to Ethiopia.* Ithaca, N.Y.: Cornell University Press.

Hann, Chris M., ed. 2002. *Postsocialism: Ideas, Ideologies, and Practices in Eurasia.* London: Routledge.

Haraway, Donna. 1997. *Modest_Witness@second_Millennium.FemaleMan_Meets_Onco Mouse.* New York: Routledge.

Hayes, Rose Oldfield. 1975. "Female Genital Mutilation, Fertility Control, Women's Roles, and the Patrilineage in Modern Sudan: A Functional Analysis." *American Ethnologist* 2:617–33.

Heckman, James J., and Jeffrey A. Smith. 1995. "Assessing the Case for Social Experiments." *Journal of Economic Perspectives* 9:85–110.

Hilgartner, Stephen. 1995. "The Human Genome Project." In *Handbook of Science and Technology Studies,* ed. Sheila Jasanoff, Gerald E. Markle, James C. Petersen, and Trevor J. Pinch, 302–15. Thousand Oaks, Calif.: Sage.

Hirsch, Jennifer. 2003. *A Courtship after Marriage: Sexuality and Love in Mexican Transnational Families.* Berkeley: University of California Press.

Hochschild, Arlie. 2000. "The Nanny Chain." *American Prospect* 11 (4).

Hondagneu-Sotelo, Pierrette. 2002. "Families on the Frontier: From *Braceros* in the Fields to *Braceras* in the Home." In *Latinos: Remaking America,* ed. Marcelo Suarez-Orozco, 259–73. Cambridge: Harvard University Press.

Horn, David. 1994. *Social Bodies: Science, Reproduction, and Italian Modernity.* Princeton: Princeton University Press.

Hosken, Fran. 1980. *Female Sexual Mutilations: The Facts and Proposals for Action.* Lexington, Mass.: Women's International Network News.

———. 1982. *The Hosken Report: Genital and Sexual Mutilation of Females.* 3rd ed. Lexington, Mass.: Women's International Network News.

Hynes, Michelle, Mani Sheik, Hoyt Wilson, and Paul Spiegel. 2002. "Reproductive Health Indicators and Outcomes among Refugee and Internally Displaced Persons in Postemergency Phase Camps." *Journal of the American Medical Association* 288 (5): 595–603.

IBGE (Instituto Brasileiro de Geografia e Estatística). 2005. "Sintese de indicadores soci-
ais: Estudos e pesquisas 2005." *Informação Demografica e Socioeconomica* (Brasilia) 17.

ICMR (International Center for Medical Research). 2006. *ICMR-DBT Guidelines for Stem Cell Research and Therapy*. New Delhi: Indian Council for Medical Research and Department of Biotechnology.

IDMC (Internal Displacement Monitoring Centre). 2006. "The Definition of an Internally Displaced Person" (http://www.internal-displacement.org).

Inda, Jonathan, and Renato Rosaldo. 2002. *The Anthropology of Globalization*. London: Blackwell.

Inhorn, Marcia C. 1994. *Quest for Conception: Gender, Infertility, and Egyptian Medical Traditions*. Philadelphia: University of Pennsylvania Press.

——. 1996. *Infertility and Patriarchy: The Cultural Politics of Gender and Family Life in Egypt*. Philadelphia: University of Pennsylvania Press.

——. 2003. *Local Babies, Global Science: Gender, Religion, and in Vitro Fertilization in Egypt*. New York: Routledge.

——. 2004. "Privacy, Privatization, and the Politics of Patronage: Ethnographic Challenges to Penetrating the Secret World of Middle Eastern, Hospital-Based in Vitro Fertilization." *Social Science and Medicine* 59 (10): 2095–2108.

——. 2005. "Fatwas and ARTS: IVF and Gamete Donation in Sunni v. Shi'a Islam." *Journal of Gender, Race, and Justice* 9 (2): 291–317.

——. 2006a. "Making Muslim Babies: IVF and Gamete Donation in Sunni versus Shi'a Islam." *Culture, Medicine, and Psychiatry* 30 (4): 427–50.

——. 2006b. "'He Won't Be My Son': Middle Eastern Muslim Men's Discourses of Adoption and Gamete Donation." *Medical Anthropology Quarterly* 20 (1): 94–120.

——. 2007. "Loving Your Infertile Muslim Spouse: Notes on the Globalization of IVF and Its Romantic Commitments in Sunni Egypt and Shia Lebanon." In *Love and Globalization: Transformations of Intimacy in the Contemporary World*, ed. Mark B. Padilla, Jennifer S. Hirsch, Miguel Muñoz-Laboy, Robert Sember, and Richard G. Parker, 139–60. Nashville, Tenn.: Vanderbilt University Press.

Inhorn, Marcia, and Aditya Bharadwaj. 2007. "Reproductively Disabled Lives: Infertility, Stigma, and Suffering in Egypt and India." In *Disability in Local and Global Worlds*, ed. B. Ingstad and S. R. Whyte, 78–106. Berkeley: University of California Press.

Inhorn, Marcia, and Frank van Balen, eds. 2002. *Infertility around the Globe: New Thinking on Childlessness, Gender, and New Reproductive Technologies*. Berkeley: University of California Press.

IPPF (International Planned Parenthood Federation). 2009. "President Barack Obama Rescinds the Global Gag Rule." Press release, January 23 (http://www.ippf.org).

Jain, Kalpana. 2002. *Positive Lives: The Story of Ashok Pillai and Others with HIV*. New Delhi: Penguin Books.

James, Stanlie M., and Claire C. Robertson, eds. 2002. *Genital Cutting and Transnational Sisterhood: Disputing U.S. Polemics*. Urbana: University of Illinois Press.

Jasanoff, Sheila. 2004. "The Idiom of Co-Production." In *States of Knowledge: The Co-production of Science and Social Order*, ed. Sheila Jasanoff, 1–12. New York: Routledge.

——, ed. 2004. *States of Knowledge: The Co-production of Science and Social Order*. New York: Routledge.

Jastram, Kate. 2003. "Family Unity: The New Geography of Family Life." Migration Information Source. Migration Policy Institute (http://www.migrationinformation .org).

Jayaraman, K. S. 2001. "India Seeks to Block Trade in Human Embryos." Science and Development Network (http://www.scidev.net).

Johnson, Paul, and Robin Williams. 2003. "Genetic and Forensics: Making the National DNA Database." *Science Studies* 16 (2): 22–37.

Johnson-Hanks, Jennifer. 2006. *Uncertain Honor: Modern Motherhood in an African Crisis*. Chicago: University of Chicago Press.

Jones, Christopher A. 2008. "Ethical and Legal Conundrums of Postmodern Procreation." *International Journal of Obstetrics and Gynecology* 100 (3): 208–10.

Jordan, Brigitte. 1997. "Authoritative Knowledge and Its Construction." In *Childbirth and Authoritative Knowledge: Cross-Cultural Perspectives*, ed. Robbie E. Davis-Floyd and Carolyn F. Sargent, 55–79. Berkeley: University of California Press.

Kahn, Susan Martha. 2000. *Reproducing Jews: A Cultural Account of Assisted Reproduction in Israel*. Durham: Duke University Press.

Kanaaneh, Rhoda Ann. 2002. *Birthing the Nation: Strategies of Palestinian Women in Israel*. Berkeley: University of California Press.

Kaplan Marcusán, Adriana. 1998. *De senegambia a Cataluña: Procesos de aculturación e integración social*. Barcelona: Fundación "la Caixa."

Kaufman, Carol E. 2000. "Reproductive Control in Apartheid South Africa." *Population Studies* 54 (1): 105–14.

Kempadoo, Kamala, ed. 1999. *Sun, Sex, and Gold: Tourism and Sex Work in the Caribbean*. Lanham, Md.: Rowman and Littlefield.

Kerrigan, Deanna, Jonathan M. Ellen, Luis Moreno, Santo Rosario, Joanne Katz, David D. Celentano, and Michael Sweat. 2001. "Adapting the Thai 100 Percent Condom Programme: Developing a Culturally Appropriate Model for the Dominican Republic." *Culture, Health, and Sexuality* 3 (2): 221–40.

——. 2003. "Environmental-Structural Factors Significantly Associated with Condom Use among Female Sex Workers in the Dominican Republic." *AIDS* 17:415–23.

Kertzer, David, and Dominique Arel. 2002. "Identity Formation and Political Power." In *Census and Identity: The Politics of Race, Ethnicity, and Language in National Censuses*, ed. David Kertzer and Dominique Arel, 1–42. Cambridge: Cambridge University Press.

Kinnaird, Vivian, Uma Kothari, and Derek Hall. 1994. "Tourism: Gender Perspectives." In *Tourism: A Gender Analysis*, ed. Vivian Kinnaird and Derek Hall, 1–34. New York: John Wiley and Sons.

Kleinman, Arthur. 1995. *Writing at the Margin: Discourse between Anthropology and Medicine*. Berkeley: University of California Press.

Kligman, Gail. 1998. *The Politics of Duplicity: Controlling Reproduction in Ceausescu's Romania*. Berkeley: University of California Press.

Klugman, Barbara. 1993. "Feminism, Population Planning, and the Provision of Contraceptives in South Africa." Paper presented at the Institute on Health and Demography in Sub-Saharan Africa, Institute for Advanced Study and Research in the African Humanities, Northwestern University, Evanston, Ill., January 14.

Knoppers, Bartha M., and Ruth Chadwick. 1994. "The Human Genome Project: Under an International Ethical Microscope." *Science* 265:2035–36.

Král, David. 2006. "Visa Policies of the European Union and the United States—Challenges for Transatlantic Partners." Prague: EUROPEUM Institute for European Policy (http://www.europeum.org).

Krause, Elizabeth L. 2004. *A Crisis of Births: Population Politics and Family-Making in Italy*. Belmont, Calif.: Wadsworth.

Krause, Sandra. 2004. "Progress, Gaps, and Challenges Ahead: An Interagency Global Evaluation of Reproductive Health for Refugees and Internally Displaced Persons." *Global HealthLink* 129:6–7, 18.

Kristeva, Julia. 1982. *Powers of Horror: An Essay on Abjection*. New York: Columbia University Press.

Kulu, Hill. 2005. "Migration and Fertility: Competing Hypotheses Re-Examined." *European Journal of Population* 21:51–87.

La Documentation Française. 2006. "La politique de l'immigration." (http://www.vie-publique.fr).

Latour, Bruno. 1993. *We Have Never Been Modern*. Cambridge: Harvard University Press.

Latour, Bruno, and Steve Woolgar. 1979. *Laboratory Life: The Social Construction of Scientific Facts*. Beverly Hills: Sage.

Legros, Françoise. 2003. "La fécondité des etrangères en France: Une stabilisation entre 1990 et 1999." *INSEE Première 898*.

Leiner, Marvin. 1994. *Sexual Politics in Cuba: Machismo, Homosexuality, and AIDS*. Boulder, Colo.: Westview Press.

Lemke, Thomas. 2001. " 'The Birth of Bio-politics': Michel Foucault's Lecture at the Collège de France on Neo-liberal Governmentality." *Economy and Society* 30 (2): 190–207.

Lester, Rebecca. 1997. "The (Dis)embodied Self in Anorexia Nervosa." *Social Science and Medicine* 44:479–89.

Levitt, Peggy, and Nina Glick Schiller. 2004. "Conceptualizing Simultaneity: A Transnational Social Field Perspective on Society." *International Migration Review* 38:1002–39.

Lewis, Linden. 2004. "Caribbean Masculinity at the Fin de Siècle." In *Interrogating Caribbean Masculinities: Theoretical and Empirical Analyses*, ed. R. E. Reddock and E. Barriteau, 244–66. Kingston: University of the West Indies Press.

Liang, Zhongtang, Kejian Tan, and Shiming Jing. 1999. "On the Adjustment of the Population Control Policy" [in Chinese]. *Learned Journal of the Party School of the CPC (the Communist Party of China) Shanxi Provincial Committee* (4): 33–36.

Libman, Howard, and Michael Stein. 2003. "Primary Care and Prevention of HIV Disease: Part I." In *HIV: First Indian Edition*, ed. Howard Libman and Harvey J. Makadon, 39–64. Philadelphia: American College of Physicians.

Lightfoot-Klein, Hanny. 1989. *Prisoners of Ritual: An Odyssey into Female Genital Circumcision in Africa*. New York: Harrington Park Press.

Ligue des droits de l'Homme. 2006. *Rapport Annuel*. (http://www.ldh-france.org/IMG).

Link, Bruce G., and Jo Phelan. 1995. "Social Conditions as Fundamental Causes of Disease." Special issue, *Journal of Health and Social Behavior*, 80–94.

Lipson, Juliene, and Patricia Omidian. 1996. "Health and the Transnational Connection: Afghan Refugees in the United States." In *Selected Papers on Refugee Issues: IV*, ed. Ann M. Rynearson and James Phillips, 130–55. Arlington, Va.: American Anthropological Association.

Liu, Xin. 2000. *In One's Own Shadow: An Ethnographic Account of the Condition of Postreform Rural China*. Berkeley: University of California Press.

Lock, Margaret. 2001. "Menopause, Local Biologies, and Cultures of Aging." *American Journal of Human Biology* 13 (4): 494–504.

Lock, Margaret, and Patricia Kaufert. 1998. Introduction to *Pragmatic Women and Body Politics*, ed. Margaret Lock and Patricia Kaufert, 1–27. Cambridge: Cambridge University Press.

——, eds. 1998. *Pragmatic Women and Body Politics*. Cambridge: Cambridge University Press.

López Juárez, Alfonso. 2003. "Programa Gente Jóven Mexfam." In *Varones adolescentes: Género, identidades, y sexualidades en América Latina*, ed. José Olavarría, 279–83. Santiago: FLACSO.

Lotfalian, Mazyar. 2004. *Islam, Technoscientific Identities, and the Culture of Curiosity*. Dallas: University Press of America.

Loyo, Gilberto. 1974. "The Demographic Problems of Mexico and Latin America." In *The Dynamics of Population Policy in Latin America*, ed. Terry L. McCoy, 183–201. Cambridge, Mass.: Ballinger.

Luraschi, Moira. 2007. *New Family Ties in a Diaspora Context: The Case of Cameroonian Migration in Italy*. Turin, Italy: University of Turin.

Lynch, Michael, and Steve Woolgar, eds. 1990. *Representation in Scientific Practice*. Cambridge: MIT Press.

MacFarquhar, Roderick. 1997. *The Origins of the Cultural Revolution*. Vol. 3, *The Coming of the Cataclysm, 1961–1966*. New York: Columbia University Press.

Mahmood, Saba. 2005. *Politics of Piety: The Islamic Revival and the Feminist Subject*. Princeton: Princeton University Press.

Malik, Sonia Aziz. 2004. "Legal Status of Female Genital Mutilation under the Sudanese Laws." MA thesis, Institute of Women, Gender, and Development Studies, Ahfad University for Women, Omdurman, Sudan.

Manchuelle, François. 1997. *Willing Migrants: Soninke Labor Diasporas, 1848–1960*. Athens: Ohio University Press.

Mankekar, Purnima. 1999. *Screening Culture, Viewing Politics: An Ethnography of Television, Womanhood, and Nation in Postcolonial India*. Durham: Duke University Press.

Marcelle, Pierre. 2005. "C'est pas la faute aux polygames." Ligue des Droits de l'Homme (http://www.ldh-toulon.net).

Marcus, George. 1998. *Ethnography through Thick and Thin*. Princeton: Princeton University Press.

Márquez, Viviane B. de. 1984. "El proceso social en la formación de políticas: El caso de la planificación familiar en México." *Estudios Sociológicos* 2:309–33.

Maternowska, M. Catherine, and Paul Farmer. 2006. *Reproducing Inequities: Poverty and the Politics of Population in Haiti*. Piscataway, N.J.: Rutgers University Press.

McCoy, Terry L. 1974. "A Paradigmatic Analysis of Mexican Population Policy." In *The Dynamics of Population Policy in Latin America*, ed. Terry L. McCoy, 377–408. Cambridge, Mass.: Ballinger.

McGinn, Therese, and Susan Purdin. 2004. "Reproductive Health and Conflict: Looking Back and Moving Ahead." *Disasters* 28 (3): 235–38.

Meirow, D., and J. G. Schenker. 1997. "The Current Status of Sperm Donation in Assisted Reproduction Technology: Ethical and Legal Considerations." *Journal of Assisted Reproduction and Genetics* 14 (3): 133–38.

Merry, Sally Engel. 2005. "Human Rights and Global Legal Pluralism: Reciprocity and Disjuncture." In *Mobile People, Mobile Law: Expanding Legal Relations in a Contracting World*, ed. Franz von Benda Beckman, Keebet von Benda Beckman, and Anne Griffiths, 215–33. Aldershot: Ashgate.

Mikell, Gwendolyn, ed. 1997. *African Feminism: The Politics of Survival in Sub-Saharan Africa*. Philadelphia: University of Pennsylvania Press.

Millar, Paul. 2001. "Non-paternity in Canadá." MA thesis, Department of Sociology, University of Calgary.

Ministère de l'Emploi et de la Solidarité. 2001. "Pour sortir de la polygamie." (http://www.social.gouv.fr).

Mompoint, Pascal. 1991. *Formation et identités en mouvement: Les femmes maliennes en France en quête d'un projet migratoire*. Paris: GRDR.

Moosa, Ebrahim. 2003. "Human Cloning in Muslim Ethics." *Voices across Boundaries* (Fall): 23–26.

Morsy, Soheir. 1991. "Safeguarding Women's Bodies: The White Man's Burden Medicalized." *Medical Anthropology Quarterly* 5 (1): 19–23.

———. 1993. *Gender, Sickness, and Healing in Rural Egypt*. Boulder, Colo.: Westview Press.

———. 1995. "Deadly Reproduction among Egyptian Women: Maternal Mortality and the Medicalization of Population Control." In *Conceiving the New World Order: The Global Politics of Reproduction*, ed. Faye Ginsburg and Rayna Rapp, 162–77. Berkeley: University of California Press.

Mudor, Ganapati S. 2001. "India to Tighten Rules on Human Embryonic Stem Cell Research." *BMJ* 323:530.

Mullings, Beverley. 1999. "Globalization, Tourism, and the International Sex Trade." In *Sun, Sex, and Gold: Tourism and Sex Work in the Caribbean*, ed. K. Kempadoo, 55–80. Boulder, Colo.: Rowman and Littlefield.

Murphy, Martin F. 1990. "Need for a Re-evaluation of the Concept 'Informal Sector': The Dominican Case." In *Perspectives on the Informal Economy*, 161–81. Lanham, Md.: University Press of America.

Musallam, Bassam F. 1986. *Sex and Society in Islam: Birth Control before the Nineteenth Century*. Cambridge: Cambridge University Press.

Mutua, Makau. 2002. *Human Rights: A Political and Cultural Critique*. Philadelphia: University of Pennsylvania Press.

Nader, Laura. 2002. *The Life of the Law—Anthropological Projects*. Berkeley: University of California Press.

Naimak, Trude Holm. 2006. *Antiretroviral Treatment in the Western Cape: A Success Story Facilitated by the Global Fund*. CSSR Working Paper no. 161. South Africa: University of Cape Town.

Nandy, Ashis. 1996. *Science, Hegemony, and Violence: A Requiem for Modernity*. Delhi: Oxford University Press.

Nasr, Vali. 2006. *The Shia Revival: How Conflicts within Islam Will Shape the Future*. New York: W. W. Norton.

Nattrass, Nicoli. 2004. *The Moral Economy of AIDS in South Africa*. Cambridge: Cambridge University Press.

——. 2006. *South Africa's "Rollout" of Highly Active Antiretroviral Therapy: A Critical Assessment*. Center for Social Science Research Working Paper no. 158. University of Cape Town.

Nee, Victor. 1989. "A Theory of Market Transition: From Redistribution to Markets in State Socialism." *American Sociological Review* 54 (5): 663–81.

——. 2001. *Introduction to China's Fertility Culture*. Beijing: China Population Press.

Nguyen, Vinh-Kim. 2005. "Antiretroviral Globalism, Biopolitics, and Therapeutic Citizenship." In *Global Assemblages: Technology, Politics, and Ethics as Anthropological Problems*, ed. Aihwa Ong and Stephen J. Collier, 124–44. Malden, Mass.: Blackwell.

——. 2010. *Republic of Therapy: Triage and Sovereignty in West Africa's Time of AIDS*. Durham: Duke University Press.

NVSS (National Vital Statistics System). 2005. "Birth: Preliminary Data for 2004." *National Vital Statistics Reports* 54 (8).

Obermeyer, Carol Makhlouf. 1999. "The Cultural Context of Reproductive Health: Implications for Monitoring the Cairo Agenda." *International Family Planning Perspectives* 25: S50–S55.

Office of the High Commissioner for Human Rights. 1990. "International Convention on the Protection of the Rights of All Migrant Workers and Members of Their Families." Adopted by General Assembly resolution 45/158 of December 18, New York (http://www2.ohchr.org).

Ong, Aihwa, 1990. "State versus Islam: Malay Families, Women's Bodies, and the Body Politic in Malaysia." *American Ethnologist* 17: 258–76.

——. 2002. "The Pacific Shuttle: Families, Citizenship, and Capital Circuits." In *The Anthropology of Globalization: A Reader*, ed. Jonathan Xavier Inda and Renato Rosaldo, 172–97. Malden, Mass.: Blackwell.

Ong, Aihwa, and Stephen J. Collier. 2005. "Global Assemblages, Anthropological Problems." In *Global Assemblages: Technology, Politics, and Ethics as Anthropological Problems*, ed. Aihwa Ong and Stephen J. Collier, 3–21. Oxford: Blackwell.

———, eds. 2005. *Global Assemblages: Technology, Politics, and Ethics as Anthropological Problems*. Oxford: Blackwell.

Ortner, Sherry B. 1995. "Resistance and the Problem of Ethnographic Refusal." *Comparative Studies in Society and History* 37 (1): 173–93.

———. 1996. *Making Gender: The Politics and Erotics of Culture*. New York: Beacon.

———. 2005. "Subjectivity and Cultural Critique." *Anthropological Theory* 5 (1): 31–52.

———. 2006. *Anthropology and Social Theory: Culture, Power, and the Acting Subject*. Durham: Duke University Press.

Padilla, Mark. 2007. *Caribbean Pleasure Industry: Tourism, Sexuality, and AIDS in the Dominican Republic*. Chicago: University of Chicago Press.

Padilla, Mark D., D. Castellanos, V. Guilamo-Ramos, A. M. Reyes, L. E. Sanchesz Marte, and M. A. Soriano. 2008. "Stigma, Social Inequality, and Sexual Risk Disclosure among Dominican Male Sex Workers." *Social Science and Medicine* 67 (3): 380–88.

Pan, Guiyu, Shengli Chen, Shi Hailong, Shikun Zhang, and Zihui Yang, eds. 2001. *Introduction to China's Fertility Culture*, vol. I and II [in Chinese]. Beijing: China Population Press.

Parker, Richard. 1986. "Masculinity, Femininity, and Homosexuality: On the Anthropological Interpretation of Sexual Meanings in Brazil." In *The Many Faces of Homosexuality: Anthropological Approaches to Homosexual Behavior*, ed. Evelyn Blackwood, 155–63. New York: Haworth Press.

———. 1987. "Acquired Immunodeficiency Syndrome in Urban Brazil." *Medical Anthropology Quarterly* 1 (2): 155–75.

———. 1992. "Male Prostitution, Bisexual Behaviour, and HIV Transmission in Urban Brazil." In *Sexual Behaviour and Networking: Anthropological and Socio-cultural Studies on the Transmission of HIV*, ed. T. Dyson, 109–22. Liege, Belgium: International Union for the Scientific Study of Population.

———. 2001. "Sexuality, Culture, and Power in HIV/AIDS Research." *Annual Review of Anthropology* 30:163–79.

Parker, Richard D., Delia Easton, and Charles H. Klein. 2000. "Structural Barriers and Facilitators in HIV Prevention: A Review of International Research." *AIDS* 14 (1): S22–S32.

Patel, Tulsi. 1994. *Fertility Behaviour: Population and Society in a Rajasthan Village*. Delhi: Oxford University Press.

Patton, Michael Quinn. 2002. *Qualitative Evaluation and Research Methods*. Newbury Park, Calif.: Sage.

Paxson, Heather. 2004. *Making Modern Mothers: Ethics and Family Planning in Urban Greece*. Berkeley: University of California Press.

Peng, Peiyun, Kuifu Yang, Jimin Liang, and Honggui Li, eds. 1996. *A Complete Compilation of Documents of China's Family Planning Program* [in Chinese]. Beijing: China Population Press.

Petchesky, Rosalind Pollack. 1984. *Abortion and Woman's Choice: The State, Sexuality, and Reproductive Freedom*. New York: Longman.

Petryna, Adriana. 2002. *Life Exposed: Biological Citizens after Chernobyl*. Princeton: Princeton University Press.

Pigg, Stacy Leigh, and Vincanne Adams. 2005. "Introduction: The Moral Object of Sex." In *Sex in Development: Science, Sexuality, and Morality in Global Perspective*, ed. Vincanne Adams and Stacy Leigh Pigg, 1–38. Durham: Duke University Press.

Ponte, Stefano, Simon Roberts, and Lance van Sittert. 2007. "'Black Economic Empowerment' (BEE), Business, and the State in South Africa." *Development and Change* 38 (5): 933–55.

Potter, Joseph E. 1999. "The Persistence of Outmoded Contraceptive Regimes: The Cases of Mexico and Brazil." *Population and Development Review* 25 (4): 703–39.

Poundstone, K. E., S. A. Strathdee, and D. D. Celentano. 2004. "The Social Epidemiology of Human Immunodeficiency Virus/Acquired Immunodeficiency Syndrome." *Epidemiologic Reviews* 26:22–35.

Preble, Elizabeth, Douglas Huber, and Ellen Piwoz. 2003. *Family Planning and the Prevention of Mother-to-Child Transmission of HIV: Technical and Programmatic Issues*. Arlington, Va.: Advance Africa.

Preloran, H. Mabel, C. H. Browner, and Eli Lieber. 2005. "Impact of Interpreters' Approach on Latinas' Use of Amniocentesis." *Health Education and Behavior* 32 (5): 599–612.

Probyn, Elspeth. 1991. "This Body Which Is Not One: Technologizing an Embodied Self." *Hypatia* 6:111–24.

Quiminal, Catherine. 1993. "Mode de constitution des ménages polygames et vécu de la polygamie en France." *Migrations Études* 41.

Rabinow, Paul. 1996. *Essays on the Anthropology of Reason*. Princeton: Princeton University Press.

———. 1999a. "Artificiality and Enlightenment: From Sociobiology to Biosociality." In *The Science Studies Reader*, ed. Mario Biagioli, 407–16. New York: Routledge.

———. 1999b. *French DNA: Trouble in Purgatory*. Chicago: University of Chicago Press.

Raissiguier, Catherine. 2003. "Troubling Mothers: Immigrant Women from Africa in France." *Jenda: A Journal of Culture and African Women Studies* 4 (http://www.jenda journal.com).

Rajasingham-Senanayake, Darini. 2004. "Between Victim and Agent: Women's Ambivalent Empowerment in Displacement." In *Refugees and the Transformation of Societies: Agency, Ethics, and Politics*, ed. Philomena Essed, Georg Frerks, and Joke Schrijvers, 151–66. New York: Berghahn Books.

Ramah, Michael, Reynaldo Pareja, and Julia Hasbún. 1992. *Lifestyles and Sexual Practices: Results of KABP Conducted among Homosexual and Bisexual Men*. Santo Domingo: USAID/AIDSCAP.

Rapp, Rayna. 1988. "Chromosomes and Communication: The Discourse of Genetic Counseling." *Medical Anthropology Quarterly* 2:143–57.

———. 2000. *Testing Women, Testing the Fetus*. New York: Routledge.

———. 2001. "Gender, Body, Biomedicine: How Some Feminist Concerns Dragged Reproduction to the Center of Social Theory." *Medical Anthropology Quarterly* 15 (4): 466–67.

Rapp, Rayna, and Faye D. Ginsburg, eds. 1995. *Conceiving the New World Order: The Global Politics of Reproduction.* Berkeley: University of California Press.

Reddock, Rhoda E. 2004. *Interrogating Caribbean Masculinities: Theoretical and Empirical Analyses.* Kingston: University of the West Indies Press.

Reed, Mary M., John M. Westfall, Caroline Bublitz, Catherine Battaglia, and Alexandra Fickenscher. 2005. "Birth Outcomes in Colorado's Undocumented Immigrant Population." *BMC Public Health* 5:100 (http://www.biomedcentral.com).

Reed-Dahanay, Deborah. 2005. *Locating Bourdieu.* Bloomington: Indiana University Press.

Rezkallah, Nadia, and Alain Epelboin. 1997. *Chroniques du saturnisme infantile, 1989–1994: Enquete ethnologique aupres de familles parisiennes originaires du Senegal et du Mali.* Paris: Editions l'Harmattan.

Richards, Martin. 2006. "Genes, Genealogies, and Paternity: Making Babies in the Twenty-first Century." In *Freedom and Responsibilities in Reproductive Choice*, ed. John Spencer and Antje Du Bois–Pedain, 53–72. London: Hart.

Richey, Lisa Ann. 2003. "HIV/AIDS in the Shadows of Reproductive Health." *Interventions in Reproductive Health Matters* 11 (22): 30–35.

———. 2005. "'Lover' 'Mother' or 'Worker': Multiple Identities in the HIV/AIDS and Reproductive Health Agenda in Tanzania." *African Journal of AIDS Research* 4 (2): 83–90.

———. 2006. "Uganda: HIV/AIDS and Reproductive Health." In *Where Human Rights Begin: Essays on Health, Sexuality, and Women, Ten Years after Vienna, Cairo, and Beijing*, ed. Wendy Chavkin and Ellen Chesler, 95–126. Piscataway, N.J.: Rutgers University Press.

———. 2008. *Population Politics and Development: From the Policies to the Clinics.* New York: Palgrave Macmillan.

Riesman, Catherine. 2000. "Stigma and Everyday Resistance Practices: Childless Women in South India." *Gender and Society* 14 (1): 111–35.

Rivkin-Fish, Michelle. 2003. "Anthropology, Demography, and the Search for a Critical Analysis of Fertility: Insights from Russia." *American Anthropologist* 105 (2): 289–301.

———. 2005. *Women's Health in Post-Soviet Russia.* Bloomington: Indiana University Press.

Robertson, Claire C. 2002. "Getting beyond the Ew! Factor: Rethinking U.S. Approaches to African Female Genital Cutting." In *Genital Cutting and Transnational Sisterhood*, ed. Stanlie M. James and Claire Robertson, 54–86. Urbana: University of Illinois Press.

Rodríguez García, Dan. 2001. "Inmigración africana hacia Europa: ¿Un proceso sin fin? El caso de Gambia." In *Ô Willaeri*, 5–7. Information Review of the Work Team on Education in West Africa (ETANE), special volume.

Rofel, Lisa. 1999. *Other Modernities: Gendered Yearnings in China after Socialism.* Berkeley: University of California Press.

Roig Vila, Marta, and Teresa Castro Martín. 2007. "Immigrant Mothers, Spanish Babies: Childbearing Patterns of Foreign Women in Spain." WP-17. Bilbao: Fundación BBVA.

Ronit, Karsten, and Volker Schneider. 1998. "The Strange Case of Regulating Lobbying in Germany." *Parliamentary Affairs* 51 (4): 559–67.

Rose, Nikolas, and Carlos Novas. 2005. "Biological Citizenship." In *Global Assemblages: Technology, Politics, and Ethics as Anthropological Problems*, ed. Aihwa Ong and Steven J. Collier, 439–63. Oxford: Blackwell.

Safa, Helen I. 1995. "Economic Restructuring and Gender Subordination." *Latin American Perspectives* 22 (spring): 32–50.

Sahlins, Marshall. 1978. *Culture and Practical Reason.* Chicago: University of Chicago Press.

Said, Edward. 1978. *Orientalism.* New York: Vintage Books.

Salama, Samir. 2007. "FNC in Heated Debate on Bill Regulating IVF Centres." *Gulf News,* July 4.

Sandbaek, Ulla Margrethe. 2004. "The Global Gag on Reproductive Health Rights." *Forced Migration Review* 19:20 (http://www.fmreview.org).

Santos, Boaventura de Sousa. 2000. "Law and Democracy: (Mis)trusting the Global Reform of Courts." In *Globalizing Institutions: Case Studies in Regulation and Innovation*, ed. Boaventura de Sousa Santos and Jane Jenson, 253–84. Aldershot: Ashgate.

Sargent, Carolyn F. 2005. "Counseling Contraception for Malian Migrants in Paris: Global, State, and Personal Politics." *Human Organization* 64 (2): 147–57.

———. 2006. "Reproductive Strategies and Islamic Discourse." *Medical Anthropology Quarterly* 20 (1): 31–49.

Sargent, Carolyn F., and Carole H. Browner. 2005. "Globalization Raises New Questions about the Politics of Reproduction." *Anthropology News*, March 2005.

Sargent, Carolyn, and Dennis Cordell. 2003. "Polygamy, Disrupted Reproduction, and the State: Malian Migrants in Paris, France." *Social Science and Medicine* 56:1961–72.

Sargent, Carolyn F., Stephanie Larchanche, and Samba Yatera. 2005. "The Evolution of Telecommunications in the Context of Transnational Migration." *Hommes et Migrations* 1256:131–40.

Sargent, Carolyn, and Lauren Gulbas. In press. "Situating Birth in the Anthropology of Reproduction." In *A Companion to Medical Anthropology*, ed. Pamela Erickson and Merrill Singer. London: Blackwell.

Scheper-Hughes, Nancy. 2000. "The Global Traffic in Human Organs." *Current Anthropology* 41 (2): 191–224.

Schneider, Jane C., and Peter T. Schneider. 1996. *Festival of the Poor: Fertility Decline and the Ideology of Class in Sicily, 1960–1980.* Hegemony and Experience. Tucson: University of Arizona Press.

Schreck, Laurel. 2000. "Turning Point: A Special Report on the Refugee Reproductive Health Field." *International Family Planning Perspectives* 26 (4): 162–66.

Schuch, Patrice. 2009. *Práticas de Justiça: Antropologia dos modos de governo da Infância e Juventude no Contexto pós-ECA.* Porto Alegre: Editora da UFRGS.

Scott, James C. 1998. *Seeing like a State: How Certain Schemes to Improve the Human Condition Have Failed.* New Haven: Yale University Press.

Scott, Joan W. 1996. *Only Paradoxes to Offer: French Feminists and the Rights of Man.* Cambridge: Harvard University Press.

Seekings, Jeremy, and Nicoli Nattrass. 2006. *Class, Race, and Inequality in South Africa.* New Haven: Yale University Press.

Serour, Gamal I. 1996. "Bioethics in Reproductive Health: A Muslim's Perspective." *Middle East Fertility Society Journal* 1 (1): 30–35.

Serour, Gamal I., and B. M. Dickens. 2001. "Assisted Reproduction Developments in the Islamic World." *International Journal of Gynecology and Obstetrics* 74 (2): 187–93.

Sewell, William H. 1992. "A Theory of Structure: Duality, Agency, and Transformation." *American Journal of Sociology* 98:1–29.

Shao, Lizi. [1954] 1996. "A Speech on the First Meeting of the Standing Committee of the First National People's Congress." In *A Complete Compilation of Documents of China's Family Planning Program* [in Chinese], ed. Peiyun Peng, Kuifu Yang, Jimin Liang, and Honggui Li, 529. Beijing: China Population Press.

Sharp, Lesley A. 2000. "The Commodification of the Body and Its Parts." *Annual Review of Anthropology* 29:287–328.

Sharpe, Neil F., and Ronald F. Carter, eds. 2006. *Genetic Testing.* Hoboken, N.J.: Wiley-Liss.

Shell-Duncan, Bettina. 2001. "The Medicalization of Female 'Circumcision': Harm Reduction or Promotion of a Dangerous Practice?" *Social Science and Medicine* 52 (7): 1013–28.

Shell-Duncan, Bettina, and Ylva Hernlund, eds. 2000. *Female "Circumcision" in Africa: Culture, Controversy, and Change.* Boulder, Colo.: Lynne Rienner.

Shi, Hailong. 2001. "A Research Report on the Activity of 'Letting New Customs of Marriage and Childbearing Flow into Myriads of Families' " [in Chinese]. *Population Research* 25 (2): 76–80.

SIECUS (Sexuality Information and Education Council of the United States). 2006. "Policy Updates, January 2006: Sauerbrey Appointed; Advocates Await First Acts and Replacement at the United Nations." (http://www.siecus.org).

Silveira, José Maria da. 2001. *Avaliação das potencialidades e dos obstáculos à comercialização dos produtos das biotecnologias no Brasil.* Brasília: Ministério de Ciência e Tecnologia.

Silvestre, E., J. Rijo, and H. Bogaert. 1994. *La neo-prostitucion infantil en Republica Dominicana.* Santo Domingo: UNICEF.

Smith, Valene L., ed. 1978. *Hosts and Guests: The Anthropology of Tourism.* Oxford: Blackwell.

Sonbol, Amira el Azhary. 1995. "Adoption in Islamic Society: A Historical Survey." In *Children in the Muslim Middle East*, ed. Elizabeth Warnock Fernea, 45–67. Austin: University of Texas Press.

Sow, Papa. 2004. "Mujeres inmigrantes y/o esposas de inmigrantes senegaleses y gambianos en Cataluña (España): Entre la vida familiar y la vida professional." *Documents d'Anàlisi Geogràfica* 43:69–88.

Spar, Debora L. 2006. *The Baby Business: How Money, Science, and Politics Drive the Commerce of Conception.* Boston: Harvard Business School Press.

State Commission of Population & Family Planning and China Population & Development Research Center (SFPC & CPIRC). 2005. *Handbook of Basic Data of Population and Family Planning* [in Chinese], Beijing: China Population Press.

Stockman, Farah, Michael Kranish, and Peter S. Canellos. 2006. "Bush Brings Faith to Foreign Aid." *The Boston Globe*, October 8.

Storrow, Richard F. 2006. "Marginalizing Adoption through the Regulation of Assisted Reproduction." *Capital University Law Review* 35 (2): 479–516.

Strathern, Marilyn. 1988. *The Gender of the Gift: Problems with Women and Problems with Society in Melanesia.* Berkeley: University of California Press.

——. 1995. "Displacing Knowledge: Technology and the Consequences for Kinship." In *Conceiving the New World Order: The Global Politics of Reproduction*, ed. Faye Ginsburg and Rayna Rapp, 346–64. Berkeley: University of California Press.

Sunder Rajan, Kaushik. 2006. *Biocapital: The Constitution of Postgenomic Life.* Durham: Duke University Press.

——. 2008. "Biocapital as an Emergent Form of Life: Speculations on the Figure of the Experimental." In *Biosociality, Genetics, and the Social Sciences: Making Biologies and Identities*, ed. Sahra Gibbon and Carlos Novas, 157–87. Oxford: Routledge.

Tabet, Stephen R., A. De Moya, K. K. Holmes, M. R. Krone, M. R. de Quinones, M. B. de Lister, I. Garris, M. Thorman, C. Castellanos, P. D. Swenson, G. A. Dallabeta, and C. A. Ryan. 1996. "Sexual Behaviors and Risk Factors for HIV Infection among Men Who Have Sex with Men in the Dominican Republic." *AIDS* 10 (2): 201–6.

Thompson, Charis. 2005. *Making Parents: The Ontological Choreography of Reproductive Technologies.* Cambridge: MIT Press.

Thorold, Crispin. 2001. "Indian Firms Embrace Biotechnology." *BBC News.* http://news .bbc.co.uk/1/hi/world/south_asia/1264569.stm.

Ticktin, Miriam. 2006. "Where Ethics and Politics Meet: The Violence of Humanitarianism in France." *American Ethnologist* 33:33–49.

Tignor, Leslie. 2005. "The Truth about UNICEF." *American Life League (ALL).* (http://www.all.org).

TNSACS (Tamil Nadu State AIDS Control Society). 2004. *PPTCT (Prevention of Parent to Child Transmission of HIV): A Report, 2003.* Chennai: TNSACS, Government of Tamil Nadu.

Tobin, Graham A., and Linda M. Whiteford. 2002. "Community Resilience and the Volcano Hazard: The Eruption of Tungurahua and the Evacuation of the Faldas, Ecuador." *Disasters: The Journal of Disaster Studies, Policy, and Management* 26 (1): 28–48.

——. 2004. "Chronic Hazards: Health Impacts Associated with On-going Ash-Falls around Mt. Tungurahua, Ecuador." *Papers of the Applied Geography Conferences* 27:84–93.

Toubia, Nahid. 1985. "The Social and Political Implications of Female Circumcision." In *Woman and the Family in the Middle East*, ed. Elizabeth Fernea, 148–59. Austin: University of Texas Press.

——. 1993. *Female Genital Mutilation: A Call for Global Action.* New York: Women, Ink.

——. 1994. "Female Circumcision as a Public Health Issue." *New England Journal of Medicine* 331 (11): 712–16.

Toubia, Nahid, and Anika Rahman. 2000. *Female Genital Mutilation: A Guide to Worldwide Laws and Policies.* London: Zed.

Tremayne, Soraya. 2006. "Not All Muslims Are Luddites." *Anthropology Today* 22 (3): 1–2.

——. 2009. "Law, Ethics, and Donor Technologies in Shia Iran." In *Assisting Reproduction, Testing Genes: Global Encounters with New Biotechnologies,* ed. Daphna Birenbaum-Carmeli and Marcia C. Inhorn, 144–63. New York: Berghahn Books.

Trouillot, Michel-Rolph. 1992. "The Caribbean Region: An Open Frontier in Anthropological Theory." *Annual Review of Anthropology* 21:19–42.

Truong, Than Dam. 1990. *Sex, Money, and Morality: The Political Economy of Prostitution and Tourism in South East Asia.* London: Zed Books.

Tsing, Anna. 2000. "The Global Situation." *Cultural Anthropology* 15 (3): 327–60.

UNAIDS/IOM (United Nations Program on HIV/AIDS/International Organization for Migration). 1998. "Migration and AIDS." *International Migration* 36 (4): 44.

UNFPA. 1999. *Reproductive Health in Refugee Situations: An Inter-agency Field Manual.* (http://www.unfpa.org/emergencies/manual/index.htm).

UNHCR. 1990. "International Convention on the Protection of the Rights of All Migrant Workers and Members of Their Families." Adopted by General Assembly resolution 45/158 of December 18.

UNHCR (United National Humanitarian Committee on Refugees). 2005. "Convention Relating to the Status of Refugees." (http://www.unhcr.org).

United Nations. 2000. "Replacement Migration: Is It a Solution to Declining and Ageing Population?" United Nations Department of Economic and Social Affairs, Population Division, United Nations. New York. UN High Commission on Refugees (http://www.un.org).

USCRI (U.S. Committee for Refugees and Immigrants). 2005. "Key Statistics." Table 1, "World Refugee Survey 2005." (http://www.refugees.org).

Van Hollen, Cecilia. 2003. *Birth on the Threshold: Childbirth and Modernity in South India.* Berkeley: University of California Press.

——. 2005. "Nationalism, Transnationalism, and the Politics of 'Traditional' Indian Medicine for HIV/AIDS." In *Asian Medicine and Globalization,* ed. Joseph Alter, 88–106. Philadelphia: University of Pennsylvania Press.

——. 2007. "Navigating HIV, Pregnancy, and Childbearing in South India: Pragmatics and Constraints in Women's Decision Making." *Medical Anthropology* 26 (1): 7–52.

Vasta, Ellie. 2008. *The Paper Market: "Borrowing" and "Renting" of Identity Documents.* Oxford Center on Migration, Policy, and Society (COMPAS) Working Paper no. 61. Oxford: University of Oxford.

Verdery, Katherine. 1996. *What Is Socialism, and What Comes Next?* Princeton: Princeton University Press.

Vertovec, Steven. 2001. "Transnationalism and Identity." *Journal of Ethnic and Migration Studies* 27:573–83.

Viveros, Mara. 2002. *De quebradores y cumplidores: Sobre hombres, masculinidades, y relaciones de género en Colombia.* Bogotá: Universidad Nacional de Colombia.

Walker, Alice. 1992. *Possessing the Secret of Joy*. New York: Harcourt Brace Jovanovich.

Walker, Alice, and Prathiba Parmar. 1993. *Warrior Marks: Female Genital Mutilation and the Sexual Blinding of Women*. New York: Harcourt, Brace.

Wallace, Rodrick, Yi-Shuan Huang, Peter Gould, and Deborah Wallace. 1997. "The Hierarchical Diffusion of AIDS and Violent Crime among U.S. Metropolitan Regions: Inner-City Decay, Stochastic Resonance, and Reversal of the Mortality Transition." *Social Science and Medicine* 44 (7): 935–47.

Wallerstein, Immanuel. 1995. "The Insurmountable Contradictions of Liberalism: Human Rights and the Rights of Peoples in the Geoculture of the Modern World-System." *South Atlantic Quarterly* 94:1161–79.

Wardlow, Holly. 2006. *Wayward Women: Sexuality and Agency in a New Guinea Society*. Berkeley: University of California Press.

Watson, James Shand. 1999. *Theory and Reality in the International Protection of Human Rights*. Ardsley, N.Y.: Transnational Publishers.

White, Tyrene. 1990. "Postrevolutionary Mobilization in China: The One-Child Policy Reconsidered." *World Politics* 43 (1): 53–76.

Whiteford, Linda M. 2009. "Failure to Protect, Failure to Provide: Reproductive Rights in Refugee Shelters." In *Global Health in Times of Violence*, ed. Paul Farmer, Barbara Rylko-Bauer, and Linda Whiteford, 89–112. Santa Fe, N.M.: School for Advanced Research Press.

Whiteford, Linda M., and Lenore Manderson. 2000. *Global Health Policies, Local Realities: Leveling the Playing Field*. Boulder, Colo.: Westwood Press.

Whiteford, Linda M., and Marilyn Poland. 1989. *New Approaches to Human Reproduction: Social and Ethical Dimensions*. Boulder, Colo.: New Westview Press.

Whiteford, Linda M., and Graham Tobin. 2004. "Saving Lives, Destroying Livelihoods: Emergency Evacuation and Resettlement Policies." In *Unhealthy Health Policies: A Critical Anthropological Examination*, ed. Arachu Castro and Merrill Singer, 189–202. Walnut Creek, Calif.: AltaMira Press.

Wildman, Sarah. 2004. "Abort Mission." *American Prospect* 15 (1), (http://www.prospect.org).

Williams, Raymond. 1973. *The Country and the City*. London: Chatto and Windus.

Wilson, Peter J. 1969. "Reputation and Respectability: A Suggestion for Caribbean Ethnology." *Man* 4:70–84.

Wingate, Martha S., and Greg R. Alexander. 2006. "The Healthy Migrant Theory: Variations in Pregnancy Outcomes among U.S.-Born Migrants." *Social Science and Medicine* 62 (2): 491–98.

Wolf, Eric. 1982. *Europe and the People without History*. Berkeley: University of California Press.

Yan, Hairong. 2003. "Neo-liberal Governmentality and Neo-humanism: Organizing Suzhi/Value Flow through Labor Recruitment Networks." *Cultural Anthropology* 18 (4): 493–523.

Yang, Kuifu, Jimin Liang, Shengli Chen, and Lixia Mo. 2000. *A Concise Dictionary of Population Knowledge* [in Chinese]. Beijing: China Population Press.

Yang, Kuifu, Jimin Liang, and Fan Zhang. 2001. *A Concise Chronological Outline of the Major Events of China Population and Family Planning* [in Chinese]. Beijing: China Population Press.

Yao, Xinwu, and Yin Hua, eds. 1994. *Basic Data of China's Population* [in Chinese]. Beijing: China Population Publishing House.

Yelvington, Kevin. 1993. "Gender and Ethnicity at Work in a Trinidadian Factory." In *Women and Change in the Caribbean: A Pan-Caribbean Perspective*, ed. Janet Momsen, 263–77. Bloomington: Indiana University Press.

Yu, Xuejun. 2002. "An Assessment of the Size and Structure of China's Population Based on the Fifth National Census" [in Chinese]. *Population Research* 26 (3): 9–15.

Zatz, Mayana. 2000. "Projeto Genoma Humano e Etica." *São Paulo em Perspectiva* 14 (3): 47–52.

Zhong, Zuowen, Linsong Lai, and Xiuqin Shi. 1998. "On the 'Two Transitions' of the Family Planning Work." *Journal of Nanjing College for Population Programme Management* 14 (4): 42–46.

Zuhur, Sherifa. 1992. "Of Milk-Mothers and Sacred Bonds: Islam, Patriarchy, and New Reproductive Technologies." *Creighton Law Review* 25:1725–38.

Contributors

ADITYA BHARADWAJ is lecturer in the School of Social and Political Science, University of Edinburgh. His principal research interest is in the global spread of new reproductive, genetic, and stem cell biotechnologies. He coauthored *Risky Relations: Family, Kinship, and the New Genetics* (Berg, 2006), is the lead author of *Local Cells, Global Science: The Proliferation of Stem Cell Technologies in India* (Routledge, 2009), and is currently completing *Conceptions: Infertility and Procreative Modernity in India* (Berghahn Books, forthcoming).

CAROLINE H. BLEDSOE is Melville J. Herskovits Professor of African Studies and professor of anthropology at Northwestern University in Evanston, Illinois. Her interests include demography and family organization in Africa and the West African diaspora in Europe.

CAROLE H. BROWNER is professor in and chair of the Department of Anthropology at the University of California, Los Angeles, where she is also a professor of women's studies and in the David Geffen School of Medicine. Her monograph *Neurogenetic Diagnoses: The Power of Hope and the Limits of Today's Medicine* (with H. M. Preloran) was published in 2010 by Routledge.

JUNJIE CHEN has a Ph.D. in sociology from Peking University in China, and has published a monograph and many articles in Chinese on China's rural transformation and demographic issues. He is completing his Ph.D. in sociocultural anthropology at the University of Illinois at Urbana, Champaign, with a dissertation based on extensive fieldwork on population policy in rural northeast China supported by the Wenner-Gren Foundation. Portions of his dissertation in progress have received the David M. Schneider Award (American Anthropological Association), the Theodore C. Bestor Prize (Society for East Asian Anthropology/American Anthropological Association), the Graduate Student Paper Award (Council on Anthropology and Reproduction/American Anthropological Association), and the Percy Buchanan Prize (Midwest Conference on Asian Affairs/Association for Asian Studies).

AIMEE R. EDEN is a Ph.D. candidate in applied anthropology at the University of South Florida, where she is also working on her MPH in maternal and child health. She holds a masters degree in international development from Ohio University, and is a returned Peace Corps volunteer (Kazakhstan). She has conducted research domestically and internationally on reproductive and maternal-child health, breastfeeding, perceptions of race and ethnicity among health researchers, transnational migration of health workers, legal approaches to cases of abused and neglected children in Florida, and the impact of accelerated academic programs on underrepresented groups in Florida.

SUSAN L. ERIKSON, a medical anthropologist, is assistant professor of global health in the Faculty of Health Sciences at Simon Fraser University, near Vancouver, British Columbia, Canada. Her research focuses on using ethnography to understand both the personal experiences and institutional arrangements of health practices in Germany and Sierra Leone.

DIDIER FASSIN is James Wolfensohn Professor of Social Science at the Institute for Advanced Study of Princeton and director of studies in anthropology at the École des Hautes Études en Sciences Sociales. He directs the Interdisciplinary Research Institute for Social Sciences (CNRS–Inserm–EHESS–University Paris North). His field of interest is political and moral anthropology, including inequalities and discrimination, health, and humanitarianism. His recent publications include *De la question sociale à la question raciale?* (with Eric Fassin, Édiciones La Découverte, 2006), *Les politiques de l'enquête: Épreuves ethnographiques* (editor, with Alban Bensa, Édiciones La Découverte, 2008), *When Bodies Remember: Experience and Politics of AIDS in South Africa* (California, 2007), and *The Empire of Trauma: An Inquiry into the Condition of Victimhood* (with Richard Rechtman and Rachel Gomme, Princeton, 2009).

CLAUDIA LEE WILLIAMS FONSECA is professor of anthropology at the Federal University of Rio Grande do Sul (Brazil) and the Universidade Nacional de San Martin (Argentina). She has published extensively on subjects concerning kinship, gender, and anthropology of law.

ELLEN GRUENBAUM is professor and head of the Department of Anthropology at Purdue University. Her research has focused on the cultural contexts of women's reproductive health and female genital cutting practices, especially in Sudan.

MATTHEW GUTMANN is vice president for international affairs and professor of anthropology at Brown University. His books include *The Meanings of Macho: Being a Man in Mexico City* (California, 1996 [2006]), *Fixing Men: Sex, Birth Control, and AIDS in Mexico* (California, 2007), and *Breaking Ranks: Iraq Veterans Speak Out against the War* (with Catherine Lutz, California, 2010).

MARCIA C. INHORN is the William K. Lanman Jr. Professor of Anthropology and International Affairs and chair of the Council on Middle East Studies (CMES) in the MacMillan Center for International and Area Studies at Yale University. Her research focuses on infertility and assisted reproductive technologies in the Muslim Middle East and Arab America. She has published three books on this topic, as well as six edited volumes in the areas of science and technology studies (STS), gender and feminist theory (including masculinity studies), religion and bioethics, globalization and global health, cultures of biomedicine and ethnomedicine, and stigma and human suffering.

MARK B. PADILLA is assistant professor in the Department of Health Behavior and Health Education and adjunct assistant professor of anthropology at the University of Michigan. He conducts ethnographic research primarily on gender, sexuality, and HIV/AIDS among vulnerable populations in both the Caribbean and the United States. His work on Dominican male sex workers, tourism, and HIV earned him the Ruth Benedict Award (2008) from the Society of Lesbian and Gay Anthropologists and the John Money Award (2009) from the Society for the Scientific Study of Sexuality.

RAYNA RAPP is professor of anthropology at New York University. Her research focuses on the intersections of gender, reproduction, health, and studies of science and technology. She wrote the prize-winning monograph *Testing Women, Testing the Fetus: The Social Impact of Amniocentesis in America* (Routledge, 1999) and edited *Conceiving the New World Order: The Global Politics of Reproduction* (with Faye Ginsburg, California, 1995) and *Toward an Anthropology of Women* (Monthly Review Press, 1975).

LISA ANN RICHEY is professor of international development studies in the Department of Society and Globalisation, Roskilde University, Denmark. She is the author of *Population Politics and Development: From the Policies to the Clinics* (Palgrave Macmillan, 2008) and coauthor of *Brand Aid: Shopping Well to Save the World* (Minnesota, 2011). Her work is on international development, AIDS treatment, and Africa.

CAROLYN F. SARGENT is professor of anthropology and women, gender, and sexuality studies at Washington University in St. Louis. Her most recent research explores the intersections between French immigration policies, Islam, and reproductive strategies among Malian migrants in Paris. She is the author of *Maternity, Medicine, and Power* (California, 1989) and coeditor of *Childbirth and Authoritative Knowledge* (California, 1997), *Small Wars, Gender and Health, Gender in Cross-Cultural Perspective* (California, 1998), and *Medical Anthropology: Contemporary Theory and Method* (1996, Greenwood/ Praeger).

PAPA SOW is a Marie Curie Research Fellow at the Centre for Research in Ethnic Relations at the University of Warwick, UK, and at the Institut Fondamental d'Afrique Noire at the Université Cheikh Anta Diop in Senegal. He specializes in studies of transnationalism and gender among Gambian and Senegalese immigrants in Spain and France.

CECILIA VAN HOLLEN is associate professor of anthropology in the Maxwell School for Citizenship and Public Affairs at Syracuse University. Her book *Birth on the Threshold: Childbirth and Modernity in South India* (California, 2003) received the Association for Asian Studies 2005 A. K. Coomaraswamy Book Prize for the best book in South Asia Studies.

LINDA WHITEFORD is associate vice president of Global Strategies in the Office of the President, and also associate vice president for academic affairs and strategic initiatives in the Office of the Provost, at the University of South Florida. She is a medical anthropologist whose work has taken her to Ecuador, Mexico, the Dominican Republic, Cuba, Guatemala, Costa Rica, Nicaragua, Bolivia, Cameroon, China, Malaysia, England, Scotland, and Argentina to investigate water scarcity and vector-borne diseases, maternal-child and reproductive health, and most recently human health during and following disasters such as volcanic eruptions.

Index

A, Dr., 118–19, 120–21

Abdal Galil, Sudan, 103–4

abducted children, 248n10

Abel (legal case), 144

abortion: amniocentesis decisions and, 223n1; choice of, 27; displaced women and, 227–28; global gag rule and, 229–30; human rights and, 235–36; Ingrid (study subject) and, 24; out-of-plan pregnancies and, 44; precluded, 85; Vatican opposition to, 232

abstinence-only programs, 230–31

Accoyer, Bernard, 247n5

A Crisis of Births (Krause), 3

Adams, Vincanne, 6

adoption, 116, 132, 243, 245

adultery, 130–31, 198–99

Africa. *See* specific countries

African immigrants: family reunification policies and, 5; genetic testing of, 244–45; polygamy and, 247n5

African Union Mission in Sudan (AMIS, AU), 229

agency: autonomy and, 201; choice and constraint and, 156, 217–18; conceptualization of, 1, 13–16; destructive acts and, 13, 224, 233–34, 237; and efforts to end female genital cutting (FGC), 8, 97; global ethnography, 8, 224–37; immigration policies and, 175–91, 192–203; of men, 159–74; political nature of re-

production and, 3, 29, 37, 192, 204–23; population movements and, 224–37; social policy adjustments, 149, 152; structure-agency dyad, 7–8, 26–27, 182, 218; of women, 199, 201, 202, 233–34

age pyramids, 177

agnatic relations, 116

Ain Shams University (Cairo), 131

Al-Azhar, 128–30, 132

Algeria, 239–41, 243

alpha-fetoprotein (AFP), 37n2, 223n2

altruism, 121–24

American Life League, 231–32

Amnesty International, 229, 235

amniocentesis: abortion decisions and, 223n1; acceptance rates in study of, 207–8; Elisa (study participant) and, 208–9; genetic consultations and, 206–7; Hector (study participant) and, 208–9; inconclusive results from, 23; interpreter approach and, 211–12; Lia (study participant) and, 209; life stress and, 223n4; Lucia (study participant) and, 214–15; male partner influence and, 207–9, 217; Marta (study participant) and, 215–16; miscommunication sources and, 205; Pedro (study participant) and, 209; quantitative correlates of acceptance, 207; Rocio (study participant) and, 213

Ana (interpreter), 213

ancestor worship, 43
anchor babies, 182–83
Anderson, Benedict, 247n4
Ansar al-Sunna, 100, 107
anticircumcision laws, 99
antiretroviral drugs (ARV), 20; choice of,
   78–79; providing, in Ivory Coast, 71
Arche de Zoé association, 248n10
ARV team meetings, 74–77
assimilation and integration, 202
assisted reproductive technologies (ART):
   global movements and, 9; Islam and,
   126–37
asylum, 176
asylum seekers, numbers, 232–33
authoritative approach interpreters, 211–
   15, 217

B, Dr., 118–20
backwardness, 41–43
Baños, Ecuador, volcano eruption, 224
Beijing, Fourth World Conference on
   Women, 48, 57, 65
Beirut, reproductive tourism, 136
"best interests of the child," 183–84
big wombs (da duzi), 45
bioavailability, 113
biocommerce in India, 15–16, 111–12
biological citizens, 11–12, 70, 80
biological filiation, 243–44
biopolitics, 248n12
biosociality, 74–75, 123
birth control pill, 58
birth defects, 78
Birthing the Nation (Kanaaneh), 3
Birth on the Threshold (Van Hollen), 3
birth quota, 44
birth rate control, 58
birth-to-abortion ratios, 44
"black welfare mothers," 247n7
Boca Chica, Dominican Republic, 162, 164
body commodification, 15–16
body not reified, 15

Borai, Shaykh al-, 106
Bosnia, 229
Bourdieu, Pierre, 14
brand loyalty, 36
Brazil: Civil Code of, 143; kinship notions
   in, 112; Paternity Law of, 142; paternity
   testing in, lack of control over, 150–51;
   social justice in, 141; state power in area
   of reproduction and, 10
breast-feeding, 89–90
British National DNA Database, 153n8
Bundesausschuss: access to meetings of,
   37n9; influenced by manufacturers, 36;
   makeup of, 33–34; medical legislator
   and, 32–33
Burawoy, Michael, 7, 28
Bush, George W., 229–30

Cairo, Egypt, International Conference on
   Population and Development, 57, 65, 105
California, fetal diagnosis in, 206–7
Cameroonians: in Germany, 5, 176, 184–
   85, 190n19; Italy and, 190n20
capitalist market economy, 46–47
casa-calle (home-street) distinction, 160
Catherine (patient), 78–79
Catholicism, 59, 62–63; amniocentesis
   and, 208–9; interpretation of, 66
CC, Dr. (obstetrician), 31
census, 10–11, 46
cesarean birth, 88
Chad, 229, 235, 248n10
child-bearing and stress, 225
child rearing, division of labor, 57
children, providing for, 166
"child substitution," 240
child trafficking, 240
China: abortion and sterilization rumors
   in, 230; capitalist market economy and,
   46–47; census of 2000, 46; fertility culture in, 49–50; medical team visits and,
   50; modernization agenda and reproductive practices in, 19–20; notions of

economic prosperity linked to birth regulation, 47

Efavirenz, 78, 82n14

egg donation, 134, 136

Egypt: in vitro fertilization (IVF) and, 130–31; Ministry of Health, 130–31; reproductive tourism in, 9

Egyptian Medical Syndicate, 130

elective filiation, 243–44

Elisa (study participant), 208–9

embryo donation, 134

embryonic stem cells (ESC): biotechnology rise and, 113; ethical guidelines on procurement of, 117, 123–24; IVF payment exchanged for, 120; provenance of stem cell lines, 116–17; quality control and, 121

embryos: fears of low quality of, 119, 120; supply chain and, 115, 117–18

emergency contraception (EC), 227, 232, 235–36

emergency shelters, 225–26

Empez, Núria, 183

empowerment and anti-FGC work, 107

England, immigration to, 187

eradication, 97, 103

Erikson, Susan: model of global ethnography, 19; perspective on global ethnography, 7, 8

Erode, India, 88

Estriol, 223n2

ethnocentric Western hegemony, 97–98

European Union: citizen favoritism and, 188; family reunification policies and, 180, 189n5. *See also* specific countries

excision (FGC), 101

exploitation, 114, 121, 123

Faith (patient), 77

"faith-based initiative," 231

"fake mother," 240, 242

family planning: contraception vs., 77; Western, anti-Islam perception of, 105

family reunification policies, 5, 156; Denmark and, 190n9; DNA paternity testing and, 180; European Union and, 180; foster children and, 180; France and, 194, 242; human rights and, 178–79; occupancy of reunification positions and, 186; quantitative values and, 181; transnational mobility and, 187; youth influx and, 177

family size, 61, 63, 105, 115

Farmer, Paul, 3

farmland redistribution, 46

fatherless children, 140

Fatma (mother), 239–44

fatwas, 127–28; Ayatollah Khamanei, 133; Al-Azhar, 128–30, 132

favorcitos, 211–12

female contraceptive culture, 55–56, 64–65

female genital cutting (FGC), 8, 21; anticircumcision laws and, 99; family reunification and, 200; forms of, 100–101, 108–9; prioritization of fight against, 107; religious arguments against, 104, 106–7

female sterilization, 65

feminine spaces, 171

fertility culture, 49–50

fertility rate control, 58

fetal diagnosis: in California, 206–7; routine in prenatal care, 205, 217; state-mandated, 5, 156, 206–7

fieldwork vs. official claims, 50–51

filiation, 141, 243–44

Fofanna, Mr. (case study), 199–201

Foucault, Michel: on emergence of the modern state, 11; on racism, 248n12

Four Modernizations, 41

Fourth World Conference on Women, 48, 57, 65

France: DNA paternity testing in, 149–50, 240, 248n9; family reunification policies in, 194, 200, 242; Medal of the

French Family and, 247n6; mystery child and, 239–45; polygyny of immigrants in, 190n10, 195; pronatalism and, 241–42; racial ideal and, 241–42; riots and, 242; *trente glorieuses*, 193

fuwu (high-quality medical services), 37

Gambian families in Spain, 176, 185–87; traditional family patterns of, 188

Gambian migrants, 156

Garia Wahid, Sudan, 102–3

gastarbeiter (guest worker) period, 176

GE, ultrasound imaging, 34

gender: context-dependent phenomenon, 173; context-specific actions, 172; cross-culturally variable, 173; dichotomous constructs of, 160; meanings and practice of flexible, 171–72; power, linkage to, 160; set of cultural practices, 159; social contexts of, 174

gender binaries, 160–61

genetic consultations, 206–7; Lucia (study participant), 214–15; male partner influence and, 207–9, 217; Marta (study participant) and, 215–16; Rocio (study participant), 213; Rosalia (study participant) and, 209–11

German Federal Statistical Office figures, 184–85

German Society for Gynecology and Obstetrics (DGGG), 34–35

Germany: asylum and, 176; Cameroonian immigrants and, 5, 176, 184–85, 190n19; East Germany, 37n7; *gastarbeiter* (guest worker) period in, 176; history and process of medical regulation in, 37n7; immigration policies in, 176–77; Motherhood Guidelines and, 31–32; *Mutterpass* and, 23; prenatal care in, 19, 26; residency of immigrant spouses in, 184, 190n18; ultrasound imaging in, 8, 29–30; West Germany, 27, 30, 37n7; women and abortion in, 27

getaway vacation, symbolic meaning, 164

Giddens, Anthony, 14

Gini coefficient, 73

Ginsburg, Faye, 2–3

Global AIDS Bill, 230–31

global assemblage, 9–10; use of, in meshing qualitative and quantitative data, 28–29

global ethnography, 7–8; aggregating process, 27–29

global gag rule, 229–31

globalization, perspective used, 6–7

González-López, Gloria, 66, 170

Good Manufacturing Process (GMP), 125n2

Greenhalgh, Susan, 3

grounded globalizations, 28

HAART coverage, 72–73, 79, 81n5

habitus and identity, 14

Hadith on female genital cutting (FGC), 100–101, 109n1

Han, resistance to one-child policy, 43

haram (morally unacceptable), 132

healthcare and transnational existence, 178

health insurance, 89, 215

Hector (study participant), 208–9

Helms, Jesse, 229

Helms Amendment of 1973, 229

Henry, Doug, 233

Heshima Clinic, 74–75, 81n2

"high migration potential" countries, 178

HIV/AIDS, 54; behavioral outcomes and, 172; breast-feeding and, 89–90; cesarean birth and, 88; drugs and, 78, 82n14, 91, 94, 95n6; duplicity in relationships and, 86; as family issue, 21, 87, 90–92, 94–95; global assemblage and, 9–10; interventions and, lack of, 167; Majeed, 86; mother-to-child transmission of, 88–89, 91, 94; partner testing for, 87; risk patterns and, 168; risky so-

Introduction to China's Fertility Culture (Pan et al.), 49

in vitro fertilization (IVF), 111–12; cost of, 119; Egypt and, 130–31; governmental regulation of, 127; incest potential with, 131; *sharia* in, 112, 130; third-party donors for, 129

Iran, 134

Irma (interpreter), 215–16

Islam: adoption, 243–44; contraception, views on, 197–99; gendered views of, 203; law and, 130, 137n2; Shia Islam, 133–36; Sunni Islam, 128–32; Sunni-Shia sectarian divide, 127

Islamic Organization for Medical Sciences (IOMS), 129

Islamism (political Islam), 96–97; pursuit of, in Sudan, 99–100

Italy and Cameroonian immigrants, 190n20

IUDS, 44, 56, 58; *metas* (contraceptive prevalence targets), 65

Jagger, Mick, 147

Jair (legal case), 148

Jayanthi (patient), 90–92

Johnson-Hanks, Jennifer, 15

judicial services, 141

K, Dr. (obstetrician), 23–24

kefala (guardianship), 240–41, 243–44

Kelly (genetic counselor), 213

Kenana Arabs, 102–3

Khamanei, Ayatollah Ali Hussein, 133

Khartoum, Sudan, 101

khifad (reduction), 101

khitan (cutting), 101

kinship: redefinition of, 111; in vitro fertilization (IVF) and, 116

kinship not intrinsically desirable, 92

Kligman, Gail, 3, 4

Kosovo refugee camps, 232

Kouchner, Bernard, 248n10

Krankenkassen, 32, 37n8

labor migration and HIV/STI risks, 171, 174

Larcher, Gerard, 202

Lebanon, 135–36; reproductive tourism in, 9, 136

levirate, 116

Lia (study participant), 209

life expectancy in Mexico, 60

life stress and amniocentesis, 223n4

lineage, 131

lobbying, 36

local, the: transnational privileged over, 98; understanding of, 12–13

local biologies, 29; and global assemblage, 9

local-global schema, 27

local moral worlds, 128, 132

Lock, Margaret, 9

Loi Pasqua (Pasqua Law), 190n10, 195

London, immigrants, 187

Lorraine (legal case), 145–46, 148

Loyo, Gilberto, 64

Lucia (study participant), 214–15

Lucirene (legal case), 148

luohou (backwardness), 41–43

machismo, 61, 149, 152, 171

Majeed, 86

male spaces, 171

male sterilization, 56

Malian immigrants, 199–201; contraception, views on, 197–98

Manchelle, François, 193

Manchu resistance to one-child policy, 43

Mankekar, Purnima, 13

marabout, 199

Mariani, Thierry, 244

Marie Stopes International (MSI), 228, 230

market economy, ideal, 51

marriageability, 101–2, 104

marriages, 152n6; incentives for, 106; protection from early marriage, 190n9;

marriages (*cont.*)
  Spain and, 190n25; trend away from, 146

Marseille, France, 239

Marta (study participant), 215–16

Martín (study participant), 166

Marxist theory, 246

masculinity: children and, providing for, 166; economic changes and, 161; HIV/STI risks and, 161; not machismo, 171; reputation and, 171; respectability and, 171; shaping of reproductive health and, 160

Maternowski, Catherine, 3

Mbeki, President, 72

Medal of the French Family, 247n6

medical profiling, 56

men: barriers to responsible reproduction and, 20; contraception choices for, 56; family planning and, 57; lack of organizations for, 54; lack of trust for, 54, 58; monolithic view of, 61; prevention of pregnancy and, 15, 20; reproductive health of, 58–59

men who have sex with men (MSM): elevated risk for HIV for, 167; inadequate label for, 165; literature focus on, 168

metas (contraceptive prevalence targets), 65

Mexfam, 63

Mexican immigrants and amniocentesis decisions, 5, 156, 204–23

Mexico: men and reproduction in, 15, 20; monolithic view of men in, 61; mortality rates in, 60; population growth rates in, 65; Sanitary Code of, 60–61; women giving birth on U.S. soil and, 182–83

Mexico City policy (of the United States), 229–30

midwives' opinions on immigrants, 196–97

migrant tourism workers, 159–74

migration for work, 164

Mikell, Gwendolyn, 97–98

missionary approach interpreters, 211–13, 217

modernity pursued by China, 38–40, 51

Mohamed (child), 239–41, 243

monogamy and family reunification, 180, 184–87, 190n10

monthly periods, inspection of, 43

Moosa, Ebrahim, 129

morning-after pill emergency contraception, 232

Moroccan youths in Spain, 176, 180, 183–84, 190nn16–17

mortality rates in Mexico, 60

motherhood, honesty questioned, 148

Motherhood Guidelines, 31–32

Mount Tungurahua, 224–25

multiple marker screening, 223n2

Muslim women and female genital cutting (FGC), 21

mut'a marriage, 133

Mutterschaftsrichtlinien, 31–32

"Mystery Child from Marseille," 239

Namakkal, India, 88, 93

Nandy, Ashis, 113

narrative, individual, extrapolating to global ethnography, 25–26

nasab (lineage), 131

National AIDS Control Organization (NACO), 84

National Islamic Front, 98

national-transnational dualism, 241

Nevirapine, 78, 82n14, 84, 94, 95n6

New Delhi, India, 115

nongovernmental organizations (NGOs): birth attendant recruitment and, 109n2; global assemblage and, 9; global gag rule and, 229–31; in Mexico, 15, 54; Moroccan youths in Spain and, 184; reproductive health initiatives and, 104; reproductive health services in emer-

gencies and, 228, 230–31; in South Africa, 74, 81n6; in Sudan, 109n2
non-nucleoside reverse transcriptase inhibitors (NNRTI), 82n14
nonpaternity, 149
Novas, Carlos, 11–12
nurses' reaction to HIV-positive patients, 88–89, 91

Oaxaca de Juárez, Mexico, 58; men and reproduction, 15, 20
Obama, Barack, 230
observation instrument, 207, 218–21; interpreters involved, 207, 221–22
obstetricians as consumers, 35
Oferta Sistemática, 55, 65
Omdurman, Sudan, 101
one-child policy, 41; softening of, 46; violation of, 43–44
Ong, Aihwa, 9
Orlando (study participant), 162
Ortner, Sherry: nature of identity and agency, 14; perspective on global ethnography, 7
Other, the: Chinese rural identity and, 39, 51; creation of, 42–43
otherness, 181

parent-child relationship definitions, 180
partible self, 181
Pasqua Law (Loi Pasqua), 190n10, 195
paternity, 134; social relation vs. biological fact of, 145
Paternity Law (Brazil), 142
paternity testing: consensual principles (Human Genome Project) of, 151; divorce and, 149; ethics of, not debated, 151; France and, 149–50; honesty questioned in, 148; kinship notions and, 112; refutation of paternity and, 143, 152n3; state power in area of reproduction and, 10; TV shows and, 147
patrilineal ideology, 43, 46, 131–32

Paxson, Heather, 3
Pedro (study participant), 209
peer pressure, 101–2
Pelé, 147
personal choice, 53
personalismo, 212
pharaonic circumcision, 100, 102–4
phenotypic similarity, 136
Phillips, ultrasound imaging, 34
Phumla (patient), 76–77
Pigg, Stacy, 6
"Politics of Reproduction" (Ginsburg and Rapp), 2–3
polyandry, 133
polygamy, 134, 247n5; African immigrants and, 242; West African immigrants and, 156, 185–87, 195, 202
population control, 58, 104–5, 115; West African immigrants and, 196–97
population growth rates: annual goals for, 40–41, 52n3, 52n5; in Mexico, 65
postdiagnostic abortion, 37n6
practice theory, 14–15
pregnancy as health problem, 33
pregnancy surveillance (Schwangerschaftskontrolle), 33
prenatal care: fetal diagnosis in, 204–23; in Germany, 19, 26; lack of emphasis on, 205
prenatal diagnostic technologies, use of vs. experience of, 26–27
prenatal genetic consultations, observation instruments, 207, 218–22
Prevention of Mother-to-Child Transmission of HIV (PMTCT) program, 75, 79; renamed in India, 87
Prevention of Parent to Child Transmission of HIV (PPTCT) program: HIV testing, informed consent for, 85–86; India, 84, 87; not universally implemented, 94; participating hospitals, 93
professionalism, 215
pro-life organizations, 231–32

promiscuity, 146–47

pronatalism, 59–61, 117, 126, 241–42

"Proposal for a Council Directive on the Right to Family Reunification," 189n5

prostitution, 174n3, 199–200; and paternity tests, 139

quotas, 65

racial ideal, 241–42

racism, 248n9, 248n12

Rahad Irrigated Scheme, 102

RAINBO, 98

rape: global acknowledgment of, 228; inevitability of, after emergencies, 227, 229; Kosovo refugee camps and, 232; lack of consideration for, in U.S. aid policies, 230–31; penalties for, 54; tool of conflict and, 229

Rapp, Rayna, 2–3

Reagan, Ronald, 229

refugee camps, nonhomogenous population, 235

refugees, 226; numbers of, 232–33; and reproductive healthcare, 157, 224–237

Refugee Women and Reproductive Health Care: Reassessing Priorities (Women's Commission for Refugee Women and Children), 228

refutation of paternity, 143, 152n3

regimes of value, 71

regional masculinities, 170, 172–74; HIV/STI risks, 12–13, 155, 161; reputation, 171; respectability, 171

regional patriarchies, 170

Reichstag, 28

Reliance Life Sciences, 125n1

Reproducing Jews: A Cultural Account of Assisted Conception in Israel (Kahn), 3

reproduction: biological vs. elective, 244; as production of culture, 2–3; why study, 2–5

reproductive disruption, 117, 119, 124–25

reproductive futures, 247n7

reproductive health, 58–59; Global AIDS Bill, 231; lack of access to, 226–27; shaped by masculinity, 160

Reproductive Health in Refugee Sitations: An Inter-agency Field Manual, 228, 232

Reproductive Health Response in Conflict (RHRC), 228

reproductive rights, 58–59; therapeutic citizen, 80–81

reproductive tourism, 9, 136

reverse transcriptase, 82n14

RHRC, 230

riots, 194, 202, 242

risk groups, 167

risky social contexts, 167, 169, 174n4

River Crossing, Liaoning, China, 38–39

Rocio (study participant), 213

rollout rates, 72–73

roof tiles as symbol of family integrity, 45

Rosalia (study participant), 209–11

Rose, Nikolas, 11

Roux, Paul, 80

rural women: Chinese modernization agenda, 19–20; "failure" of, 48, 50

Saadawi, Nawal El, 97

Sahlins, Marshall, 14

salmah (uncircumcised), 101

salud reproductiva (reproductive health), 58–59

sanitary citizens, 11

Sanitary Code, 60–61

Santo Domingo, Dominican Republic, 162, 164

Saraswati (patient), 84–86, 88–90, 92

Sarkozy, Nicolas, 202

Sauerbrey, Ellen, 231

Schengen Agreement of 1985, 178

Schwangerschaftskontrolle (pregnancy surveillance), 33

Self, creation of, 42–43

Senegal, 107

Senegal River Valley region, 193–94
serial monogamy, 186–87, 190n19
Serour, Gamal, 130–31
sex: as commodity, 164; for resources, 230–31
sexual abstinence, 198
sexual behavior, not congruent with sexual identity, 172
sexual escapism, 164, 169
sexual identity, not congruent with sexual behavior, 172
sexuality, cross-culturally variable, 173
sexual labor, 155
sexually transmitted infections (STIS), 54; economic disparities and, 168; labor migration and, 171, 174; marital risk and, 172; multilevel explanation for, 173; regional masculinities and, 12–13, 155, 161; risk groups for, 167
sexual pleasure, 106–7
sexual violence: inevitable after emergencies, 227, 229
sex worker, inadequate label, 165
sex workers: bribes to police from, 174n3; literature focus on, 168
shame, 235
sharia, 137n2; assisted reproductive technologies (ART) and, 130; in vitro fertilization (IVF) and, 112
sharia circumcision, 100
shehui fuyang fei (Social Nurturance Fee), 52n7
Shia Islam, 133–36
Siemens Medical Solutions, 28; "branding" of doctors and, 36; demonstration of ultrasound technology and, 34; marketing managers interview and, 35
Sierra Leone, 233
silk and paper flower assembly, 47–48, 52n6
single motherhood, 134
site, concept of, 15
Sittalbanat, Dr., 100

"Smaller families live better," 61, 63
Small Shock Brigades, 45
social contexts, 174, 174n4; home community and, 172; tourism area and, 172
social inequalities, 169
social issues, 235
social justice, 141
Social Nurturance Fee (shehui fuyang fei), 52n7
Soninke, 193
sorcery, 201
South Africa: HIV/AIDS in, 9–10, 20; population movements and, 81n8; Western Cape of, 73, 81n7
South India, 10
Spain: Gambian immigrants in, 156, 185–87; immigration policies of, 177; international human rights and, 179; marriages in, 190n25; Moroccan youths in, 176, 180, 183–84, 190n16, 190n17
Spanish Childhood Protection System, 183
Spanish Municipal Register, 185
sperm donation, in Iran, 134
spina bifida: no test for, 37n2; ultrasound imaging and, 23–24
Sri Lanka, 234
state, the: creation of cultural identities and, 10–11; reification of, 39; roles of, 113; use of term, 10–12
static binaries, moving beyond, 7–8
"stratified reproduction," 247n7
structural violence, 168
structure-agency dyad, 7–8, 26–27, 182, 218
subcontractor work, 47–48
Sudan: anticircumcision laws, 99; end of civil war, 101; female genital cutting (FGC), 8, 21; female genital cutting forms, 108–9; traditions suppressed, 98–99
Sudanese Communist Party, 98
Sudanese Women's Union, 98
Sudan Medical Association, 103

Western Cape, South Africa, 69, 71–74, 81n8

West Germany: history and process of medical regulation in, 37n7; ultrasound imaging and, 30; women and abortion in, 27. *See also* Germany

Williams, Raymond, 41

women: agency and autonomy, 199, 201–2, 233–34; not protected, 227; refugees and IDPs, percentage of, 226; wage work, 161

Women's Health in Post-Soviet Russia (Rivkin-Fish), 3

women's issues, 235

worker hostels, 194, 196, 198, 200

World Health Organization (WHO): cate-gories of FGC, 101, 108–9; reproductive health policies of, following emergencies, 228

Xoliswa (patient), 76

Yassa (case study), 200–201

Yehia, Mohamed, 131

Yue, Zhejiang, China, 39, 44

Zabarma, 102

zero immigration proposals, 195

zero population growth, 41

Zidovudine, 91, 95n6

zina (adultery), 129, 133–34

CAROLE H. BROWNER is professor and chair of the Department of Anthropology at the University of California, Los Angeles, where she is also a professor of women's studies and in the David Geffen School of Medicine.

CAROLYN F. SARGENT is professor of anthropology and women, gender, and sexuality studies at Washington University in Saint Louis.

Library of Congress Cataloging-in-Publication Data
Reproduction, globalization, and the state : new theoretical and ethnographic perspectives / Carole H. Browner and Carolyn F. Sargent, editors.
p. cm.
Includes bibliographical references and index.
ISBN 978-0-8223-4941-9 (cloth : alk. paper)
ISBN 978-0-8223-4960-0 (pbk. : alk. paper)
1. Reproductive rights. 2. Human reproduction—Moral and ethical aspects.
3. Human reproduction—Political aspects. 4. Human reproduction—Religious aspects.
I. Browner, C. H. (Carole H.), 1947– II. Sargent, Carolyn Fishel, 1947– III. Title.
HQ766.R477 2011
306.874—dc22   2010038074